Functional Occlusion
in Restorative Dentistry
and Prosthodontics

Functional Occlusion
in Restorative Dentistry
and Prosthodontics

Edited by

Iven Klineberg
AM RFD BSc MDS PhD FRACDS FICD FDSRCS (Lond, Edin)
Professor, Head of Discipline of Oral Rehabilitation, Nobel
Biocare Chair of Oral Rehabilitation, Faculty of Dentistry,
Westmead Hospital, University of Sydney,
New South Wales, Australia

Steven E. Eckert
DDS MS FACP
Professor Emeritus, Mayo Clinic, College of Medicine,
Rochester, Minnesota, USA

Foreword by

George Zarb
CM, BChD, MS, DDS, MS, FRCD(C)
Emeritus Professor, University of Toronto
Editor-in-Chief, International Journal of Prosthodontics

ELSEVIER
MOSBY   Edinburgh   London   New York   Oxford   Philadelphia   St Louis   Sydney   Toronto   2015

3251 Riverport Lane
St. Louis, Missouri 63043

FUNCTIONAL OCCLUSION IN RESTORATIVE DENTISTRY
AND PROSTHODONTICS

ISBN: 978-0-723438090

Library of Congress Cataloging-in-Publication Data

Functional occlusion in restorative dentistry and prosthodontics / edited by Iven Klineberg, Steven E. Eckert; foreword by Professor George Zarb.
        p.; cm.
Includes bibliographical references.
ISBN 978-0-7234-3809-0 (hardcover : alk. paper)
I. Klineberg, Iven, editor.   II. Eckert, Steven E., editor.
[DNLM: 1. Dental Occlusion.   2. Dental Implantation–methods.   3. Prosthodontics–methods.
4. Temporomandibular Joint–physiopathology.   WU 440]
RK651
617.6′9–dc23

2015015057

Executive Content Strategist: Kathy Falk
Content Development Manager: Jolynn Gower
Senior Content Development Specialist: Brian Loehr
Publishing Services Manager: Julie Eddy/Jeff Patterson
Project Manager: Sara Alsup
Design Direction: Teresa McBryan
Text Designer: Ashley Miner

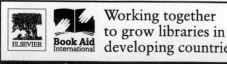

CONTENTS

FOREWORD

The topic of Occlusion has tended to languish at the bottom of the scientific heap. It either struggled to sustain a position as a stand-alone clinical academic entity in dental school curricula, or else fell between the cracks of discipline-driven territorial conflicts. It consequently tended to fare better in continuing education programs where gifted and assertive dentists often packaged their empirical clinical experiences and observations in cult-like offerings. The net outcome of these educational agendas was to lose sight of the relatively recent scientific method's challenge to traditional perceptions—to question and refine past convictions on Occlusion's true significance, irrespective of their presumed or contrived scientific pedigree.

A few books sought to place Occlusion in its deserved scientific context; and I continue to believe that the one Norman Mohl, Gunnar Carlsson, John Rugh and I co-edited in 1988 was a particularly good start. However, three decades of compelling scientific advances have profoundly changed the dental professional landscape e.g. Osseointegration, CAD/CAM influenced bio-technology, pain management, neuroplasticity etc, and what is now needed is a newer and more robust consideration of Occlusion's expanded biological context.

This book certainly provides it!

It is a welcome reminder that while still a relatively young science, the study of Occlusion does not preclude the virtues of synthesizing clinical observations and experiences to ensure that they are reconcilable with scientifically based insights and explanations; and more especially when confronted with unresolved clinical issues. It also reminds us that any health discipline that neglects addressing concerns derived from clinical observations risks usurping its claim to scientific advancement. The two Editors' insistence that occlusion changes as chronology, diseases and therapeutic interventions place demands on muscles and bones that require a far more complex understanding of biological processes, is both compelling and challenging. Moreover, their recruitment of uniquely qualified colleagues to advance their scholarly objective via this book's message proves to be a brilliant initiative. The profession owes this text's authors—indeed the entire team—a sincere vote of gratitude for a rational and nondoctrinaire approach to a topic whose relevance has been frequently under-estimated.

George Zarb CM, BChD, MS, DDS, MS, FRCD(C)
Emeritus Professor, University of Toronto
Editor-in-Chief, International Journal
of Prosthodontics

This book is an up-to-date statement on occlusion and its implications for contemporary dental practice and prosthodontics. It provides an insight into a new dimension for prosthodontic practice with the introduction of the crucial role of the occlusion of the teeth and mastication for maintenance of cognition and higher-level cognitive skills. This is a new paradigm: one that emphasizes the singular importance of maintaining an occlusion with teeth ideally or through rehabilitation for function and expands the importance of prosthodontics and the general well-being of individuals.

The book also stands at the crossroads as dentistry and prosthodontics, having embraced biology as the fundamental construct within which case management is considered as well as the far-reaching implications of the principles of implant dentistry utilizing osseointegration for implant rehabilitation in treatment planning and decision-making, are to be fundamentally transformed within the digital revolution. Industry has progressively introduced computer technology to enhance production, accuracy, precision, and efficiency. Clinical science has been the beneficiary of these changes. In prosthodontics, the digital revolution is already gaining traction, and the visionary implications of the digital workflow will continue this transformation. The availability of computer-aided design and computer-aided manufacture (CAD/CAM) has had a major impact on restorative dental practice, linked with the availability of contemporary ceramic materials. CAD/CAM applications for inlays, onlays, and, more recently, full-coverage restorations are being embraced progressively in clinical practice. The introduction of the chair-side CEREC (Sirona, Bensheim, Germany) CAD/CAM system was of considerable interest to dental practitioners; however, the early versions of the system provided a poor marginal fit of restorations, and it has taken over a decade for the technology to develop to the point where it can generate the desired restoration accuracy for practice (Tsitrou et al. 2007, Lee et al. 2008). Contemporary CAD/CAM now generates marginal accuracy and marginal gap that improve upon the traditional lost-wax technique (Almasri et al. 2011) as the crucial feature for optimizing clinical restorative outcomes (Renne et al. 2012).

Given that three-dimensional (3D) images of patients are nearly ubiquitous, the ability to combine these images with recordings of the natural dentition and opposing tooth surfaces portends near-natural replication of tooth anatomy in static and dynamic conditions. Predictably accurate imaging of tooth preparations followed by accurate milling of restorations can be anticipated with enhanced prognosis as well, as a direct product of the quality of tooth preparation.

More recent extensions of this technology into many fields have impacted dentistry and introduced the concept of the virtual articulator. Software development for virtual treatment planning for implant placement allows the interface between a 3D radiographic image, such as computerized tomography (CT) or volumetric cone beam CT of jaw bone anatomy, and software systems (such as Nobel Biocare—with progressive developments from Nobel Guide, Nobel Clinician to Nobel Connect, and an alternative in SimPlant) for manipulation of virtual implant placement to optimize 3D location within available bone. The template developed as an imaging guide contains possible location markers for implants derived from a diagnostic preparation of the potential final restorations, as determined and guided by the 3D images.

Computer-aided planning has also been embraced to facilitate complex craniofacial surgery. Computer software is used as a virtual articulator, and planning is undertaken on a computer. Traditionally, as with implant placement, the initial preparation of gypsum casts, articulated with the patient's transfer records (facebow and maxillomandibular record), can be analyzed and altered on the casts to provide a defined plan for each patient.

A 3D imaging and computer simulation study (Schendel & Jacobson 2009), applied contemporary software with imaging interpretation to develop what the authors described as a patient-specific reconstruction along with a virtual patient record. The authors reported that the precision was significantly improved over traditional 2D imaging and articulated study-cast analysis. A further study by Ghanai et al. (2010) compared the traditional technique of using plaster models, transfer records, and an articulator with computer-assisted 3D surgical planning and development of a virtual technique. A validation tool was developed to assess the virtual and traditional techniques. Data indicated that the virtual approach resulted in outcomes that were at least as accurate as the traditional technique while overcoming the need for study-cast analysis and transfer recording for articulator mountings, with their associated inaccuracies.

The book is presented in four sections:

Section 1 covers biological considerations of the occlusion. Comprehensive overviews of the neurophysiological mechanisms by Barry Sessle and periodontal biology by Stefan Heinz and Sašo Ivanovski give important statements on the biological framework. This is complemented by occlusion and health (Iven Klineberg), occlusion and adaptation to change (Sandro Palla), jaw movement and its control (Greg Murray), and anatomy and pathophysiology of the temporomandibular joints (Sandro Palla).

Section 2, on assessment, includes chapters on occlusal form and clinical specifics (Iven Klineberg), treatment planning and diagnostics (Iven Klineberg), and transfer records, articulators, and study casts (Rob Jagger and Iven Klineberg).

Section 3, on oral implant occlusion, includes chapters on the physiological considerations of oral implant function (Krister Svensson and Mats Trulsson), cclusion and principles of oral implant restoration (John Hobkirk), and implant rehabilitation and clinical management (Steven Eckert).

Section 4, on clinical practice and occlusion management, provides specific clinical approaches for patient care and includes chapters on temporomandibular joint disorders (Gunnar Carlsson), jaw muscle disorders (Merete Bakke), occlusion and periodontal health (Jan De Boever and AnnMarie De Boever), occlusion and orthodontics (Ali Darendeliler and Om Karbanda), occlusion and fixed prosthodontics (Terry Walton), occlusion and removable prosthodontics (Rob Jagger), maxillofacial prosthetics and occlusion (Rhonda Jacob), occlusal splints and management of the occlusion (Tom Wilkinson), and occlusal adjustment in occlusion management (Anthony Au and Iven Klineberg).

Iven Klineberg
Steven E. Eckert

REFERENCES

Almasri R, Drago CJ, Seigel SC, et al: Volumetric misfit in CAD/CAM and cast implant frameworks: a university laboratory study, *J Prosthodont* 20:267–274, 2011.

Ghanai S, Marmulla R, Wiechnik J, et al: Computer-assisted three-dimensional surgical planning: 3D virtual articulator: technical note, *Int J Oral Maxillofac Surg* 39:75–82, 2010.

Lee KB, Park CW, Kim KH, et al: Marginal and internal fit of all-ceramic crowns fabricated with two different CAD/CAM systems, *Dent Mater J* 27:422–426, 2008.

Renne W, McGill ST, Forshee KV, et al: Predicting marginal fit of CAD/CAM crowns based on the presence or absence of common preparation errors, *J Prosthet Dent* 108:310–315, 2012.

Schendel SA, Jacobson R: Three-dimensional imaging and computer simulation for office-based surgery, *J Oral Maxillofac Surg* 67:2107–2114, 2009.

Tsitrou EA, Northeast SE, van Noort R: Evaluation of the marginal fit of three margin designs of resin composite crowns using CAD/CAM, *J Dent* 35:68–73, 2007.

ACKNOWLEDGMENT

The editors wish to acknowledge the assistance and commitment of Mrs. Rita Penos, of Sydney, Australia, who worked with Iven Klineberg on the project from the start and has assisted in meeting time lines, interacting with authors and managing the progressively increasing database to the conclusion.

CONTRIBUTORS

Anthony Au, BDS, MDSc, FRACDS, FICD, MRACDS(Pros)
Clinical Associate Professor, Faculty of Dentistry, University of Sydney, Sydney, New South Wales, Australia

Merete Bakke, DDS, PhD, DrOdont
Associate Professor, Department of Odontology, University of Copenhagen, Copenhagen, Denmark

Gunnar E. Carlsson, LDS, OdontDr/PhD, DrOdonthc, FDSRDS (Eng)
Professor Emeritus, Institute of Odontology, University of Gothenburg, Gothenburg, Sweden

M. Ali Darendeliler, BDS PhD, DipOrtho
Professor and Chair of Orthodontics, Faculty of Dentistry, University of Sydney, Sydney, New South Wales, Australia

AnnMarie De Boever, DDS
Department of Fixed Prosthodontics and Periodontology, Faculty of Medicine and Health Sciences, Ghent University, Ghent, Belgium

Jan De Boever, DDS, DrMedDent, PhD
Professor Emeritus, Department of Fixed Prosthodontics and Periodontology, Faculty of Medicine and Health Sciences, Ghent University, Ghent, Belgium

Steven E. Eckert, DDS, MS, FACP
Professor Emeritus, Mayo Clinic, College of Medicine, Rochester, Minnesota, USA

Stefan A. Hienz, DMD, PhD
Associate Professor Periodontology, Program Director MClinDent Implantology, Regenerative Medicine Center, Griffith Health Institute, School of Dentistry and Oral Health, Griffith University, Queensland, Australia

John A. Hobkirk, BDS, PhD, DrMedhc, FDSRCS (Ed), FDSRCS (Eng)
Professor Emeritus, Prosthetic Dentistry, Eastman Dental Institute, Faculty of Medical Sciences, University College, University of London, UK

Sašo Ivanovski, BDSc, BDentSt, MDSc (Perio), PhD, FICD
Professor of Periodontology, School of Dentistry and Oral Health, Griffith Health Institute, Griffith University, Queensland, Australia

Rhonda F. Jacob, DDS, MS
Formerly Professor of Maxillofacial Prosthodontics, MD Anderson Cancer Center, Houston, Texas, USA

Rob Jagger, BDS, MScD, FDSRCS
Consultant Senior Lecturer, Bristol Dental School, University of Bristol, UK

Om Prakash Kharbanda, BDS, MDS, MOrth, RCS (Edin), M MEd (Dundee)
Professor and Head, Division of Orthodontics and Dentofacial Deformities, Centre for Dental Education and Research, All India Institute of Medical Sciences, New Delhi, India

Iven Klineberg, AM, RFD, BSc, MDS, PhD, FRACDS, FICD, FDSRCS (Lond, Edin)
Professor, Head of Discipline of Oral Rehabilitation, Nobel Biocare Chair of Oral Rehabilitation, Faculty of Dentistry, Westmead Hospital, University of Sydney, New South Wales, Australia

Greg M. Murray, BDS, MDS, PhD
Professor, Faculty of Dentistry, University of Sydney, New South Wales, Australia

Sandro Palla, Prof Dr Med Dent
Professor Emeritus, Clinic of Masticatory Disorders, Removable Prosthodontics and Special Care Dentistry, Center for Dental Medicine, University of Zurich, Switzerland

Barry J. Sessle, BDS, MDS, BSc, PhD, DSc (hc)
Professor and Canada Research Chair, University of Toronto, Toronto, Canada

Krister G. Svensson, DDS, MSc, PhD
Assistant Professor, Department of Dental Medicine, Section for Oral Rehabilitation, Karolinska Institute, Stockholm Sweden

Mats Trulsson, DDS, OdontDr/PhD
Professor and Head, Department of Dental Medicine, Karolinska Institute, Stockholm, Sweden

Terry Walton, BDS, MDSc, MS (Mich), FRACDS
Clinical Professor, Faculty of Dentistry, University of Sydney; Specialist Private Practitioner, Sydney, New South Wales, Australia

Tom Wilkinson, BDS, MSc, MDS, GradDip (Orofacial Pain)
Private Practitioner, Specialist Prosthodontist Practice limited to Orofacial Pain and Temporomandibular Disorders, Adelaide; Clinical Senior Lecturer University of Adelaide, South Australia, Australia

Thomas J. Vergo, Jr DDS, FACD, FAAMP
Professor Emeritus, Department of Restorative Dentistry, Tufts University School of Dentistry, Boston, Massachusetts, USA

SECTION | 1 |

Biological Considerations

CHAPTER 1

The Biological Basis of a Functional Occlusion: The Neural Framework

Barry J. Sessle

CHAPTER OUTLINE

SYNOPSIS

This chapter outlines the neural framework that determines and influences the occlusal interface. This framework includes also the neural underpinning of our ability to learn to adapt our masticatory behavior to an altered intraoral state produced by pain or changes to the occlusal interface following loss of teeth or their replacement by dental rehabilitative procedures.

CHAPTER POINTS

- The neural framework pertinent to a functional occlusion and occlusal rehabilitative approaches includes the peripheral and central nervous system (CNS) processes underlying orofacial perceptual, emotional and cognitive behaviors and the control of the orofacial musculature, as well as the adaptive potential of these peripheral and central components.
- Receptors in and around the teeth and in other orofacial tissues provide the CNS with feedback and feedforward sensory information that is used for these CNS processes.
- The excitability of the central components of the orofacial sensory and motor systems is subject to neural and nonneural modulatory influences in the CNS that underlie different behavioral states and that use a variety of endogenous chemical mediators.
- Chewing, swallowing, and other orofacial sensorimotor functions depend on brainstem neural circuits (e.g., central pattern generators), as well as on modulatory influences from higher brain centers such as the facial sensorimotor cortex.

- The effects of orofacial trauma and standard dental or oral and maxillofacial clinical procedures involving injury of orofacial tissues are not only limited to the face and mouth per se but also induce neuroplastic changes in the CNS.
- Injury or inflammation of orofacial tissues can increase the excitability of not only nociceptive afferents (i.e., peripheral sensitization) but also nociceptive neurons transmitting pain-related information in the CNS (i.e., central sensitization).
- Peripheral sensitization and central sensitization reflect neuroplastic changes that are normally reversible after a transient, uncomplicated injury or inflammation, but can sometimes persist and lead to a chronic pain state.
- Neuroplastic changes may also occur in the facial sensorimotor cortex and related CNS regions because of intraoral alterations producing pain or dental occlusal changes.
- Some of these neuroplastic changes may have detrimental effects on cognition, memory, and sensorimotor control, but others may reflect positive dynamic constructs that are crucial for adaptation and learning of new motor skills and for behavior that is appropriate to the altered intraoral sensory environment.

Dentists usually think of the biological framework of the dental occlusion in terms of the teeth and the biomechanical factors that result in the teeth coming into functional contact (e.g., the bony base, cuspal inclines, and structural features of the temporomandibular joint [TMJ]). These are certainly important, and this part of the framework can be disrupted in the case of disorders or diseases affecting these tissues (e.g., periodontitis and TMJ arthritis), and thus compromise the occlusion. These particular contributing factors are covered in Chapters 2, 13 and 15. The focus of this chapter is on the neural framework that is also particularly pertinent to a functional occlusion. This framework includes the peripheral sensory and motor components of the masticatory system, the peripheral and central nervous system (CNS) processes underlying orofacial perceptual, motivational, affective, and cognitive behaviors and the control of the orofacial musculature, and the adaptive potential of these peripheral and central components. These neural processes provide the neural framework for the occlusion and for occlusal rehabilitative approaches. The neural framework itself interacts with other physiological influences (e.g., endocrine, metabolic, and immunological) that form part of the biological basis of a functional occlusion, and it can also be influenced by genetic and environmental elements that include local factors (e.g., mechanical trauma, tissue loading, and disease), as well as other "life events" (e.g., psychological stress and socioeconomic conditions). Along with changes in the neural framework, these various influences may themselves affect the functional reserve of the masticatory system and may function as risk or predisposing factors that can foster or compromise the adaptive capacity of the system. These adaptive processes are especially pertinent to intraoral alterations associated with both pain and changes to the occlusal interface.

Given these various considerations, the chapter reviews in sequence the peripheral mechanisms and the CNS mechanisms that provide the neural framework. Moreover, the chapter outlines their involvement in adaptive mechanisms when the dental occlusion or related intraoral structures have been altered.

PERIPHERAL MECHANISMS: SENSORY PROCESSES

The orofacial tissues, such as the teeth, facial skin, TMJ, and associated musculature, are richly innervated by primary afferent (sensory) nerve fibers mainly of the trigeminal nerve. These afferents terminate in the tissues as specialized or nonspecialized endings, which are sometimes referred to as receptors. Nearly all of these afferents have their primary afferent cell bodies in the trigeminal ganglion, but in the case of the afferents associated with stretch-sensitive receptors called muscle spindles, in the jaw-closing muscles, and with some periodontal mechanoreceptors, their primary afferent cell bodies are located within the CNS, in the trigeminal mesencephalic nucleus. These various primary afferents provide the

CNS with sensory information that is used for perceptual, motivational, affective (e.g., emotional), and cognitive functions, as well as crucial peripheral feedback and feedforward information needed for the fine control of orofacial sensorimotor functions (for a review, see Dubner et al. 1978, Lund et al. 2009, Sessle 2006, 2009).

Many orofacial tissues are innervated by large-diameter, fast-conducting primary afferents (A-beta and A-delta fibers) that terminate in the tissues as low-threshold receptors and are activated by nonnoxious mechanical stimuli, such as tactile, pressure, and stretch stimuli. They typically have epithelial or connective tissue cell specializations embracing the afferent endings and endowing the endings with biomechanical features accounting for their high sensitivity to low-threshold mechanical stimuli applied to the tissues in which the afferents terminate. Low-threshold mechanoreceptors in the periodontal tissues of each tooth, for example, are activated by such mechanical stimuli applied to the tooth (e.g., when the tooth makes contact with opposing teeth) but they may also be activated during tooth movement. The analogous specialized endings in oral mucosa, facial skin, and TMJ may also act as mechanoreceptors when the tissues are mechanically stimulated or can function as proprioceptors that provide sensory information from these tissues when they are activated during orofacial muscle contractions, jaw or tongue movements, or TMJ condylar movements. This property may be especially important for the control of facial and jaw-opening muscles because, in contrast to most other skeletal muscles, including the jaw-closing muscles in primates and subprimates, as well as the tongue muscles in primates, these muscles have few or no muscle spindles and Golgi tendon organs (see Dubner et al. 1978, Sessle 2006, 2009). These specialized muscle or tendon receptors respond, respectively, to muscle stretch and contractile tension developed by the muscle.

Small-diameter, slow-conducting primary afferents (e.g., A-delta and C fibers) with free nerve endings acting as nociceptors also exist within the orofacial tissues. Moreover, as noted later, they carry into the brainstem nociceptive afferent information from their nociceptive afferent endings that is used for motor control and perceptual processes, such as pain (see Dubner et al. 1978, Sessle 2000, 2006).

Some small-diameter afferents instead have terminal endings that act as thermoreceptors. The orofacial region is further characterized by specialized chemoreceptive endings in taste buds; their small-diameter afferent inputs to the CNS are involved in taste sensory and affective functions but may also influence the patterns of mastication (Neyraud et al. 2005).

Activation of the various low-threshold receptors in oral mucosa, facial skin, periodontium, TMJ, muscle, etc. can result in the generation of nerve impulses (action potentials) in their associated primary afferents. These impulses are conducted along the afferents into the CNS and thereby provide sensory information used for motor (e.g., reflex), as well as perceptual and other responses related to tactile or nonnoxious thermal stimulation of intraoral and cutaneous tissues, nonnoxious joint position and movement, muscle stretch, and tension (see Dubner et al. 1978, Sessle 2000, 2006). Some low-threshold nonnociceptive TMJ afferents respond to condylar movement, but other nonarticular receptors (e.g., jaw-closing muscle spindles and some skin and intraoral mechanoreceptor afferents) may, as noted previously, also be activated during jaw movements, and so by their movement-evoked activity, these nonarticular afferents may contribute to jaw position sense (kinesthesia) and motor control. TMJ and jaw-closing muscle mechanoreceptors also have been shown to contribute, along with periodontal mechanoreceptors, to interdental size discrimination (i.e., the ability to discriminate the size of objects between opposing teeth).

The properties of periodontal mechanoreceptors are reviewed extensively in Chapter 10, and thus will only be outlined briefly here. As noted previously, periodontal low-threshold mechanoreceptors contribute to interdental size discrimination and to our perception of tactile stimulation of teeth because they code the spatiotemporal features of forces applied to the teeth (e.g., as a result of tooth-food, tooth-tooth, or tooth-tongue contact). This sensory information is processed in the CNS and used not only for the perception of these forces but also for motor control. For example, the information is important in the regulation of the level and direction of the forces applied to the teeth by the contraction of the masticatory muscles to assist in positioning food between the teeth before biting or during chewing. It is also important for adjusting and adapting the motor programs used to split and crush food during biting and chewing so that jaw muscle activity is adjusted to the hardness of the food and bite force parameters are optimized for the location of the food relative to the teeth. It is not surprising then that patients who have implant-supported prostheses to replace lost teeth have decreased control over bite force and other aspects of mastication because they lack such precise information from the periodontal mechanoreceptors of these teeth as a result of the periodontal receptors being destroyed or no longer able to provide this information. However, some residual control does remain; although the types and locations of the receptors involved in the sensory and motor responses and sensorimotor control when implant-supported prostheses are stimulated are unclear (see Jacobs & van Steenberghe 2006).

In the case of orofacial nociceptors, the activation of these nociceptive endings because of a noxious stimulus applied to an orofacial tissue can lead to the generation of action potentials in their associated A-delta and C-fiber afferents. Moreover, these nociceptive afferent inputs projecting via the trigeminal ganglion to the CNS can lead to the perceptual, reflex, and other behavioral responses that characterize pain (Dubner et al. 1978, Lam et al. 2005, Sessle 2000, 2009, Dostrovsky et al. 2014). The nociceptive afferent endings can be activated by chemicals (e.g., K^+, prostaglandins, and bradykinins) released from cells or vessels damaged by the noxious stimulus. The afferent endings can also manifest a prolonged increased excitability (termed *nociceptor* or *peripheral sensitization*) under certain conditions involving the teeth or other orofacial tissues. Further details of this hyperexcitability of the nociceptive afferent endings and of clinically relevant factors that can also modulate the excitability are provided below.

CENTRAL MECHANISMS

Brainstem Sensory Nuclei and Pathways

As noted previously, most primary afferents that supply peripheral tissues in the face and mouth have their primary afferent cell bodies in the trigeminal ganglion; from the ganglion, the central (proximal) component of each primary afferent projects into the

brainstem and synapses onto second-order neurons within the trigeminal brainstem sensory nuclear complex (Dubner et al. 1978, Sessle 2000, 2006, Dostrovsky et al. 2014). The adjacent solitary tract nucleus receives not only cranial nerve VII, IX, and X visceral afferents (e.g., those supplying lingual, laryngeal, and pharyngeal taste buds) but also receives some trigeminal afferent inputs. The trigeminal brainstem sensory nuclear complex can be subdivided into the principal or main sensory nucleus and the spinal tract nucleus. The latter comprises three subnuclei (oralis, interpolaris, and caudalis; Fig. 1-1), and its most caudal component, the subnucleus caudalis, is a laminated structure that resembles the spinal dorsal horn and indeed extends into the cervical spinal cord where it merges with the spinal dorsal horn. There are intrinsic connections between neurons in the different components of the trigeminal brainstem complex but the axons of many neurons in the four components of the complex project to areas such as the ventrobasal thalamus, periaqueductal gray, pontine parabrachial area, or brainstem reticular formation. Thereby, these neurons contribute to ascending nociceptive or nonnociceptive pathways involved in somatosensory functions or modulation of these functions, but some of the connections to the reticular formation and other parts of the brainstem are used in autonomic reflex responses (e.g., salivation and cardio-respiratory changes) to orofacial stimuli. Further, some neurons in all components of the complex and in areas adjacent to it (e.g., supratrigeminal nucleus) serve as interneurons in orofacial or cervical muscle reflex pathways (that are briefly reviewed in the following).

The low-threshold mechanosensitive trigeminal primary afferents terminate mainly in the rostral components of the trigeminal brainstem complex and in laminae III-VI of subnucleus caudalis. Some trigeminal nociceptive cutaneous and intraoral afferents, including dental pulp afferents, also terminate in some of these rostral components, but most trigeminal nociceptive afferents terminate in subnucleus caudalis, particularly in its laminae I, II, V, and VI (Dubner et al. 1978, Sessle 2000, 2006, Dostrovsky et al. 2014). Although its predominant input is from trigeminal primary afferents, the trigeminal brainstem complex (especially its subnucleus caudalis) may also receive afferent inputs from other cranial nerves (e.g., VII, IX,

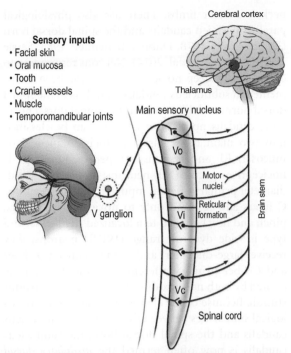

Sensory inputs
- Facial skin
- Oral mucosa
- Tooth
- Cranial vessels
- Muscle
- Temporomandibular joints

FIG 1-1 Major Somatosensory Pathway from the Orofacial Region Most primary afferents in the trigeminal (V) nerve have their cell bodies in the V ganglion and project to second-order neurons in the V brainstem sensory nuclear complex. This complex comprises the main sensory nucleus and the spinal tract nucleus; the latter has three subnuclei: oralis (*Vo*), interpolaris (*Vi*), and caudalis (*Vc*). These neurons may project to neurons situated in higher levels of the brain (e.g., in the thalamus) or in brainstem regions such as reticular formation or in the cranial nerve motor nuclei. Not shown are the projections of some cranial nerve VII, IX, X, and XII and cervical nerve afferents to the complex and the projections of many V, VII, IX, and X afferents to the solitary tract nucleus. (Reproduced from Sessle 2000, with permission.)

X, and XII), as well as from upper cervical nerves; these convergent input patterns are relevant to mechanisms underlying pain spread and referral (see the following section).

Properties of Low-Threshold Mechanoreceptive Brainstem Neurons

By way of their receipt of low-threshold mechanosensory primary afferent inputs from localized regions of the face and mouth and their projections to the thalamus, many second-order neurons in the rostral components of the trigeminal brainstem complex are essential brainstem neural elements relaying so-called fine touch (see Dubner et al. 1978, Sessle 2006). Nonetheless, some neurons at all levels of the complex can also transmit detailed somatosensory information about tactile stimuli delivered to localized orofacial regions. The localized orofacial region, which when stimulated can activate a neuron, is termed the neuron's *receptive field* (RF). The response properties of the tactile-transmission neurons, the so-called low-threshold mechanoreceptive (LTM) neurons, allow for the precise coding of orofacial mechanical (i.e., tactile) stimuli. For example, the LTM neurons show progressively increased (graded) responses as the area of stimulation of their localized RF or the stimulus intensity is gradually increased. Their activation is brought about by the release of excitatory neurotransmitters (e.g., the excitatory amino acid glutamate) from the brainstem endings of the LMT afferents that are excited by the RF stimulation. The neurotransmitters are synthesized in the cell bodies of the afferents in the trigeminal ganglion, and, when released in the brainstem, they act on ion channels and membrane receptors of the LTM neurons to activate the neurons.

These functional properties of LTM neurons ensure that tactile information derived from orofacial mechanoreceptors is securely transmitted through the trigeminal brainstem complex to the higher levels of the brain (e.g., thalamus and cerebral cortex), which process this detailed information of the modality and spatiotemporal features of a tactile stimulus applied to a part of the face or mouth. The processing of this information at these higher brain levels results in our ability to perceive the modality, location, duration, and intensity of the stimulus, but the information also is used for cognitive, emotional, and motivational functions, as well as for motor control. Many of the LTM neurons in the trigeminal brainstem complex serve, for example an important function in both mechanosensation from the teeth and in sensorimotor control. They relay the sensory information that they receive from the mechanosensitive periodontal afferents to higher levels of the CNS involved in perception and in the control of sensorimotor functions, and some of this information is in addition passed to brainstem areas that are also involved in sensorimotor (reflex) control (see the following discussion).

There are other types of low-threshold neurons in the trigeminal brainstem complex (Dubner et al. 1978, Trulsson & Essick 2004). Some are excited by jaw, tongue, or condylar movements, through afferent inputs from low-threshold mechanoreceptors in the TMJ or stretch-sensitive muscle receptors that are activated by the movements. These particular neurons appear to contribute to sensory pathways ascending to higher brain centers (e.g., to thalamus and cortex) or to brainstem circuits underlying the reflex regulation of masticatory muscle activity. Other neurons, especially those in trigeminal subnucleus caudalis, respond exclusively and with great sensitivity to innocuous cooling or warming stimuli applied to orofacial tissues and are important for the relay to the higher brain centers of detailed spatiotemporal information (e.g., location, duration, and intensity) about thermal stimuli applied to the face or mouth.

It should also be noted that not all of the afferent inputs to the neurons are of an excitatory nature associated with activation of the LTM neurons. Some inputs access and activate inhibitory circuits within and outside the trigeminal brainstem complex and these inhibitory circuits project to the neurons and can reduce or even completely suppress the activity of the neurons. These inhibitory effects reflect so-called afferent or segmental inhibition.

Properties of Nociceptive Brainstem Neurons

As already mentioned, most small-diameter nociceptive primary afferents terminate in trigeminal subnucleus caudalis, where they release neurochemicals (synthesized in their cell bodies in the trigeminal ganglion), such as glutamate and the neuropeptide substance P (Sessle 2000, 2006, Lam et al. 2005, Dostrovsky et al. 2014). These chemical mediators act on the ion channels and membrane receptors of caudalis second-order neurons to excite the neurons (e.g., the neurokinin receptor subtype NK-1 is activated by substance P, and the N-methyl-D-aspartate [NMDA] receptor, an ionotropic excitatory amino acid receptor subtype, as well as non-NMDA receptors, are activated by glutamate).

There are parallels in structure, afferent inputs, cell types, and projection sites between the subnucleus caudalis and the spinal cord dorsal horn, which is the integral relay in the spinal cord of nociceptive signals conducted by afferents supplying nociceptors in the neck, trunk, or limbs. There are also physiological parallels between caudalis and the spinal dorsal horn (Dubner et al. 1978, Dubner & Bennett 1983, Sessle 2000, Dostrovsky et al. 2014). Neurons responding to cutaneous or deep noxious stimuli have been documented in subnucleus caudalis, as well as in the spinal dorsal horn, and, like those in the spinal dorsal horn, these caudalis nociceptive neurons can be classified into two main types based on their cutaneous (or mucosal) RF and response properties. One type is nociceptive-specific (NS) neurons; they receive small-diameter primary afferent inputs from A-delta and/or C fibers and respond only to noxious stimuli (e.g., pinch and heat) applied to a localized RF. The second type is wide dynamic range (WDR) neurons; they receive large-diameter and small-diameter A-fiber and C-fiber primary afferent inputs and so can be excited by both nonnoxious (e.g., tactile) and noxious stimuli. Because of the close functional and morphological similarities between the trigeminal subnucleus caudalis and the spinal dorsal horn, the subnucleus caudalis is now often termed the *medullary dorsal horn*.

These nociceptive neurons, like LTM and other low-threshold neurons in the trigeminal brainstem complex, are subject to afferent (segmental) inhibitory influences evoked by some afferent inputs. These inhibitory influences have clinical relevance because they may come into play in situations whereby pain may be attenuated by tactile or proprioceptive afferent inputs evoked by rubbing an injured tissue and by clinical procedures that also evoke afferent inputs (e.g., acupuncture and transcutaneous electrical nerve stimulation [TENS]). They also involve inhibitory circuits and associated chemical mediators through which many centrally acting algesic drugs may exert control over pain (see also the following discussion).

It is also noteworthy that many of the properties of these nociceptive neurons are retained in different behavioral states, although state of consciousness and level of attention can influence the excitability of the neurons (e.g., their responses to orofacial stimuli may be depressed during certain sleep stages). Further, many WDR and NS neurons receive convergent inputs from afferents supplying superficial (e.g., skin, mucosa) and deep (e.g., TMJ, muscle, tooth pulp) tissues and are involved in relaying deep, as well as superficial, orofacial pain; some of the convergent afferent inputs may only be manifested (unmasked) in pathophysiological conditions such as those reflecting central sensitization and pain referral (see the Neuroplastic Changes in Nocueptive Neurons: Central Sensitization section). In addition, some WDR and NS neurons occur in the more rostral components (e.g., subnuclei oralis and interpolaris) of the trigeminal brainstem complex, but their role in orofacial-pain mechanisms is not fully clear (Sessle 2000).

Thalamic and Cerebral Cortical Sensory Areas and Pathways

The projections to the thalamus from neurons in the trigeminal brainstem complex can result in the activation of neurons in parts of the lateral thalamus (e.g., the ventrobasal complex in animals; also known as the ventroposterior thalamic nucleus in humans), the thalamic posterior nuclear group, and the medial thalamus (see Dubner et al. 1978, Sessle 2000, 2006). These thalamic areas contain many LTM neurons, as well as some thermosensitive and nociceptive (WDR and NS) neurons that receive orofacial somatosensory information relayed through the trigeminal brainstem complex. Some neurons instead receive gustatory information relayed to them via the solitary tract nucleus. Many of the ventrobasal somatosensory neurons are relay neurons projecting directly to neurons in the overlying somatosensory cerebral cortex, and they have functional properties consistent with a principal role in the sensory-discriminative aspects of touch, temperature, and pain. For example, like WDR and NS neurons in subnucleus caudalis, the ventrobasal thalamic nociceptive neurons have a RF within a localized part of the orofacial region and have graded responses to orofacial stimuli. However, nociceptive neurons in the medial thalamus generally have a more extensive RF, as well as other properties and connections (e.g., with anterior cingulate cortex; see the following discussion), indicating that their role is related more to the affective or motivational dimensions of pain.

In the so-called facial primary somatosensory cortex (SI), there are many LTM neurons, each with a localized cutaneous or intraoral RF and having graded responses to tactile stimuli. Thus these neurons are implicated in the cortical processing underlying the localization and intensity and temporal coding of orofacial tactile stimuli including those applied to dental tissues (see Dubner et al. 1978, Sessle 2006, Avivi-Arber et al. 2011). The SI area also contains some thermosensitive neurons implicated in orofacial temperature sensibility, as well as some WDR and NS neurons. The latter have properties that are generally similar to those of the subnucleus caudalis and ventrobasal nociceptive neurons, consistent with a role for them in pain localization and stimulus intensity and temporal coding (i.e., the sensory-discriminative dimension of pain). Nociceptive neurons are also present in other cortical regions, such as the anterior cingulate cortex and the insula, and they have properties implicating them in the affective or motivational dimensions of pain. The relevance of these cortical features to human pain processes is evident from recent brain imaging studies showing that noxious stimulation in humans can activate the somatosensory cortex, anterior cingulate cortex, and insula; these areas may also be activated in chronic pain states (May 2008, Davis & Stohler 2014).

Low-intensity stimulation of jaw, tongue, or facial muscle afferent inputs can also activate some neurons in the ventrobasal thalamus or facial SI or primary motor cortex (MI; Sessle 2006, Avivi-Arber et al. 2011). These sensory inputs to the facial SI and MI, along with those from more superficial receptors (e.g., cutaneous and periodontal), are important in mandibular kinesthesia and interdental size discrimination and in providing sensory feedback from orofacial receptors that may be used in the cortically mediated control of orofacial motor function. Sensory inputs to the facial SI and MI also appear to arise from stimulation of implant-supported prostheses, and are likely relevant to the concept of "osseoperception" (Klineberg & Murray 1999, Jacobs & van Steenberghe 2006).

Brainstem Motor Nuclei and Reflex Pathways

Orofacial muscles and movements require sophisticated and adaptive neural circuits providing for their control and for their integration with associated motor behaviors such as respiration. These circuits include various sensory nuclei and motor nuclei arranged into distinct neuronal pools in the brainstem that receive inputs from orofacial afferents and higher CNS regions that regulate the activity of the neuronal pools (see Dubner et al. 1978, Sessle 2009, Avivi-Arber et al. 2011). The motor supply to the orofacial muscles originates from brainstem motoneurons in the cranial nerve motor nuclei; these include (1) the motoneurons of the trigeminal motor nucleus that through their motor axons (alpha efferents) provide the motor innervation of most jaw muscles, (2) the motoneurons of the facial motor nucleus that supply the muscles of facial expression, (3) the motoneurons of the hypoglossal nucleus that innervate the intrinsic and extrinsic tongue muscles, and (4) the motoneurons of the nucleus ambiguus that mainly supply muscles of the palate, larynx, and pharynx. The motoneurons supplying these various muscles receive afferent inputs from receptors that are activated by tactile, thermal, or noxious orofacial stimuli or by those that signal taste, joint position, or muscle stretch.

Other than the trigeminal mesencephalic nucleus through which some primary afferent (muscle, spindle, and periodontal) inputs project to jaw-closing motoneurons in the trigeminal motor nucleus, most of the orofacial afferent inputs to the brainstem motoneurons are indirect because they involve interneurons that receive the afferent inputs and relay them to the relevant motoneurons (see Lund et al. 2009). The trigeminal brainstem complex and the solitary tract nucleus are major interneuronal sites, but other important interneuronal sites include the intertrigeminal nucleus, the supratrigeminal nucleus, as well as components of the medial and especially lateral reticular formation that lie immediately adjacent to the trigeminal brainstem complex and the solitary tract nucleus. These sites provide part of the neural circuitry and processes constituting the central pattern generators (CPGs) that are so crucial in the initiation and control of complex orofacial functions such as chewing and swallowing (see Dubner et al. 1978, Jean 2001, Lund et al. 2009). The interneuronal regions also provide a neural substrate that allows for the initiation or modulation of brainstem reflexes by receiving and integrating afferent inputs evoked by stimuli applied to various orofacial tissues. The afferent inputs to these interneuronal sites are capable not only of evoking brainstem-based reflex changes in orofacial muscles, but the afferent signals are also relayed from the brainstem to higher brain centers

that, through their descending projections back down to the interneurons, CPGs or motoneurons, are involved in sensorimotor control of the muscles. Through these various brainstem connections and higher brain center influences, the orofacial afferent inputs can activate or inhibit the cranial nerve motoneurons supplying the orofacial muscles. Brainstem circuits also underlie the autonomic reflex changes in heart rate, blood pressure, breathing, and salivation noted previously. Moreover, some may contribute to complex behaviors that can be evoked by nonnoxious or noxious stimulation of orofacial tissues.

In view of the large array of muscles in the orofacial region and the great diversity of receptors and afferent inputs, the number of orofacial reflexes is also vast. For example, stretch of a jaw-closing muscle (e.g., masseter) evokes a myotatic stretch reflex (termed the jaw-closing or jaw-jerk reflex) in the stretched muscle. This reflex involves the stretch-induced activation of muscle spindle afferents in the jaw muscle, which, as indicated previously, have their primary afferent cell bodies in the trigeminal mesencephalic nucleus; the stretch-evoked impulses are conducted along the afferents through this nucleus and into their central axons projecting to and monosynaptically activating jaw-closing motoneurons in the trigeminal motor nucleus that supply the stretched muscle (Dubner et al. 1978, Sessle 2006). The jaw-opening reflex and the reflex effects of stimulation of periodontal receptors are two other examples of jaw reflexes involving brainstem circuits. This stimulation activates afferent inputs that can evoke a brief excitatory reflex in the jaw-opening muscles (e.g., anterior digastric), but a transient inhibitory reflex involving one or more so-called silent periods in the antagonistic jaw-closing muscles can also occur. These reflex effects appear to reflect brainstem neural circuits that serve a protective or regulatory function, for example, to help control for excessive bite force during jaw-closing movements or to allow for a protective jaw opening if the individual encounters an intraoral noxious stimulus (e.g., a fishbone while eating fish). However, animal experiments have also revealed that the application of algesic chemicals (e.g., hypertonic saline, glutamate, mustard oil, and capsaicin) to the TMJ, muscle, tooth, or another orofacial tissue can result in prolonged increases in electromyographic (EMG) activity of both the jaw-opening and jaw-closing muscles (Lam et al. 2005, Sessle 2000, 2006). These particular reflex effects involve activation of nociceptive endings in these tissues, and their nociceptive afferent input into the trigeminal brainstem complex produces activation of interneurons, especially in the subnucleus caudalis, that project directly or indirectly to the jaw-opening and -closing motoneurons in the trigeminal motor nucleus. Several chemical mediators and receptor mechanisms (e.g., NMDA, opioids, and GABA) in the caudalis and the motor nucleus are involved in the circuitry for activation or modulation of the reflex effects. Such co-contraction of the jaw-opening and the jaw-closing muscles may be a mechanism providing for a "splinting" effect to limit jaw movements in pathophysiological conditions (e.g., pain) affecting deep tissues such as the TMJ and muscles. In addition, nociceptive activity can influence higher brain centers involved in sensorimotor control, such as the sensorimotor cortex, and provide additional pathways by which pain-related sensory inputs can influence masticatory muscle function. The following considers these descending influences in more detail.

Descending Influences on Sensory and Motor Processes

The activity of the interneurons and motoneurons, like that of the neurons in the trigeminal brainstem complex and solitary tract nucleus that project to higher brain centers, can vary depending on the behavioral state (e.g., the level of consciousness, arousal, attention, sleep). In addition to the afferent and segmental modulatory influences mentioned previously, there are modulatory influences of an excitatory or inhibitory nature that are exerted on the neurons by descending projections to them from various cortical and subcortical structures involved in such behavioral states and other functions (Dubner et al. 1978, 2013, Sessle 2000, 2009, Avivi-Arber et al. 2011; Fig. 1-2). These descending modulatory influences include those originating from higher brain centers, such as several regions of the cerebral cortex (e.g., the sensorimotor cortex, cortical premotor and supplementary motor areas, and cortical masticatory and swallowing areas), the amygdala and other parts of the limbic system, lateral hypothalamus, basal

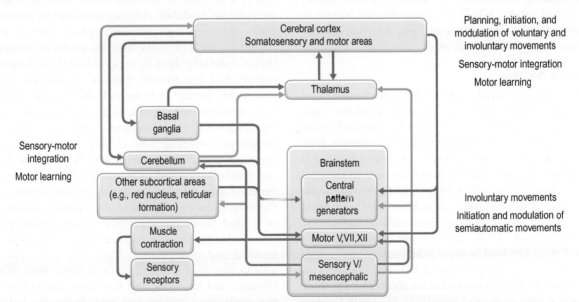

FIG 1-2 Illustration of the Main Connections of the Orofacial Sensorimotor System There are extensive excitatory and inhibitory interconnections between the different cortical and subcortical regions. The central pattern generators provide the programmed output to cranial nerve motoneurons supplying the muscles active in chewing (the "chewing center") and swallowing (the "swallowing center"). (Reproduced from Avivi-Arber et al. 2011, with permission.)

ganglia, anterior pretectal nucleus, and red nucleus, as well as regions in the brainstem, such as the CPGs, cerebellum, and raphe system. Through these descending excitatory or inhibitory influences, the descending projections can exert control over the spatiotemporal coding properties of the LTM and nociceptive neurons, relaying sensory information to higher brain centers, over the CPGs and those interneurons involved in orofacial sensorimotor functions, and over the brainstem motoneurons themselves supplying the orofacial musculature. These modulatory influences exert their effects by releasing several excitatory or inhibitory neurochemicals (e.g., opioids, GABA, serotonin [5-HT], and norepinephrine) that act upon these neuronal elements, and thereby they can initiate, guide, or regulate orofacial sensorimotor functions. The importance of their role is reflected in the orofacial sensory or motor deficits that can arise following damage or other alterations to some of the regions, giving rise to these descending influences (e.g., some abnormal sensorimotor functions, such as those seen in oral dyskinesia and sleep bruxism, may be partly due to an imbalance in dopamine in parts of the basal ganglia). Three other specific descending modulatory influences are now briefly outlined (raphe, CPGs, and sensorimotor cortex) to exemplify the importance of these descending influences in orofacial sensorimotor functions.

Raphe System

The periaqueductal gray (PAG) and rostroventral medial medulla (RVM) are components of the raphe system, an important intrinsic CNS for modulation of several functions including pain. For example, both PAG and RVM project to the trigeminal brainstem complex, and stimulation of certain parts of the PAG or RVM can markedly suppress the activity of caudalis nociceptive neurons, as well as reflex and other behavioral responses to noxious orofacial stimuli (see Dubner et al. 1978, 2013, Sessle 2000). Chemical mediators involved in these inhibitory effects include opioids (e.g., enkephalins), 5-HT, and GABA. This system contributes to our innate ability to exert some control over pain, and variability in its effectiveness is probably a factor explaining why persons vary in their ability to withstand pain. There is also evidence that some pain-relieving approaches utilizing activation of afferent inputs (e.g., acupuncture and

TENS) involve at least in part, recruitment of this intrinsic pain-inhibitory system, and that some analgesic drugs (e.g., opiates) exert their effects by acting upon components of the system. However, some parts of the system have instead a facilitatory influence over nociceptive transmission, so the role of the raphe system in pain modulation is quite complex (see Dubner et al. 2013). Further, alterations to the modulatory influences from the PAG or RVM may be involved in producing chronic pain states (May 2008, Dubner et al. 2013).

Central Pattern Generators

Another important set of influences is the CPGs for chewing, swallowing, and other analogous complex sensorimotor behaviors. They receive, directly or via interneurons, afferent inputs from orofacial tissues and from higher brain centers, and after processing these afferent and descending inputs, the CPGs send signals to the cranial nerve motoneurons to produce or regulate chewing, swallowing, and other orofacial sensorimotor functions (see Dubner et al. 1978, Jean 2001, Lund et al. 2009, Sessle 2006, 2009). In the case of the CPG for mastication (the "chewing center"), this is a network of neurons in the brainstem that generate or modulate chewing movements through their excitatory and inhibitory projections to the motoneurons. The CPG uses its orofacial afferent inputs, especially those from periodontal mechanoreceptors and jaw muscle spindles, in concert with descending inputs to it from higher brain regions (e.g., sensorimotor cortex), to provide guidance and modification of the movements (Fig. 1-2). Thus the stereotyped opening and closing jaw movements typical of chewing are patterned by the CPG, but they can also be varied and programmed, for example, to function in an integrated manner with movements of the tongue and cheeks so as to allow for repositioning of a food bolus and for alterations in masticatory force, velocity, and jaw displacement as the bolus is crushed and manipulated. These processes explain why factors such as the number of teeth, food composition and hardness, and bite force can influence the masticatory process and provide for the breakdown of the bolus to a size suitable for swallowing. By monitoring the intraoral sensory inputs that it receives from the teeth, tongue, cheeks, etc. and that are evoked during different phases of this process, the CPG can also modulate these sensory inputs. It can provide a form of central control that may inhibit afferent inputs to the motoneurons that would otherwise produce undesirable perturbations and reflexes that might disrupt the ongoing masticatory process. However, it may not inhibit nociceptive afferent inputs but it allows them to access the masticatory motoneurons and thereby provides protection of the masticatory apparatus. A common example of this central control in operation involves the jaw-opening reflex noted earlier; the CPG may not suppress nociceptive afferent inputs during chewing. Rather, it allows for the interruption of chewing and for the jaw-opening reflex to be elicited by a noxious stimulus, such as the example given earlier of a fish bone piercing the oral mucosa when an individual is eating fish. In such an instance, it is important for chewing to be halted to prevent further damage to the mucosal tissues. In the case of the CPG for swallowing (the "swallow center"), it involves brainstem neurons within and adjacent to the solitary tract nucleus. The output of these swallow CPG neurons provides the time-locked, patterned drive to the different cranial nerve motoneuron pools supplying the many muscles participating in swallowing. The swallow CPG neurons are triggered into action by afferent inputs especially from the pharynx and larynx, but unlike the CPG for chewing, which is sensitive to both sensory inputs and CNS controls, the CPG for swallowing is relatively insensitive to sensory feedback or descending controls once the swallow has started (Dubner et al. 1978, Jean 2001).

Sensorimotor Cortex

The sensorimotor area of the cerebral cortex plays an integral role in sensorimotor control, through its regulatory influences on both sensory and motor pathways in the CNS. The sensorimotor cortex includes the primary somatosensory cortical area (SI) and the primary motor cortical area (MI). Both the SI and MI are somatotopically organized such that their medial parts deal with respectively somatosensory or motor functions of the trunk and limbs, whereas the lateral parts of the SI and MI deal with orofacial sensory functions or motor functions. Accordingly, the latter are referred to collectively as the face sensorimotor cortex (see Avivi-Arber et al. 2011). Lateral to and indeed overlapping the lateral

boundary of face SI and face MI is a region termed the *cortical masticatory area* or, more appropriately, the *cortical masticatory and swallow cortex* because this area is involved in the initiation or modulation of both chewing and swallowing. One clinical example of the importance of these cortical regions is the loss of sensorimotor control of orofacial movements needed for speech, chewing, or swallowing that can follow a stroke, affecting the face sensorimotor cortex or the cortical masticatory and swallow cortex (see Martin 2009).

Techniques such as cortical surface electrical stimulation, intracortical microstimulation (ICMS), transcranial magnetic stimulation (TMS), brain imaging, or cortical neural recordings have provided insights into the functions of the face sensorimotor cortex including the cortical masticatory and swallow cortex. The major role of facial MI is in the initiation, control, and execution of orofacial movements, but it also may contribute to the learning of new motor skills and the adaptation to altered sensory inputs, such as might occur with changes to the dental occlusion through loss of teeth, dental restorations, orthodontically induced tooth movement, etc. (see Avivi-Arber et al. 2011). Through the direct and indirect descending projections of face-MI neurons to brainstem interneurons and to the motoneurons supplying the orofacial muscles, face MI is involved in the bilateral control of "elemental" movements of the face, jaw, and tongue (e.g., tongue protrusion and jaw opening). Along with the cortical masticatory and swallow cortex, its projection targets include the CGPs and thereby it can regulate "semiautomatic" movements such as chewing and swallowing, which in the past have been thought to be mainly controlled by brainstem regulatory circuits (e.g., CPGs). Despite its name, face MI is not purely "motor" because, like face SI, its neurons receive sensory inputs (relayed to it via the brainstem and thalamus or face SI) from muscle, facial skin, teeth, and other orofacial tissues, and it may use this sensory information in the control of the orofacial musculature (e.g., to regulate bite force or vertical dimension of the jaw). In the case of face SI, its neurons have a major role in somatosensory functions such as touch, by virtue of their processing of orofacial somatosensory inputs that they receive via the brainstem and thalamus. However, face SI also makes an important contribution to oroface sensorimotor control through its interconnections with face MI and its descending projections that modulate the brainstem and thalamic neurons transmitting sensory information evoked by orofacial stimuli including those occurring during ongoing movements (see Avivi-Arber et al. 2011).

EFFECTS OF OCCLUSAL AND OTHER INTRAORAL CHANGES ON SENSORY AND MOTOR CONTROL MECHANISMS

Intraoral pain and alterations to the dental occlusion or other intraoral tissues not only may activate orofacial afferent endings as well as cause a host of morphological and functional changes in other cellular elements of the tissues, but may also induce neuroplastic changes in the afferent endings and in the central elements (trigeminal brainstem complex, thalamus, and cerebral cortex) of the orofacial sensorimotor system. The following outlines the effects of occlusal and other intraoral changes on sensorimotor functions and their underlying mechanisms.

Peripheral Effects

Changes to the dental occlusion as well as alterations to other orofacial tissues can modify the properties of the trigeminal LTM primary afferents supplying these tissues. Injury of peripheral tissues (including nerves) can also influence the excitability of the peripheral endings of nociceptive afferents (Lam et al. 2005, Sessle 2011, Iwata et al. 2011, Dostrovsky et al. 2014). The injury can result in inflammation and involve chemical mediators released from the damaged cells or blood vessels. Some of these mediators, such as prostaglandins, can produce overt activation of the nociceptive endings, but others can modulate the excitability of the endings. Some mediators are neurochemicals (e.g., glutamate, substance P, calcitonin gene-related peptide [CGRP]) that are released from nociceptive afferent endings following damage or inflammation of the peripheral tissue (Fig. 1-3). These neurochemicals may act on platelets, macrophages, mast cells, and other cells of the immune system to cause them to release inflammatory mediators such as serotonin (5-HT), histamine, bradykinins, and cytokines, as well other mediators (e.g.,

opioids such as the enkephalins). Thus, a "neurogenic inflammation" may be produced, so named because it is initially generated by substances released from the nociceptive afferent endings. In addition, the mediators may also act on membrane receptors and ion channels on the nociceptive afferent endings that selectively interact with each mediator; for example, 5-HT acts on 5-HT receptors; the enkephalins on opioid receptors; glutamate on glutamatergic receptors; and histamine on histamine receptors. Some of the mediators (e.g., enkephalins) decrease the excitability of the nociceptive afferent endings. However, many mediators increase their excitability, and this so-called peripheral sensitization (see Lam et al. 2005, Dostrovsky et al. 2014) is reflected in spontaneous activity of the afferent endings, as well as in their increased responsiveness to subsequent noxious stimuli. It also induces lowered activation thresholds that are decreased to such an extent that the nociceptive afferent endings may develop responsiveness to nonnoxious stimuli. These physiological changes contribute, respectively, to the spontaneous pain, hyperalgesia (increased sensitivity to noxious stimuli), and allodynia (pain produced by normally nonnoxious a stimulus) that are features of acute pain. The mediators may also diffuse through the damaged and inflamed tissues and influence the excitability of adjacent nociceptive endings; this represents a peripheral process contributing to the spread of pain. As the tissues heal, normally the peripheral sensitization gradually subsides, but if the peripheral sensitization persists, it can contribute to the spontaneous pain, allodynia, hyperalgesia, and pain spread typical of many chronic pain states such as arthritis.

There are also sex differences in the effects of some of the mediators, and the excitability of the nociceptive afferent endings can be modulated by circulating hormones such as estrogens (Lam et al. 2005, Cairns et al. 2014). These features are thought to be peripherally based processes contributing to the well-documented sex differences in pain and to the female predominance of many chronic pain states. Also of clinical relevance are findings that the activation or sensitization of the nociceptive afferent endings can be modulated by some antiinflammatory or analgesic drugs (e.g., the analgesic effect of aspirin can largely be explained by its peripheral action on prostaglandin synthesis). In addition, substances (e.g.,

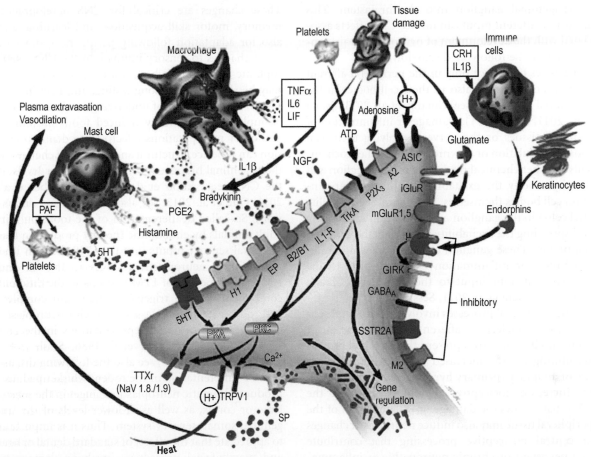

FIG 1-3 Mediators Involved in Inflammation-Related Peripheral Sensitization of Nociceptive Afferent Nerve Endings in Orofacial Tissues Inflammation leads to numerous chemicals being released from macrophages, mast cells, immune cells, and injured cells. By acting upon ion channels or membrane receptors on the nociceptive afferent endings, these mediators may alter the sensitivity of the endings. Some of the mediators can increase the excitability of the nociceptive afferent endings (i.e., peripheral sensitization), others may exert inhibitory effects. Several of these mediators are shown. ASIC, acid-sensing ion channel; CRH, corticotrophin-releasing hormone; GIRK, G-protein-coupled inward rectifying potassium channel; 5-HT, serotonin; iGluR, ionotropic glutamate receptor; IL-1β, interleukin-1-beta; IL-6, interleukin-6; LIF, leukemia inhibitory factor; μ, mu-opioid receptor; M_2, muscarinic receptor; mGluR, metabotropic glutamate receptor; NGF, nerve growth factor; PAF, platelet-activating factor; PGE_2, prostaglandin E_2; PKA, protein kinase A; PKC, protein kinase C; SSTR2A, somatostatin receptor 2A; TNF-α, tumor necrosis factor alpha; TrkA, tyrosine kinase receptor A; TRPV1, transient receptor potential vanilloid 1; TTXr, tetrodotoxin-resistant sodium channel. (Reproduced from Meyer et al. 2006, with permission.)

noradrenaline) released from the sympathetic efferents that innervate many peripheral tissues can also modulate the excitability of the nociceptive afferents and thereby contribute to the pain seen in conditions such as complex regional pain syndrome.

Damage of peripheral afferents themselves may lead to nerve sprouting into the peripheral tissues or to afferent fiber changes that are associated with so-called ectopic or aberrant afferent discharges. The discharges are conducted along the afferent fibers via

15

the trigeminal ganglion into the brainstem. This abnormal afferent input can induce CNS effects associated with the development of neuropathic pain conditions (see the following discussion).

Changes occur not only in the peripheral afferent fibers themselves but also in their cell bodies in the trigeminal ganglion (see Chiang et al. 2011, Iwata et al. 2011, Sessle 2011). Damage or inflammation of orofacial tissues or the nerves supplying them can cause upregulation or downregulation of neurochemicals or other chemical mediators in the ganglion and thereby modify the excitability of the afferent ganglion cell bodies themselves. Nonneural cells (satellite glial cells) in the ganglion are involved in influencing and spreading the excitability changes in the ganglion cell bodies. These ganglion changes following orofacial injury or inflammation can contribute to the abnormal afferent input to the brainstem (Chiang et al. 2011, Iwata et al. 2011, Sessle 2011).

The peripheral processes involving peripheral sensitization of nociceptive afferent endings at the site of injury itself appear to represent the principal process accounting for the increased pain sensitivity at the site of an injury (primary hyperalgesia). Nevertheless, the increased nociceptive afferent barrage into the CNS that follows the damage or inflammation of the peripheral tissue may also induce neuroplastic changes in central nociceptive processing that contribute to a persistent or chronic neuropathic or inflammatory pain state. As noted later, this process is termed *central sensitization* and is particularly involved in so-called secondary hyperalgesia, whereby increased pain sensitivity occurs well beyond the site of tissue injury. In addition, the peripheral damage may be associated with CNS neuroplastic changes in LTM neurons processing tactile information, as outlined in the following.

Central Effects
Neuroplastic Changes in Low-Threshold Mechanoreceptive Neurons

In addition to the afferent, segmental, and descending modulatory influences described earlier, another form of modulation of the spatiotemporal coding characteristics of the LTM neurons is reflected in the neuroplasticity of these neurons. The term *neuroplasticity* refers to the brain's remarkable ability to undergo structural and functional changes throughout life.

These changes are critical for CNS development, memory, motor skill acquisition, and learning, and also for adaptation following peripheral trauma or other changes to sensory inputs into the CNS. Neuroplastic changes may have fast onset or slow onset, may be short lived or long lasting, and may involve several different types of underlying mechanisms. For example, orthodontically induced tooth movement and other manipulations affecting the dental occlusion can produce structural and functional changes in the trigeminal brainstem complex or higher levels of the CNS (e.g., Kubo et al. 2007, Avivi-Arber et al. 2011, Oue et al. 2013; see also the following discussion). So-called deafferentation of the tooth pulp in adult animals by endodontic therapy produces a loss of dental sensory inputs into the CNS that can lead to profound neuroplastic changes in the RF and response properties of LTM neurons in the different components of the trigeminal brainstem complex, and tooth extraction is associated with neuroplastic changes in the orofacial representations in the face sensorimotor cortex (Hu et al. 1986, Sessle 2000, Avivi-Arber et al. 2011; see also the following discussion). Deafferentation of the rodent whisker pad also produces dramatic neuroplastic changes in the sensorimotor cortex, as well as in lower levels of the trigeminal somatosensory system. Thus it is important to appreciate that the effects of standard dental or oral and maxillofacial procedures involving damage to tissues are not only limited to the face or mouth per se but also induce neuroplastic changes in the brain. Such changes are especially evident in the trigeminal nociceptive system in the CNS, as outlined in the following.

Neuroplastic Changes in Nociceptive Neurons: Central Sensitization

Neuroplasticity is evident in the nociceptive pathways in the CNS because of injury or inflammation of peripheral tissues. In the trigeminal system, neuroplasticity of caudalis nociceptive neurons may be induced either by increased nociceptive afferent input into the CNS (e.g., by direct stimulation of peripheral nerves by a neuropathic injury or by inflammation) or by a decreased afferent input (e.g., through nerve damage resulting in deafferentation). The neuroplasticity can be reflected in a heightened excitability of the central nociceptive neurons, which may be accompanied by pain. It is considered a reflection of a centrally based "functional plasticity" or "central sensitization" of the nociceptive neurons (Sessle 2000, 2011, Iwata et al. 2011).

The neuroplastic changes underlying central sensitization occur in acute pain states following injury or inflammation and also appear to be important in the development of chronic pain conditions, thereby providing justification for the emerging view that chronic pain is a neurological disease or disorder in itself. The central sensitization may result in part from an unmasking and increased efficacy of the extensive array of convergent afferent inputs that are a feature of many of the WDR and NS neurons. Disinhibition involving a counteraction in the CNS of some of the descending inhibitory influences may also contribute to the central sensitization, as may enhancement of descending facilitatory influences (Dubner et al. 2013, 2014). Increases in nociceptive neuronal spontaneous activity and responses to noxious stimuli and a decreased activation threshold are cardinal features of central sensitization that contribute respectively to the spontaneous pain, hyperalgesia, and allodynia that characterize many clinical cases of persistent pain following injury or inflammation (Sessle 2000, 2011, Iwata et al. 2011, Dostrovsky et al. 2014). Central sensitization may also include an increase in the RF size of nociceptive neurons that results from the unmasking of some of the convergent afferent inputs to the neurons. This feature of centrally sensitized nociceptive neurons is thought to be a major contributor to the pain spread and referrals that are seen clinically in many orofacial inflammatory or neuropathic pain states.

Several neuropeptides (e.g., CGRP and substance P) and excitatory amino acids (e.g., glutamate) released from the central endings of the primary afferents onto the WDR and NS neurons in the brainstem are involved in the production of trigeminal central sensitization (Sessle 2000, 2011, Iwata et al. 2011, Dostrovsky et al. 2014). For example, glutamate and substance P respectively activate NMDA and NK-1 receptors on the neurons, thereby initiating intracellular changes that lead to an increased excitability of the neurons (i.e., central sensitization). Several other chemicals released from the primary afferent endings or from adjacent neurons, as well as from descending projections to the WDR and NS neurons or from nearby nonneural cells (glia; see also the following discussion), may modulate these central effects; these chemical mediators include opioids (e.g., enkephalins), GABA, ATP, and 5-HT.

It is important to appreciate that while central sensitization, like peripheral sensitization, is usually reversible after a transient, uncomplicated trauma or inflammation associated with an acute pain, it nonetheless can sometimes persist and lead to pain that can last for hours, days, weeks, or even longer. Why central sensitization can resolve after most injuries but be maintained in others is unclear, but genetic factors may contribute.

Both the development and the maintenance of central sensitization also depend on the functional integrity of nonneural cells, namely glial cells. Recent studies of trigeminal central sensitization in animal models of acute or chronic orofacial pain have revealed that damage or inflammation of dental and other orofacial tissues, or trigeminal nerve injury, leads to an upregulation in the trigeminal subnucleus caudalis of two types of glial cells (astroglia and microglia) along with central sensitization of caudalis WDR and NS neurons and pain behavior; further, blockade of the glial cell activation can overcome both the caudalis central sensitization and the pain behavior (see Chiang et al. 2011, Iwata et al. 2011, Sessle 2011). Glial cells thus offer a novel target for the development of new therapeutic approaches to control pain.

Central sensitization induced by alterations to afferent inputs underscores the fact that the afferent inputs and the nociceptive circuitry in the CNS are not "hard-wired" but are indeed plastic. In other words, neuroplastic changes can occur in the RF and response properties of the nociceptive neurons because of damage of trigeminal nerves or injury or inflammation of other peripheral tissues, including trauma associated with an occlusal interference or injury induced during dental or oral and maxillofacial procedures (Sessle 2000, 2011, Iwata et al. 2011, Cao et al. 2013, Dubner et al. 2013, 2014). Further, central sensitization in trigeminal nociceptive pathways is not limited to the subnucleus caudalis. It also occurs in nociceptive neurons in subnucleus oralis of the trigeminal brainstem complex, as well as in higher brain regions such as the ventrobasal thalamus (see Sessle 2000, 2011). Nonetheless, the importance of the subnucleus caudalis is underscored by evidence that the subnucleus caudalis is responsible for the expression of central sensitization in these structures by way of its projections to both oralis and ventrobasal thalamus. Further, increases in jaw muscle activity reflexively evoked by deep craniofacial noxious stimuli often accompany the trigeminal central sensitization process; these motor responses are also dependent on the functional integrity of caudalis because they involve reflex interneurons in the subnucleus caudalis (see Sessle 2000, 2006). They likely contribute to the altered or limited jaw movements that are characteristic of many orofacial-pain states (e.g., Temporomandibular disorders).

Neuroplastic Changes in Central Nervous System Circuits Involved in Cognition, Memory, and Related Functions

It is well known that loss of teeth can negatively affect the masticatory ability, speech, and quality of life of patients (Feine & Carlsson 2003; see Chapters 3 and 4). Recent studies suggest cognitive and memory impairment may be associated with tooth loss or related changes in mastication, diet, etc. (e.g., Grabe et al. 2009, Okamoto et al. 2010, Weijenberg et al. 2011, Noble et al. 2013). These findings are supported by brain imaging and other findings in humans of changes in cortical and subcortical regions involved in orofacial sensorimotor functions, learning, and memory (e.g., Momose et al. 1997, Yan et al. 2008, Weijenberg et al. 2011). Animal studies also provide support in showing that a reduced vertical dimension (caused by grinding occlusal surfaces) or tooth loss may cause an alteration in chewing ability that is associated with reduced learning ability and spatial memory in rodents. These changes may be accompanied by alterations in stress hormone levels and in cell density and underlying neurochemical processes (e.g., cholinergic) in the hippocampus, which is an integral CNS region for memory (see Onozuka et al. 1999, Kubo et al. 2007, Oue et al. 2013, Iida et al. 2014).

Neuroplastic Changes in Face Sensorimotor Cortex

There is emerging evidence that alterations to orofacial tissues, including dental occlusal changes and the rehabilitative procedures (e.g., implants, bridges, and dentures) used to address these changes, may lead to neuroplasticity in not only CNS circuits underlying orofacial somatosensory functions, learning, and memory, as noted previously, but also CNS regions involved in orofacial sensorimotor functions such as the face sensorimotor cortex (see Avivi-Arber et al. 2010a,b, 2011, Weijenberg et al. 2011). The findings are particularly pertinent to the clinically important question of why is it that some patients can adapt to dental occlusal changes (e.g., tooth loss) or rehabilitative procedures (e.g., dentures or dental implants) and learn quickly how to function again appropriately, whereas other patients cannot? In addition, how do these rehabilitative procedures functionally produce their therapeutic effects? At least part of the answers to these questions lies in the ability of the fundamental features of the face sensorimotor cortex to undergo neuroplastic changes that allow for the acquisition of new motor skills or adaptation to an altered intraoral environment.

Neuroplasticity of the face sensorimotor cortex in this context may reflect beneficial adaptive modifications, as, for example, when an infant encounters novel sensory and motor experiences and develops new motor skills (e.g., crawling, walking, and chewing), when a person learns to play a new sport or musical instrument, or when a patient regains lost sensorimotor functions during recovery from injury to peripheral tissues or to the CNS. Neuroplasticity may, however, also reflect behavioral maladaptation that may be associated with a variety of persistent sensorimotor dysfunctions, such as phantom pain following peripheral limb injury, focal hand dystonia in keyboard musicians, or persistent disrupted chewing or swallowing following brain injuries such as stroke (see May 2008, Martin 2009, Avivi-Arber et al. 2011).

Brain imaging and cortical TMS studies in humans suggest that neuroplasticity may occur to a varying extent in the facial sensorimotor cortex and other areas with which it is functionally connected that may reflect the variability between individuals in chewing patterns and the state of the dentition (see Momose et al. 1997, Yan et al. 2008, Avivi-Arber et al. 2011). Human and animal studies have also revealed that learning of a new orofacial motor skill or manipulations of orofacial sensory inputs are associated with neuroplasticity of the facial sensorimotor cortex that is reflected as changes in cortical excitability, neuronal properties, and organizational features of somatosensory representations in facial SI or motor representations in facial MI (see Avivi-Arber et al. 2011). For example, training humans for less than 1 hour in a novel tongue-protrusion task is sufficient for a significant expansion to occur in the human MI tongue representation defined by TMS or brain imaging, as well as a decreased TMS-evoked threshold for tongue muscle activation, and an increased amplitude of TMS-evoked tongue motor potentials. Likewise, training monkeys in an analogous novel tongue-protrusion task is associated with (1) a significant increase in the proportion of discrete ICMS-defined motor output zones of the monkey's facial MI that project to the brainstem and produce tongue protrusion, (2) increases in the proportion of MI and SI neurons showing tongue protrusion-related activity, and (3) an increase in the proportion of neurons receiving lingual tactile sensory inputs. Also of interest from these studies is the finding that when acute intraoral pain was experimentally induced in the human subjects, both the facial-MI neuroplasticity and the tongue motor skill performance were markedly impaired, consistent with animal studies showing that noxious intraoral stimulation reduces facial-MI excitability. This may explain why persons in pain have difficulty in learning a new sensorimotor behavior or adapting to an altered oral environment.

Face sensorimotor-cortex neuroplasticity can also be induced by other intraoral changes, including trigeminal nerve trauma and alterations to the dental occlusion (see Avivi-Arber et al. 2011). For example, modifying the dental occlusion and vertical dimension of the jaw of rats by trimming the mandibular incisors out of occlusion with their maxillary counterparts, by inducing tooth movement with orthodontic appliances, by extracting incisor or molar teeth, and by placement of dental implants in the extraction sites, is associated with significant neuroplastic changes in jaw or tongue motor representations in the face sensorimotor cortex (e.g., Avivi-Arber et al. 2010a,b, 2011, Fig. 1-4). Changes to teeth are also associated with neural changes in subcortical structures, as noted previously.

Positive adaptive behaviors can occur when the dental occlusion is modified, when orofacial pain occurs, when intraoral nerves are damaged, or when dental rehabilitative procedures are carried out.

Nonetheless, maladaptive behaviors and development of chronic pain or sensorimotor disturbances may sometimes result in such circumstances, and may compromise even the best-intentioned rehabilitative approaches. The recent findings documenting cortical and subcortical neuroplasticity provide a new conceptualization of how to understand and explain clinical outcomes resulting from alterations to the dental occlusion and other orofacial tissues. For example, the findings indicate that even subtle changes to tooth form can lead rapidly to neuroplastic changes in orofacial somatosensory or motor representations in the face sensorimotor cortex and other parts of the CNS that are critically involved in somatosensory function and masticatory control. The neuroplasticity appears to reflect dynamic, adaptive constructs that underlie our ability to learn new motor skills, but are also responsive to intraoral sensory alterations such as pain or changes to the occlusal interface. Thus facial-MI and facial-SI neuroplasticity appears critical for adaptation and learning of new motor skills and for behavior that is appropriate to the altered intraoral sensory environment. It is still not completely clear what cellular mechanisms underlie the neuroplasticity in the CNS, which of the neuroplastic changes represent positive or negative adaptive processes, and how the adaptive capacity of the face sensorimotor cortex and other related CNS regions can be targeted to enhance rehabilitative procedures to exploit these mechanisms in humans suffering from chronic pain or sensorimotor disorders affecting the orofacial region. Further investigations to clarify the cerebral cortical, and subcortical, processes underlying the behavioral responses to intraoral alterations and the adaptive mechanisms associated with these changes are crucial for understanding how humans learn, or relearn, oral sensorimotor behaviors or adapt or not to an altered oral environment, including that reflecting prosthetically based rehabilitative procedures.

SUMMARY

This chapter has emphasized the neural framework for a functional dental occlusion, as well as CNS mechanisms that come into play in situations associated with pain or with changes to the occlusal interface following loss or alterations of teeth and

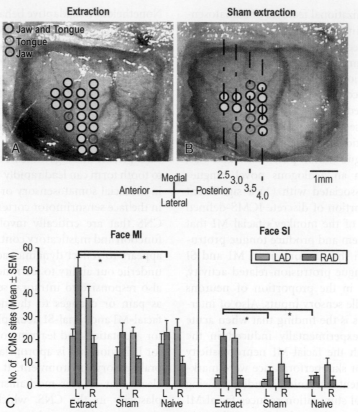

FIG 1-4 Effects of Dental Occlusal Changes Produced by Tooth Extraction on the Jaw and Tongue Motor Representations in Face Sensorimotor Cortex of a Rat A and **B** show surface views of the cortical sites from which jaw and tongue muscle activities could be evoked by intracortical microstimulation (ICMS, 60 µA) at anterior-posterior planes 2.5, 3.0, 3.5, and 4.0 mm (anterior to bregma) and within the left cortex of a rat that 1 week earlier had its incisor extracted, and of a rat that 1 week earlier had undergone sham extraction. Scale bar = 1 mm. **C** notes the number of sites from which ICMS within the left (L) and right (R) face primary motor cortex (MI) and face primary somatosensory cortex (SI) could evoke EMG responses in the left and right anterior digastric muscles (LAD and RAD). There were significantly larger numbers of LAD and RAD sites within the contralateral face MI (ANOVA, Bonferroni: $P < 0.0001$). Within the left facial MI, the number of RAD sites was significantly larger in rats of the extraction group than in rats of the sham-extraction group and a group of naive rats (*ANOVA: $P < 0.0004$. Bonferroni: $P < 0.0015$ and 0.0016, respectively). (Adapted from Avivi-Arber et al. 2010b, with permission.)

rehabilitative procedures to restore the occlusion. The neural pathways and neural and nonneural processes underlying orofacial touch and pain have been outlined, including the role of peripheral sensitization and CNS neuroplasticity expressed as central sensitization in acute and chronic pain conditions. The brainstem neural circuits and higher brain centers involved in chewing, swallowing, and other orofacial sensorimotor functions were also outlined, including the descending influences of these higher brain centers

that can modulate the processes involved in orofacial touch and pain and sensorimotor functions, and thereby underlie several therapeutic approaches used to control pain or sensorimotor dysfunction. Particular attention was paid to the contribution of the face sensorimotor cortex in these descending influences and its role in orofacial sensorimotor control. Studies in humans or laboratory animals have documented that face SI and MI make important contributions to not only the control of elemental and learned orofacial movements but also mastication and swallowing. Reports show that changes to the dental occlusion associated with a reduction in chewing activity may lead to detrimental changes in CNS regions involved in cognition, memory, and sensorimotor control. Particularly, the neuroplasticity of the face sensorimotor cortex in association with oral motor skill acquisition and following intraoral alterations was noted (e.g., noxious stimulation, dental occlusal changes, and nerve trauma). These cortical changes reflect dynamic and adaptive events modelled by behaviorally significant experiences that include orofacial pain and alterations to the occlusal interface, and they are crucial for our ability to learn and adapt to an altered or restored intraoral environment.

ACKNOWLEDGMENTS

The author acknowledges gratefully the secretarial assistance of Susan Carter and Fong Yuen. His own cited studies were supported by the US National Institutes of Health, the Canadian Research Chair programme, the Canadian Foundation for Innovation, and the Canadian Institutes for Health Research.

REFERENCES

Avivi-Arber L, Lee J-C, Fung M, et al: Neuroplasticity of face motor cortex following molar teeth extraction and implant treatment, *Abstr Soc Neurosci* #284.9, 2010a.

Avivi-Arber L, Lee JC, Sessle BJ: Effects of incisor extraction on jaw and tongue motor representations within face sensorimotor cortex of adult rats, *J Comp Neurol* 7:1030–1045, 2010b.

Avivi-Arber L, Martin R, Lee JC, et al: Face sensorimotor cortex and its neuroplasticity related to orofacial sensorimotor functions, *Arch Oral Biol* 56(12): 1440–1465, 2011.

Cairns BE, Ren K, Tambeli CH: Recent advances in orofacial musculoskeletal pain mechanisms. In Sessle BJ, editor: *Orofacial Pain. Recent Advances in Assessment, Management and Understanding of Mechanisms*, Washington, DC, 2014, IASP Press, pp 351–372.

Cao Y, Wang H, Chiang C-Y, et al: Pregabalin suppresses nociceptive behavior and central sensitization in a rat trigeminal neuropathic pain model, *J Pain* 14:193–204, 2013.

Chiang C-Y, Dostrovsky JO, Iwata K, et al: Role of glia in orofacial pain, *Neuroscientist* 17:303–320, 2011.

Davis KD, Stohler CS: Neuroimaging and orofacial pain 2014. In Sessle BJ, editor: *Orofacial Pain. Recent Advances in Assessment, Management and Understanding of Mechanisms*, Washington, DC, 2014, IASP Press, pp 165–184.

Dostrovsky JO, Sessle BJ, Lam DK: Inflammatory and cancer-related orofacial pain mechanisms: insights from animal models. In Sessle BJ, editor: *Orofacial Pain. Recent Advances in Assessment, Management and Understanding of Mechanisms*, Washington, DC, 2014, IASP Press, pp 305–330.

Dubner R, Bennett GJ: Spinal and trigeminal mechanisms of nociception, *Annu Rev Neurosci* 6:381–418, 1983.

Dubner R, Iwata K, Wei F: Trigeminal neuropathic pain models in animals. In Sessle BJ, editor: *Orofacial Pain, Recent Advances in Assessment, Management and Understanding of Mechanisms*, Washington, DC, 2014, IASP Press, pp 331–350.

Dubner R, Ren K, Sessle B: Sensory mechanisms of orofacial pain. In Greene CS, Laskin DM, editors: *Treatment of TMDs: Bridging the Gap Between Advances in Research and Clinical Patient Management*, Hanover Park, 2013, Quintessence, pp 3–16.

Dubner R, Sessle BJ, Storey AT: *The Neural Basis of Oral and Facial Function*, New York, 1978, Plenum Press. 483 pp.

Feine JS, Carlsson G: *Implant Overdentures as Minimum Standard of Care*, Hanover Park, 2003, Quintessence. 162 pp.

Grabe HJ, Schwahn C, Voelzke H, et al: Tooth loss and cognitive impairment, *J Clin Periodonto* 36:550–557, 2009.

Hu JW, Dostrovsky J, Lenz Y, et al: Tooth pulp deafferentation is associated with functional alterations in the properties of neurons in the trigeminal spinal tract nucleus, *J Neurophysiol* 56:1650–1668, 1986.

Iida S, Hara T, Araki D, et al: Memory-related gene expression profile of the male rat hippocampus induced by teeth extraction and occlusal support recovery, *Arch Oral Biol* 59:133–141, 2014.

Iwata K, Imamura Y, Honda K, et al: Physiological mechanisms of neuropathic pain: the orofacial region, *Int Rev Neurobiol* 97:227–250, 2011.

Jacobs R, Van Steenberghe D: From osseoperception to implant-mediated sensory-motor interactions and related clinical implications, *J Oral Rehabil* 33:282–292, 2006.

Jean A: Brain stem control of swallowing: neuronal network and cellular mechanisms, *Physiol Rev* 81:929–969, 2001.

Klineberg I, Murray G: Osseoperception: sensory function and proprioception, *Adv Dent Res* 13:120–129, 1999.

Kubo K-Y, Yamada Y, Iinuma M, et al: Occlusal disharmony induces spatial memory impairment and hippocampal neuron degeneration via stress in SAMP8 mice, *Neurosci Lett* 414:188–191, 2007.

Lam DK, Sessle BJ, Cairns BE, et al: Neural mechanisms of temporomandibular joint and masticatory muscle pain: a possible role for peripheral glutamate receptor mechanisms, *Pain Res Manag* 10:145–152, 2005.

Lund JP, Kolta A, Sessle BJ: Trigeminal motor system. In Squire L, editor: *Encyclopedia of Neuroscience*, vol 9, Oxford, 2009, Academic Press, pp 1167–1171.

Martin RE: Neuroplasticity and swallowing, *Dysphagia* 24:218–229, 2009.

May A: Chronic pain may change the structure of the brain, *Pain* 137:7–15, 2008.

Meyer RA, Ringkamp M, Campbell JN, et al: Peripheral mechanisms of cutaneous nociception. In McMahon SB, Koltzenburg M, editors: *Wall and Melzack's Textbook of Pain*, ed 5, Amsterdam, 2006, Elsevier, pp 3–34.

Momose T, Nishikawa J, Watanabe T, et al: Effect of mastication on regional cerebral blood flow in humans examined by positron-emission tomography with 15O-labelled water and magnetic resonance imaging, *Arch Oral Biol* 42(1):57–61, 1997.

Neyraud E, Peyron MA, Vieira C, et al: Influence of bitter taste on mastication pattern, *J Dent Res* 84:250–254, 2005.

Noble JM, Scarmeas N, Papapanou PN: Poor oral health as a chronic, potentially modifiable dementia risk factor: Review of the literature, *Curr Neurol Neurosci Rep* 13:384, 2013.

Okamoto N, Morikawa M, Okamoto K, et al: Relationship of tooth loss to mild memory impairment and cognitive impairment: Findings from the fujiwara-kyo study, *Behav Brain Funct* 6:77, 2010.

Onozuka M, Watanabe K, Mirbod SM, et al: Reduced mastication stimulates impairment of spatial memory and degeneration of hippocampal neurons in aged SAMP8 mice, *Brain Res* 826:148–153, 1999.

Oue H, Miyamoto Y, Okada S, et al: Tooth loss induces memory impairment and neuronal cell loss in app transgenic mice, *Behav Brain Res* 252:318–325, 2013.

Sessle BJ: Acute and chronic craniofacial pain: brainstem mechanisms of nociceptive transmission and neuroplasticity, and their clinical correlates, *Crit Rev Oral Biol Med* 11:57–91, 2000. Online version available at: http://cro.sagepub.com/content/11/1/57.full .pdf+html. Accessed 5 June 2014.

Sessle BJ: Mechanisms of oral somatosensory and motor functions and their clinical correlates, *J Oral Rehabil* 33:243–261, 2006.

Sessle BJ: Orofacial motor control. In Squire L, editor: *Encyclopedia of Neuroscience*, vol 7, Oxford, 2009, Academic Press, pp 303–308.

Sessle BJ: Peripheral and central mechanisms of orofacial inflammatory pain, *Int Rev Neurobiol* 97:179–206, 2011.

Weijenberg RAF, Scherder EJA, Lobbezoo F: Mastication for the mind-the relationship between mastication and cognition in ageing and dementia, *Neurosci Biobehav Rev* 35:483–497, 2011.

Yan C, Ye L, Zhen J, et al: Neuroplasticity of edentulous patients with implant-supported full dentures, *J Oral Sci* 116(5):387–393, 2008.

CHAPTER 2

Periodontal Microbiology and Immunobiology

Stefan A. Hienz and Sašo Ivanovski

SYNOPSIS

As the microbiology and immunobiology of periodontal disease has continued to evolve, several changes to our understanding of health and disease have emerged. One cornerstone of this evolution has been the increased understanding of the microbiology characterizing health and disease of the periodontium. Another involves the continued progress in determining the complexity of the human inflammatory response to the periodontal biofilm, leading to a better understanding of the key innate and adaptive immune mechanisms. This knowledge has produced a "blue-print" of the host-microbial interactions that occur in the periodontium, elucidating how the host responds to commensal and pathogenic bacteria, succeeding to achieve a balance in most but resulting in disease in some cases (Ebersole et al. 2013). An understanding of the normal structure and function of the periodontium provides the basis for making clinical decisions aimed at maintaining periodontal health.

CHAPTER POINTS

- Bacterial colonization of the tooth surface begins with highly specific interactions between oral bacteria, mostly *Streptococcus* species, and the tooth pellicle.
- Historically, several hypotheses have been suggested to explain microorganisms as possible etiological agents for periodontal disease.
- Periodontitis is currently characterized as a microbial-shift disease, resulting from a change in the microorganisms that are present during the transition from periodontal health to periodontal disease.
- Normal periodontium is comprised of four principal components: gingiva, periodontal ligament, cementum, and alveolar bone.

- These components play an active role in the innate host defense by responding to bacteria in an interactive manner.
- An imbalance or disruption in the expression of inflammatory mediators in response to a microbial challenge contributes greatly to the destruction of the periodontal tissues.
- The identification of the toll-like receptor family of receptors that recognize microorganisms has contributed to the realization that both commensal and periopathogenic bacteria can activate innate immune responses.

MICROBIOLOGY

In 1683 Antoine van Leeuwenhoek examined his own gingival tooth scrapings using his improved microscope and reported seeing "animalcules." His discovery provided the groundwork for a better understanding of periodontal microbiology, and to date, more than 700 microbial species are estimated to coexist in the oral cavity (Paster et al. 2001, 2006).

Biofilms

Recent estimates suggest that 60% to 85% of all microbial infections involve biofilms developed on natural tissues or artificial devices (Peyyala & Ebersole 2013, Peyyala et al. 2012). Historically, biofilms were described as sessile communities of microbes, characterized by cells that are irreversibly attached to a substratum and coaggregate with each other. Generally, they are embedded in a matrix of extracellular polymeric substances. Furthermore, the initial bacterial adherence and biofilm accretion are considered to proceed in two steps, with attachment to a surface followed by cell-to-cell adhesion (Fig. 2-1). This is followed by maturation of the biofilm that frequently is represented by stratification of bacteria within the biofilms and finally dispersal from the sessile community (Peyyala & Ebersole 2013).

Colonization of the tooth surface begins with highly specific interactions between oral bacteria, mostly *Streptococcus* species, and the tooth pellicle. The pellicle is a thin layer of both saliva and gingival crevicular fluid that coats the dentin surface of the tooth. Oral bacteria have evolved highly specific adhesions to pellicle proteins and carbohydrates. This is similar to specific adhesins found in other commensal and pathogenic bacteria that display highly specific tissue tropisms (Curtis et al. 2011). After early colonizers have established themselves on the tooth surface through host-derived pellicle interactions, these bacteria themselves then serve as additional binding sites for intermediate and late colonizers. This process, which has been eloquently studied and described by Kolenbrander's group, reveals that each step in dental plaque biofilm formation is highly specific and represents coevolution between different oral bacterial species and the host (Curtis et al. 2011, Kolenbrander et al. 2010, Socransky & Haffajee 2005).

Possible Etiological Agents for Periodontal Disease

Historically, several hypotheses have been suggested to explain microorganisms as possible etiological agents for periodontal disease.

Nonspecific Plaque Hypothesis

The resolution of gingival inflammation after the physical removal of dental plaque in a model system referred to as experimental gingivitis led to the formulation of the "nonspecific" plaque hypothesis (Theilade et al. 1966, Theilade 1986, Loesche 1976, Loe et al. 1965). This concept was based on the notion that the destruction of periodontal tissues is proportionally related to the amount of dental plaque and the toxins it releases. If only small amounts of plaque were present, the host would be able to deal with the microbial challenge and no periodontal destruction would ensue, with disease occurring only when plaque accumulates beyond a certain pathogenic threshold (Box 2.1).

In the presence of a uniform host response, these findings were incongruent with the idea that all plaque was equally pathogenic, which thus led to the development of the "specific plaque" hypothesis.

Specific Plaque Hypothesis

The specific plaque hypothesis was first proposed at the turn of the twentieth century, but it was largely overlooked until it reemerged in the 1970s, following experiments in which periodontal disease could be transmitted in experimental animals (Keyes & Jordan 1964, Jordan et al. 1972). Later, the identification of

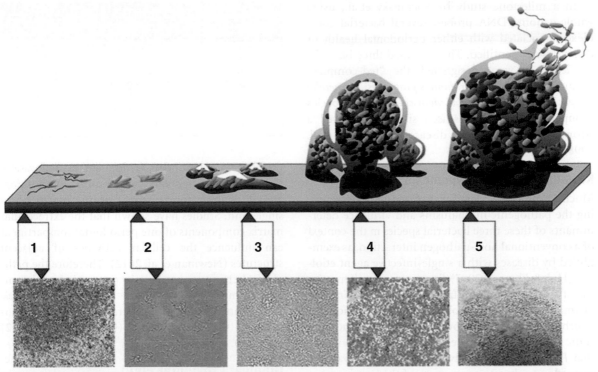

FIG 2-1 Five Stages of Biofilm Development Stage 1, initial attachment; stage 2, irreversible attachment; stage 3, maturation I; stage 4, maturation II; stage 5, dispersion. Each stage of development in the diagram is paired with a photomicrograph of a developing *Pseudomonas aeruginosa* biofilm. All photomicrographs are shown to same scale. (From http://upload.wikimedia.org/wikipedia/commons/4/4a/Biofilm.jpg.)

BOX 2.1 "NON-SPECIFIC" PLAQUE HYPOTHESIS SHORTFALLS

The concept of a "nonspecific" plaque hypothesis came short of explaining why (Socransky & Haffajee 1994, Bartold & Van Dyke 2013):

- Some patients accumulated high levels of plaque and did not show any sign of disease.
- Some sites are more affected by disease than adjacent ones are, despite having similar loads of plaque.
- In some patients, with very little visible detectable plaque, the manifestation of disease was more of an aggressive or advanced form.

---

bacteria, such as *Actinobacillus actinomycetemcomitans* (today *Aggregatibacter actinomycetemcomitans*) (Norskov-Lauritsen & Kilian 2006) as specific pathogens in aggressive periodontitis fueled the search for specific microorganisms associated with the various forms of periodontal disease (Slots 1976, Newman et al. 1976). Subsequently, by investigating the development of dental plaque as it matures, clear changes in its composition were noted in which the presence of gram-negative, obligate anaerobic species was associated with an increase in periodontal pocket probing depths (Socransky et al. 1998, Bartold & Van Dyke 2013).

Microbial Shift

Similarly to other polymicrobial diseases, periodontitis is now characterized as a microbial-shift disease, owing to a well-characterized change in the microorganisms that are present (from mostly gram-positive to mostly gram-negative species) during the transition from periodontal health to periodontal disease (Marsh 1994, Darveau 2010). Undoubtedly, the nature of the host response plays a role in contributing to this microbial shift.

In a milestone study by Socransky et al., using whole-genome DNA probes, several bacterial complexes associated with either periodontal health or disease were identified. This included three bacterial species that were designated the "red-complex" periopathogens: *Porphyromonas gingivalis*, *Tannerella forsythia*, and *Treponema denticola*. These species grouped together in diseased sites and showed a strong association with disease (Socransky et al. 1998).

Keystone-Pathogen Hypothesis

Much research has been directed toward understanding the pathogenic mechanisms and virulence determinants of these three bacterial species in the context of a conventional host-pathogen interaction, as exemplified by diseases with a single-infective agent etiology (Holt & Ebersole 2005). Support for the alternative hypothesis that periodontal pathogens transform the normally symbiotic microbiota into a dysbiotic state, which leads to a breakdown in the normal homeostatic relationship with the host, comes from evidence that *P. gingivalis* has evolved sophisticated strategies to evade or subvert components of the host immune system (e.g., toll-like receptors [TLRs] and complement), rather than acting directly as a proinflammatory bacterium (Hajishengallis & Lambris 2011). In other words, *P. gingivalis* could be a keystone pathogen of the disease-provoking periodontal microbiota (Hajishengallis et al. 2012).

The keystone hypothesis is supported by a study in the mouse model. This study showed that, at very low colonization levels (<0.01% of the total bacterial count), *P. gingivalis* induces periodontitis accompanied by significant alterations in the number and community organization of the oral commensal bacteria. This supports the notion that low-abundance biofilm species can create an environment that leads to inflammatory periodontal disease by influencing the commensal microbiota and the complement system (Hajishengallis & Lamont 2012, Hajishengallis et al. 2011).

IMMUNOLOGY

The normal periodontium provides the support necessary for teeth in their function. It is comprised of four principal components: gingiva, periodontal ligament, cementum, and alveolar bone. Each of these

---

BOX 2.2 UNIQUENESS OF THE ORAL EPITHELIUM

The oral cavity with its oral epithelium represents the only site in the entire body in which the epithelial barrier is breached by a nonshedding hard tissue. To achieve and maintain homeostasis within the oral cavity, distinct immune response systems contributing to the control of microbial colonization have evolved.

---

periodontal components is different in its location, tissue architecture, and biochemical composition, and all of these components function together as a single unit. Studies have shown that the extracellular matrix components of one periodontal compartment can influence the cellular activities of adjacent structures (Newman et al. 2012). Therefore the pathological changes occurring in one periodontal component may have significant ramifications for the maintenance, repair, or regeneration of other components of the periodontium (Newman et al. 2012) (Box 2.2).

Gingival Crevicular Fluid

The gingival tissues and gingival crevicular fluid have been shown to contain a complex array of immune components that not only irrigate the gingival sulcus but also are released into the oral cavity (Ebersole 2003, Ebersole et al. 2013). Gingival crevicular fluid (GCF) has been shown to be derived from gingival capillary beds (serum components) and from both resident and emigrating inflammatory cells. This fluid contains an array of innate, inflammatory and adaptive immune molecules and cells whose role is to contribute to the interaction of host and bacteria in this ecological niche (Ebersole et al. 2013). Analysis of GCF has identified cell and humoral responses in both healthy individuals and those with periodontal disease. The cellular immune response includes the release of cytokines in GCF, but there is no direct evidence of a relationship between specific cytokines and disease. Nevertheless, interleukin-1 alpha (IL-1α) and IL-1β are known to increase the binding of PMNs and monocytes and macrophages to endothelial cells and to stimulate the production of prostaglandin E_2 (PGE$_2$), the release of lysosomal enzymes, and bone resorption (Gupta 2013). Preliminary evidence also indicates the presence of interferon-α in

GCF, which may have a protective role in periodontal disease because of its ability to inhibit the bone resorption activity of IL-1β (Gowen & Mundy 1986, Lamster & Novak 1992). The amount of GCF is greater when inflammation is present and is sometimes proportional to the severity of inflammation (Shapiro et al. 1979). GCF production is not increased by trauma from occlusion but is increased by mastication of coarse foods, tooth brushing, gingival massage, ovulation, hormonal contraceptives, and smoking (Lindhe et al. 1968, McLaughlin et al. 1993). Other factors that influence the amount of GCF are circadian periodicity and periodontal therapy (Bissada et al. 1967).

Epithelium of the Gingiva

Normal gingiva covers the alveolar bone and tooth root to a level just coronal to the cement-enamel junction. At the dentogingival junction, the marginal, or unattached, gingiva is the terminal edge of the gingiva, surrounding the teeth in a collar-like fashion. The gingival sulcus is the shallow crevice around the tooth bounded by the surface of the tooth on one side and the epithelium lining of the free margin of the gingiva on the other side (Fig. 2-2; Box 2.3).

Historically, the epithelial compartment was thought to provide only a physical barrier to infection and the underlying gingival attachment. However, it is now known that epithelial cells play an active role in the innate host defense by responding to bacteria in an interactive manner.

The Epithelium Participates Actively in Responding to Infection

- In signaling further host reactions
- In integrating innate and acquired immune responses

Overall, the functions of the epithelium are to act as a mechanical, chemical, fluid, and microbial barrier, as well as signaling to the deeper periodontal structures. Although predominantly consisting of keratocytes, there are also Langerhans cells, melanocytes, and Merkel cells that can be found carrying out these functions in the epithelium (Dale 2002, 2003). In the gingiva, Langerhans cells are dendritic cells located among keratinocytes. They belong to the mononuclear phagocyte system (reticuloendothelial system) as modified monocytes derived from the

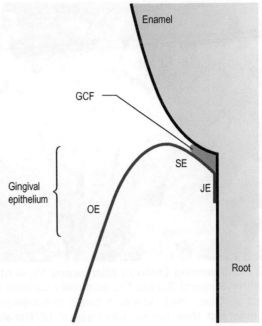

FIG 2-2 Healthy periodontal tissue contains connective tissue and bone, which support the gingival epithelium. The gingival epithelium facing the oral cavity is called oral epithelium (OE). The gingival sulcus is covered by sulcular epithelium (SE), and a specialized junctional epithelium (JE) connects it to the tooth apically. The gingival sulcus is filled with gingival crevicular fluid (GCF).

BOX 2.3 EPITHELIUM OF THE GINGIVA

The epithelium of the gingiva consists of the following:
- Oral (outer/gingival) epithelium—faces the oral cavity
- Sulcular epithelium—lines the sulcus
- Junctional epithelium (JE)—acts as a "seal" at base of the sulcus

bone marrow, and have an important role in the immune reaction as antigen-presenting cells for lymphocytes (Barrett et al. 1996).

Sulcular epithelium is extremely important because it acts as a semipermeable membrane through which injurious bacterial products pass into the gingiva and tissue fluid from the gingiva seeps into the sulcus (Fig. 2-3). Unlike the sulcular epithelium, the junctional epithelium is heavily infiltrated by

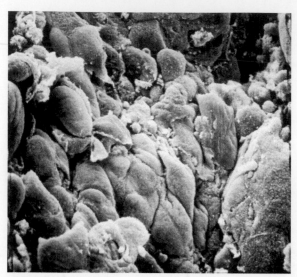

FIG 2-3 Scanning Electron Microscopic View of a Healthy Gingival Sulcus The epithelial cells form an intact surface, which acts as a barrier to subgingival bacteria and their toxins. (Courtesy of Dr Renaldo Saglie.)

BOX 2.4 CLINICAL NOTE

Clinicians must be aware of the defense mechanisms of the gingiva because dental treatment can influence gingival defenses. Routine scaling and restorative procedures that involve the subgingival region can disrupt the epithelial lining of the gingival sulcus, resulting in increased levels of inflammation, as bacteria and their products have direct contact with the underlying connective tissue. The junctional and oral sulcular epithelium have the capacity to heal and reform the epithelial barrier in 7 to 10 days following disruption, and during this time, plaque control must be optimized to limit the risk of initiating periodontal breakdown. The use of gentle minimally traumatic techniques is also important, especially when carrying prophylactic plaque removal in the absence of periodontal disease (Newman et al. 2012).

polymorphonuclear neutrophil leukocytes (PMNs), and appears to be less permeable (Bartold et al. 2000). Epithelial cells may respond to bacteria by increased proliferation, alteration of cell-signaling events, changes in differentiation and cell death, and ultimately, alteration of tissue homeostasis. They play a crucial role in intraepithelial recruitment of phagocytes and specific lymphocyte subsets and therefore control bacterial invasion into the mucosal compartments (Kornman et al. 1997, Svanborg et al. 1994).

To cope with constant microbial stimulation, the periodontium has a highly orchestrated expression of select innate host defense mediators. Coordinated expression of innate defense mediators such as interleukin-8 (IL-8), facilitate neutrophil transit through the tissue. In addition, the gingival epithelium expresses several innate host defense mediators that contribute to the clearance and killing of dental plaque bacteria, including TLRs (which recognize pathogens and commensal bacteria), β-defensins, and lipopolysaccharide-binding protein (LBP). Junctional epithelium is highly porous; cells are interconnected by a few desmosomes and the occasional gap junction, resulting in large fluid-filled, intracellular spaces (Bosshardt & Lang 2005). Further,

the junctional epithelium produces soluble CD14 (another bacterial clearance mediator) and LBP. Innate host protective mechanisms are coupled with regenerative and biomechanical signaling systems, resulting in tissue homeostasis (Darveau 2010).

In summary, epithelial tissues play a key role in host defenses, as they are the main site of initial interaction between plaque bacteria and the host. The keratinized epithelium of the sulcular and gingival epithelial tissues not only provides protection for the underlying periodontal tissue but also acts as a barrier against bacteria and their products (Bartold et al. 2000, Schroeder & Listgarten 1997, 2003). In contrast, the unique microanatomic structure of the junctional epithelium has significant intercellular spaces, is not keratinized, and exhibits a higher cellular turnover rate. These properties render the junctional epithelium permeable, allowing for inward movement of microbial products and outward movement of GCF, and the cells and molecules of the innate immune system. Further, the spaces between the cells of the junctional epithelium widen with inflammation, resulting in increased GCF flow (Bartold et al. 2000, Newman et al. 2012) (Box 2.4).

Gingival Connective Tissue

The major components of the gingival connective tissue are the following:

- Collagen fibers (approximately 60% by volume)
- Fibroblasts (5%), vessels, nerves
- Matrix (approximately 35%)

BOX 2.5 FUNCTIONS OF GINGIVAL FIBERS

The gingival fibers have the following functions (Newman et al. 2012):

- To brace the marginal gingiva firmly against the tooth
- To provide the rigidity necessary to withstand the forces of mastication without being deflected away from the tooth surface
- To provide the rigidity necessary to withstand the forces of mastication without being deflected away from the tooth surface
- To unite the free marginal gingiva with the cementum of the root and the adjacent attached gingiva

The connective tissue of the marginal gingiva is densely collagenous, containing a prominent system of collagen fiber bundles called the gingival fibers. They consist predominantly of type I collagen (Box 2.5).

Fibroblasts are the major players in the development, maintenance, and repair of connective tissue in the periodontium. They mainly synthesize and maintain the components of the extracellular matrix of the connective tissue. Historically, these cells have been seen as only passive contributors to the periodontium. However, current evidence indicates that fibroblasts can behave quite distinctly in response to cytokines and growth factors (Bartold et al. 2000). Studies have shown that lymphocyte-fibroblast interactions potentially contribute to the inflammatory reaction via the release of soluble mediators following interactive processes of an autocrine or juxtacrine nature (Bartold et al. 2000, Schroeder & Page 1972). Direct adhesive interactions of fibroblasts and lymphocytes are a possible mechanism by which lymphocytes become lodged in gingival tissues and contribute to ongoing tissue destruction (Murakami et al. 1993).

If bacteria and their products infiltrate the periodontal tissues, then dedicated "sentinel cells" of the immune system can identify their presence and signal protective immune responses. Thus, macrophages and dendritic cells express a range of pattern recognition receptors (PRRs) that interact with specific molecular structures on microorganisms called microbe-associated molecular patterns (MAMPs), to signal immune responses. Innate immune responses are therefore activated to provide immediate protection, and adaptive immunity is activated with the aim of establishing a sustained antigen-specific defense. Excessive and inappropriate immune responses lead to chronic inflammation and the concomitant tissue destruction associated with periodontal disease (Darveau 2010, Ebersole et al. 2013, Newman et al. 2012). A number of nonimmune cells in the periodontium (epithelial cells and fibroblasts) also express PRRs and may recognize and respond to MAMPs from plaque bacteria. Signaling of cytokine responses via PRRs influences innate immunity (e.g., neutrophil activity), adaptive immunity (T-cell effector phenotype), and the development of destructive inflammation (e.g., activation of osteoclasts). A number of cytokines are particularly important in innate immune signaling, and there is now good evidence that these have a role in immune responses in the periodontium. The archetypal proinflammatory cytokine is IL-1β, which exerts its action directly by activating other cells that express the IL-1R1 receptor (e.g., endothelial cells) or by stimulating the synthesis and secretion of other, secondary mediators such as prostaglandin E_2 (PGE_2) and nitric oxide (NO) (Darveau 2010, Ebersole et al. 2013, Newman et al. 2012).

Receptor-Activator of Nuclear Factor-κB Ligand

A consequence of an increase in the concentrations of inflammatory mediators is the resorption of alveolar bone, which is the trademark of periodontitis. The key mechanism that regulates the normal bone resorption and deposition activities that occur during bone remodeling is the ratio of RANKL (receptor-activator of nuclear factor-κB ligand) to OPG (osteoprotegrin), and this mechanism contributes to the bone loss observed in periodontitis (Boyle et al. 2003, Cochran 2008, Darveau 2010). RANKL is present on several cell types and it binds to RANK on osteoclast precursors, causing them to differentiate into active multinuclear cells that secrete enzymes, which degrade bone. OPG is a soluble receptor of RANKL that prevents the RANK-RANKL interaction. At high OPG concentrations, RANKL does not bind to osteoclast precursors, and bone loss is averted. OPG levels are regulated by transforming growth factor-β-related bone morphogenic proteins, whereas the synthesis of RANKL is induced by proinflammatory cytokines such as IL-1β and TNF. Therefore increases in the concentration of proinflammatory cytokines in healthy periodontal tissue can directly affect bone loss by increasing the RANKL/OPG ratio (Belibasakis 2012, Darveau 2010).

"Pathological" versus "Physiological" Bone Loss

It is likely that the fundamental biological mechanisms associated with "pathological" bone loss as a result of periodontitis are similar to those associated with "physiological" bone loss from periodontal ligament widening associated with tooth mobility. The major difference is that the pathogenic process is associated with periodontal attachment loss and apical migration of long junctional epithelium, and hence is irreversible, whereas no attachment loss is associated with tooth mobility alone, and hence the bone loss is reversible if the tooth is stabilized. This is consistent with studies that show that mobility alone in the absence of marginal inflammation does not lead to periodontal attachment loss. However, tooth mobility may accelerate attachment loss in the presence of periodontal inflammation (Polson et al. 1976a,b, Waerhaug 1970, 1979, Lindhe et al. 2008).

Adaptive Immune Responses

The importance of adaptive immune responses in periodontal pathogenesis is endorsed by histologic studies of established lesions in periodontal disease (Kornman et al. 1997). The population of leukocytes in the periodontium in gingivitis (i.e., the early stages of responses to the plaque biofilm) and in stable periodontal lesions (i.e., those at which tissue destruction is apparently not progressing) is dominated by T-cells, and these cells are clustered mainly around blood vessels. Cell surface marker studies suggest that these cells are activated but not proliferating (Gemmell et al. 2007). In addition, there is a predominance of the helper T-cell subset (i.e., CD4 expressing T-cells) over the cytotoxic T-cell subset (i.e., CD8 expressing T-cells). These T-cells are considered to be proactively maintaining tissue homeostasis in the face of the microbial challenge of the plaque biofilm (Gemmell et al. 2007; Newman et al. 2012). In contrast, in active periodontitis, B-cells and plasma cells predominate and are associated with pocket formation and progression of disease. The periodontium is often compared to other mucosal tissues and the skin in terms of its repertoire of immune cells, and it contains a number of "professional" antigen-presenting cells (Cutler & Jotwani 2006; Cutler & Teng 2007). These include B-cells, macrophages, and at least two types of dendritic cells (dermal dendritic cells and Langerhans cells). These cells naturally express major histocompatibility complex (MHC) Class II molecules necessary for antigen presentation to cognate T-cell receptors and may take up specific antigens and transport them to local lymph nodes, thereby facilitating the activation of specific effector T-cells and the generation of an antigen-specific immune response to periodontal pathogens (Cutler & Jotwani 2006). Finally, the evolution of the Human Microbiome Project has helped develop the notion that a healthy mature immune system depends on the constant intervention of beneficial bacteria (Ebersole et al. 2013). Commensals have been found to keep the immune system in balance by boosting its antiinflammatory arm (Lee & Mazmanian 2010).

SUMMARY

In summary, several advances in the past 10 years have changed our thinking about periodontal microbiology and immunology. First, it is now well recognized that the host innate immune defense system is highly active in healthy tissue, and an imbalance or disruption in the expression of inflammatory mediators contributes greatly to the destruction of the tissue and bone supporting the root structures. Second, the identification of the TLR family of receptors, which recognize microorganisms, has contributed to the realization that both commensal and periopathogenic bacteria can activate innate immune responses. Finally, the understanding that the oral microbial community is a biofilm has led to a greater emphasis on the idea that microbial community interactions may modulate the expression of host innate immune mediators.

REFERENCES

Barrett AW, Cruchley AT, Williams DM: Oral mucosal Langerhans' cells, *Crit Rev Oral Biol Med* 7:36–58, 1996.

Bartold PM, Van Dyke TE: Periodontitis: a host-mediated disruption of microbial homeostasis. Unlearning learned concepts, *Periodontol 2000* 62:203–217, 2013.

Bartold PM, Walsh LJ, Narayanan AS: Molecular and cell biology of the gingiva, *Periodontol 2000* 24:28–55, 2000.

Belibasakis GN, Bostanci N: The RANKL-OPG system in clinical periodontology, *J Clin Periodontol* 39(3):239–248, 2012.

Bissada NF, Schaffer EM, Haus E: Circadian periodicity of human crevicular fluid flow, *J Periodontol* 38:36–40, 1967.

Bosshardt DD, Lang NP: The junctional epithelium: from health to disease, *J Dent Res* 84:9–20, 2005.

Boyle WJ, Simonet WS, Lacey DL: Osteoclast differentiation and activation, *Nature* 423:337–342, 2003.

Cochran DL: Inflammation and bone loss in periodontal disease, *J Periodontol* 79:1569–1576, 2008.

Curtis MA, Zenobia C, Darveau RP: The relationship of the oral microbiota to periodontal health and disease, *Cell Host Microbe* 10:302–306, 2011.

Cutler CW, Jotwani R: Dendritic cells at the oral mucosal interface, *J Dent Res* 85:678–689, 2006.

Cutler CW, Teng YT: Oral mucosal dendritic cells and periodontitis: many sides of the same coin with new twists, *Periodontol 2000* 45:35–50, 2007.

Dale BA: Periodontal epithelium: a newly recognized role in health and disease, *Periodontol 2000* 30:70–78, 2002.

Dale BA: Fascination with epithelia: architecture, proteins, and functions, *J Dent Res* 82:866–869, 2003.

Darveau RP: Periodontitis: a polymicrobial disruption of host homeostasis, *Nat Rev Microbiol* 8:481–490, 2010.

Ebersole JL: Humoral immune responses in gingival crevice fluid: local and systemic implications, *Periodontol 2000* 31:135–166, 2003.

Ebersole JL, Dawson DR 3rd, Morford LA, et al: Periodontal disease immunology: "double indemnity" in protecting the host, *Periodontol 2000* 62:163–202, 2013.

Gemmell E, Yamazaki K, Seymour GJ: The role of T cells in periodontal disease: homeostasis and autoimmunity, *Periodontol 2000* 43:14–40, 2007.

Gowen M, Mundy GR: Actions of recombinant interleukin 1, interleukin 2, and interferon-gamma on bone resorption in vitro, *J Immunol* 136:2478–2482, 1986.

Gupta G: Gingival crevicular fluid as a periodontal diagnostic indicator. II. Inflammatory mediators, host-response modifiers and chair side diagnostic aids, *J Med Life* 6:7–13, 2013.

Hajishengallis G, Darveau RP, Curtis MA: The keystone-pathogen hypothesis, *Nat Rev Microbiol* 10:717–725, 2012.

Hajishengallis G, Lambris JD: Microbial manipulation of receptor crosstalk in innate immunity, *Nat Rev Immunol* 11:187–200, 2011.

Hajishengallis G, Lamont RJ: Beyond the red complex and into more complexity: the polymicrobial synergy and dysbiosis (PSD) model of periodontal disease etiology, *Mol Oral Microbiol* 27:409–419, 2012.

Hajishengallis G, Liang S, Payne MA, et al: Low-abundance biofilm species orchestrates inflammatory periodontal disease through the commensal microbiota and complement, *Cell Host Microbe* 10:497–506, 2011.

Holt SC, Ebersole JL: *Porphyromonas gingivalis, Treponema denticola*, and *Tannerella forsythia*: the "red complex," a prototype polybacterial pathogenic consortium in periodontitis, *Periodontol 2000* 38:72–122, 2005.

Jordan HV, Keyes PH, Bellack S: Periodontal lesions in hamsters and gnotobiotic rats infected with actinomyces of human origin, *J Periodontal Res* 7:21–28, 1972.

Keyes PH, Jordan HV: Periodontal lesions in the Syrian hamster. III. Findings related to an infectious and transmissible component, *Arch Oral Biol* 9:377–400, 1964.

Kolenbrander PE, Palmer RJ Jr, Periasamy S, et al: Oral multispecies biofilm development and the key role of cell-cell distance, *Nat Rev Microbiol* 8:471–480, 2010.

Kornman KS, Page RC, Tonetti MS: The host response to the microbial challenge in periodontitis: assembling the players, *Periodontol 2000* 14:33–53, 1997.

Lamster IB, Novak MJ: Host mediators in gingival crevicular fluid: implications for the pathogenesis of periodontal disease, *Crit Rev Oral Biol Med* 3:31–60, 1992.

Lee YK, Mazmanian SK: Has the microbiota played a critical role in the evolution of the adaptive immune system? *Science* 330:1768–1773, 2010.

Lindhe J, Attstrom R, Bjorn AL: Influence of sex hormones on gingival exudation in dogs with chronic gingivitis, *J Periodontal Res* 3:279–283, 1968.

Lindhe J, Lang NP, Karring T: *Clinical Periodontology and Implant Dentistry*, Oxford, 2008, Blackwell Munsgaard.

Loe H, Theilade E, Jensen SB: Experimental gingivitis in man, *J Periodontol* 36:177–187, 1965.

Loesche WJ: Chemotherapy of dental plaque infections, *Oral Sci Rev* 9:65–107, 1976.

Marsh PD: Microbial ecology of dental plaque and its significance in health and disease, *Adv Dent Res* 8:263–271, 1994.

Mclaughlin WS, Lovat FM, Macgregor ID, et al: The immediate effects of smoking on gingival fluid flow, *J Clin Periodontol* 20:448–451, 1993.

Murakami S, Shimabukuro Y, Saho T, et al: Evidence for a role of VLA integrins in lymphocyte-human gingival fibroblast adherence, *J Periodontal Res* 28:494–506, 1993.

Newman MG, Socransky SS, Savitt ED, et al: Studies of the microbiology of periodontosis, *J Periodontol* 47:373–379, 1976.

Newman MG, Takei H, Klokkevold PR, et al: *Carranza's Clinical Periodontology*, St Louis, 2012, Elsevier Saunders.

Norskov-Lauritsen N, Kilian M: Reclassification of *Actinobacillus actinomycetemcomitans, Haemophilus aphrophilus, Haemophilus paraphrophilus* and *Haemophilus segnis* as *Aggregatibacter actinomycetemcomitans* gen. nov., comb. nov., *Aggregatibacter aphrophilus* comb. nov. and *Aggregatibacter segnis* comb. nov., and emended description of *Aggregatibacter aphrophilus* to include V factor-dependent and V factor-independent isolates, *Int J Syst Evol Microbiol* 56:2135–2146, 2006.

Paster BJ, Boches SK, Galvin JL, et al: Bacterial diversity in human subgingival plaque, *J Bacteriol* 183:3770–3783, 2001.

Paster BJ, Olsen I, Aas JA, et al: The breadth of bacterial diversity in the human periodontal pocket and other oral sites, *Periodontol 2000* 42:80–87, 2006.

Peyyala R, Ebersole JL: Multispecies biofilms and host responses: "discriminating the trees from the forest," *Cytokine* 61:15–25, 2013.

Peyyala R, Kirakodu SS, Novak KF, et al: Oral microbial biofilm stimulation of epithelial cell responses, *Cytokine* 58:65–72, 2012.

Polson AM, Meitner SW, Zander HA: Trauma and progression of marginal periodontitis in squirrel monkeys. III. Adaption of interproximal alveolar bone to repetitive injury, *J Periodontal Res* 11:279–289, 1976a.

Polson AM, Meitner SW, Zander HA: Trauma and progression of marginal periodontitis in squirrel monkeys. IV. Reversibility of bone loss due to trauma alone and trauma superimposed upon periodontitis, *J Periodontal Res* 11:290–298, 1976b.

Schroeder HE, Listgarten MA: The gingival tissues: the architecture of periodontal protection, *Periodontol 2000* 13:91–120, 1997.

Schroeder HE, Listgarten MA: The junctional epithelium: from strength to defense, *J Dent Res* 82:158–161, 2003.

Schroeder HE, Page R: Lymphocyte-fibroblast interaction in the pathogenesis of inflammatory gingival disease, *Experientia* 28:1228–1230, 1972.

Shapiro L, Goldman H, Bloom A: Sulcular exudate flow in gingival inflammation, *J Periodontol* 50:301–304, 1979.

Slots J: The predominant cultivable organisms in juvenile periodontitis, *Scand J Dent Res* 84:1–10, 1976.

Socransky SS, Haffajee AD: Evidence of bacterial etiology: a historical perspective, *Periodontol 2000* 5:7–25, 1994.

Socransky SS, Haffajee AD: Periodontal microbial ecology, *Periodontol 2000* 38:135–187, 2005.

Socransky SS, Haffajee AD, Cugini MA, et al: Microbial complexes in subgingival plaque, *J Clin Periodontol* 25:134–144, 1998.

Svanborg C, Agace W, Hedges S, et al: Bacterial adherence and mucosal cytokine production, *Ann N Y Acad Sci* 730:162–181, 1994.

Theilade E: The non-specific theory in microbial etiology of inflammatory periodontal diseases, *J Clin Periodontol* 13:905–911, 1986.

Theilade E, Wright WH, Jensen SB, et al: Experimental gingivitis in man. II. A longitudinal clinical and bacteriological investigation, *J Periodontal Res* 1:1–13, 1966.

Waerhaug J: Pathogenesis of periodontal diseases, *Br Dent J* 129:181–182, 1970.

Waerhaug J: The angular bone defect and its relationship to trauma from occlusion and downgrowth of subgingival plaque, *J Clin Periodontol* 6:61–82, 1979.

CHAPTER | 3 |

Occlusion and Health

Iven Klineberg

SYNOPSIS

It is now apparent that occlusion and health
have greater implications for the individual
than previously acknowledged. It has been
generally recognized that being able to
chew effectively influences food selection,
which also bears directly on individual
confidence. Moreover, the accepted flow-on
benefit is that a "balanced" diet with a
broad range of dietary requirements meets
individual nutritional requirements. Recent
data from animal and clinical research have
confirmed an additional and significant
benefit to individuals, resulting in enhanced
cognition and higher-level cognitive
reasoning. However, the relative importance
of the benefit of optimizing mastication and
the occlusion compared with other factors
that influence cognition is not yet known.
Nevertheless, it is clear that the occlusion of
the teeth in both natural and restored
dentitions has effects that go far beyond the
previously accepted understanding. This
chapter explores these implications and
further supports the importance of
understanding and restoring the occlusion
as an integral component of mastication
and health.

CHAPTER POINTS

- Occlusion is important for function,
  affecting diet, nutrition, and general health.
- Occlusion contributes to optimizing
  aesthetics, speech, and nonverbal
  communication.
- Occlusion contributes to enhancing
  self-confidence, social interaction, and
  self-esteem.
- Occlusion contributes to maintaining
  cognition and higher-level cognitive skills.
- The combined benefits of occlusion
  support the fundamental importance of
  maintaining teeth and/or restoring the
  occlusion for optimizing individual
  well-being.

With the development of new technologies in oral
rehabilitation, including three-dimensional (3D)-
image manipulation in treatment planning, computer-
aided design and computer-aided manufacturing
(CAD/CAM), and the new ceramics, fundamentals of
occlusion are often overlooked. Intraoral scanning is
now available and, although not in widespread use,
it will progressively be applied for 3D planning and
scanning of restorations, full dental arches, and
jaw relationships. This innovation will transform
traditional clinical protocols and laboratory support

requirements for restorative and prosthodontic procedures.

Notwithstanding these technology advances and treatment developments, recognition of the importance of occlusion for all aspects of restorative and oral rehabilitation is crucial for best practice and optimizing patient outcomes. The importance of the occlusion is nevertheless becoming recognized as having critical significance to the individual, far beyond the commonly accepted importance of the arrangement of the teeth for aesthetics and function. The occlusion is the key to optimizing mastication, swallowing, diet, nutrition, and general health, as well as speech clarity. In addition, anterior tooth arrangement, form, color, and character enhance aesthetics, social interaction, social confidence, and quality of life. Moreover, data are emerging to support that the occlusion has an important role in cognition and the maintenance of higher-level cognitive skills.

This development represents a new paradigm for oral rehabilitation and restorative dentistry and, in particular, where oral health management requires reestablishment of tooth contacts and occlusal scheme, a topic that is emphasized by Klineberg et al. (2012) in their systematic review.

Such a paradigm shift represents a new direction for management, with renewed emphasis on the mouth and maintenance of the teeth as important for not only aesthetic enhancement, function, and nutrition but also cognition, and this is the so-called new dynamic.

This new dynamic, the additional dimension to our understanding of the teeth and the importance of the occlusion, adds to the significance of maintaining teeth for function and aesthetics, and the elevated importance of prosthodontic rehabilitation as a requirement for cognitive health.

It is well known that the benefits of oral rehabilitation include improved aesthetics, diet and nutrition, quality of life, social interaction, and psychological health. The additional dimension clearly places maintenance of teeth and the occlusion as a key element of general health.

PROSTHODONTIC REHABILITATION AND GENERAL HEALTH

Occlusion influences the ability of an individual to chew and swallow effectively and thus influences a person's diet and resulting nutrition. Given the importance of an appropriate diet for optimal nutrition, it is clear that the diet is linked with individual susceptibility to dental caries, and it contributes to obesity, heart disease, hypertension, and diabetes (Morita et al. 2006, Osterberg et al. 2007, 2008, 2010).

The occlusion may also influence an individual's susceptibility to sleep apnea if it is associated with restricted airway; this susceptibility is linked with increased risk of cardiovascular disease, especially in women (Lavie 2014).

Temporomandibular dysfunction (TMD) is a component of generalized arthritis and musculoskeletal conditions (Carlsson Chapter 13), which are not influenced by the occlusion (Stohler 2004, Michelotti et al. 2005, Clark & Minakuchi 2005, Dao 2005, Markland & Wanman 2010, Greene 2010, 2011, Turp & Schlinder 2012) but may influence functional ability.

Appropriately planned and delivered oral rehabilitation and restored occlusal features are associated with enhanced appearance, general well-being, self-confidence, improved function, and psychosocial well-being.

CLINICAL OUTCOMES

For a successful prosthodontic rehabilitation, the range of variability of individual skeletal, morphometric, and occlusal features must be recognized (Sessle 2005, Chapter 1). Adaption to restorations and prostheses is continuous and dependent on (1) psychosocial factors, (2) aesthetic acceptance and well-being, (3) functional improvement (especially mastication), and (4) neurophysiological factors through central neuroplasticity for adaptation to changes in dental status. These mechanisms underpin each patient's development of confidence and competence with their oral rehabilitation (see Chapters 1 and 4).

FACE AND MOUTH: PSYCHOSOCIAL IMPLICATIONS
Neurophysiology and Psychology

In addition to the physiological dynamics of afferent projections to the sensorimotor cortex, the mouth and face are of preeminent psychosocial importance to the individual (Fig. 3-1). Within this context and the face exposed in Western society for appearance,

Sensory homunculous

Motor homunculus

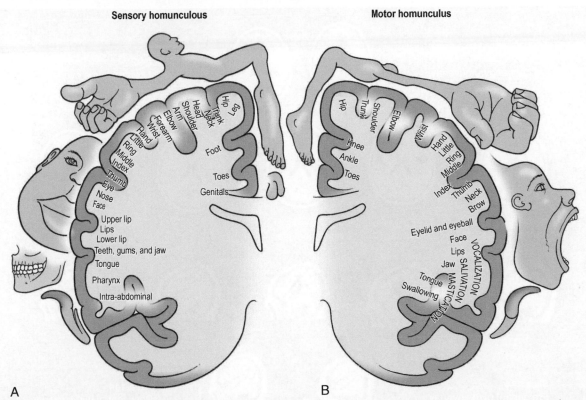

A

B

FIG 3-1 Sensorimotor representation of face and mouth. This "cortical homunculus" is the diagrammatic representation of the somatotropic distribution of sensory afferent projections to the sensorimotor cortex (SMC), with the sensory cortex (**A**) and motor output distribution (**B**). In addition to the physiological dynamics of afferent projections to SMC, the mouth and face are of preeminent psychosocial importance to the individual. Within this context and the face exposed in Western society for appearance, expression, communication, chewing, swallowing, the presence or absence of teeth, and the quality of their replacement are of paramount importance. (From Penfield & Rasmussen. The Cerebral Cortex of Man. © 1950 Gale, a part of Cengage Learning, Inc. Reproduced by permission. www.cengage.com/permissions.)

expression, communication, chewing, swallowing, the presence or absence of teeth, and the quality of their replacement are of paramount importance.

In industrialized economies, individuals prioritize aesthetics primarily and then function. Individuals have high aesthetic expectations to preserve or restore beauty, elegance, and social desirability, together with function for communication, mastication, diet, social interaction, self-esteem, and enhanced quality of life. The media has become a driver and major influence on perception of bodily appearance, with emphasis on rewards for greater physical attractiveness (Bull & Rumsey 1988, Patzer 2008). Moreover, people look longer and more often at faces perceived as "attractive" (Maner et al. 2003). It follows that seeing attractive faces recalibrates individual preferences to want similar "attractive" facial characteristics.

In nonindustrialized economies, individuals prioritize function before aesthetics out of necessity. Function is often the driver of survival, and aesthetics are regarded with modest expectations.

Occlusion and Sensorimotor Change

As part of an analysis of occlusal change and stereognosis, a study was undertaken using an occlusal overlay to increase mandibular crown length and occlusal vertical dimension (OVD) by 3 mm in the incisor region. The increase resulted in immediate changes in cortical activation, as shown in Figs. 3-2 and 3-3 (Lai et al. J Dent Res 2015).

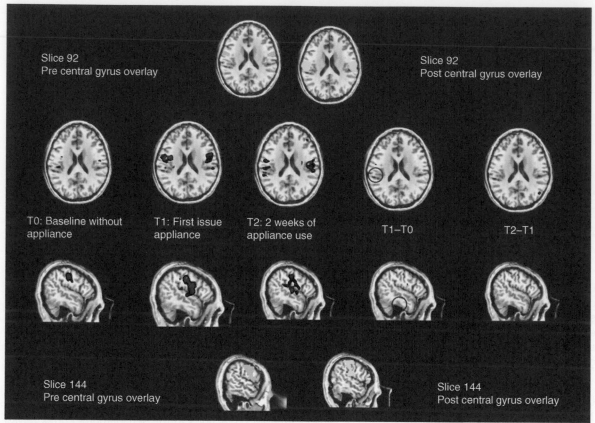

FIG 3-2 A data set of fMRI scans to show activity in the cortical areas of the precentral and postcentral gyrus indicating activity at (1) baseline, (2) issue of the appliance (T1), and (3) after 2 weeks of appliance use (T2). Colored zones indicate increased cellular activity in the sensorimotor cortex (SMC) at issue, which is sustained at 2 weeks. (Adapted from Lai et al. in press 2015.)

Interestingly, subject-group analysis showed that occlusal change resulted in immediate and significant activation of the sensorimotor cortex in both the left and right hemispheres of the brain. Areas of activation included frontal, parietal, and sublobar regions. Specific sensoricortical changes in the right and left middle temporal, medial frontal, precentral, and postcentral gyrus regions were shown to be significant in the following three specific areas:

- Medial frontal gyrus—area 6 ($p = 0.004$)
- Precentral gyrus—areas 4 and 6 ($p = 0.007$)
- Postcentral gyrus—area 3 ($p = 0.001$)

Figure 3-2 features a data set of functional magnetic resonance imaging (fMRI) scans to show activity in the cortical areas of the precentral and postcentral gyrus indicating activity at (1) baseline, (2) issue of the appliance (T1), and (3) after 2 weeks

of appliance use (T2). The colored zones indicate increased cellular activity in the sensorimotor cortex at issue, which is sustained at 2 weeks. These data provide clinical justification as a case-specific requirement to increase the OVD with fixed or removable oral rehabilitations where required.

New Prostheses

Prosthodontic treatment aims to improve quality of life by restoring function and aesthetics. Each patient's impairment is not only dependent on lack of teeth but also strongly related to perception and adaptive capability.

The role of neuroplasticity in adaptation to the rehabilitation of lost teeth and tissues was also investigated with consideration of four paradigms

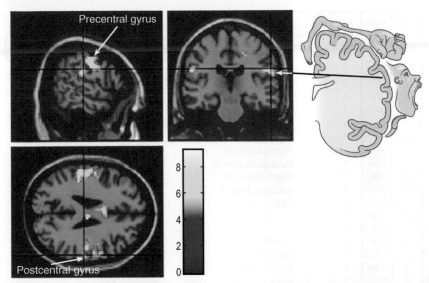

FIG 3-3 fMRI images from group analyses of 10 subjects at immediate issue of the new denture showed a significant activation in the precentral and postcentral gyrus: the upper-left sagittal, lower-horizontal, and upper-right frontal slice images each indicate sensorimotor activation. The activation pattern during the task performed (lip pursing) corresponds with the lip area of the sensory homunculus. A conjunction analysis showed statistically consistent areas activated over time. The percentage of BOLD signal values of the precentral gyrus and postcentral gyrus confirm change with time, indicating immediate plasticity. (Adapted from Luraschi et al. 2013, with permission.)

(Klineberg et al. 2012, Luraschi et al. 2013, Chapters 1 and 4), as follows:

- *Psychophysical*—occlusal thickness perception for oral stereognosis
- *Cortical*—fMRI changes with clenching, tapping, and lip pursing
- *Physical*—bite force and chewing efficiency
- *Psychological profile*—use of Symptom Checklist 90 Revised (SCL-90-R; Fig. 3-4), Oral Health Related Quality of Life (OHRQoL), and prosthesis satisfaction with Visual Analogue Scale (VAS) assessments (Fig. 3-5)

The use of VAS assessment in monitoring prosthesis acceptance is a valuable component of case management. The example given is from Feine and Lund (2006), reporting on data where VAS was used to assess patient satisfaction with their prostheses concerning (1) general satisfaction, (2) physical satisfaction, and (3) psychological satisfaction. The relative values along each line from totally dissatisfied or uncomfortable to completely satisfied or comfortable, provides objective and patient-specific feedback on the use of prostheses and its effect on patients. It is a valuable means of monitoring treatment outcomes.

fMRI from subject group analyses at immediate issue of new dentures showed significant activation in the precentral and postcentral gyrus.

The activation pattern during the task performed (lip pursing, Fig. 3-2) corresponded with the lip-mouth area of the sensory homunculus, and the area activated was shown to be statistically consistent over time. Together with blood oxygen level dependent (BOLD) signal values of the precentral gyrus and postcentral gyrus representations, these consistent changes indicated an immediate plasticity response to the fitting of new prostheses.

PSYCHOLOGICAL FACTORS

Clinical success must include the psychological construct within which treatment is planned and delivered, through the use of specific questionnaires, which could include, the SCL-90-R and Research Diagnostic Criteria for Temporomandibular Disorders (RDC/TMD, Dworkin & Le Resche 1992) (Figs. 3-4 to 3-6), or the recent revision Diagnostic Criteria for Temporomandibular Disorders (DC/TMD) for clinical and research applications as recommendations from

DRN			Gender	Female	Age	

Questions					
Q1s	4	Q31d	4	Q61l	2
Q2a	4	Q32d	2	Q62p	2
Q3o	4	Q33a	4	Q63h	0
Q4s	3	Q34i	4	Q64	3
Q5d	4	Q36l	4	Q65o	0
Q6i	1	Q37i	2	Q66	4
Q7p	4	Q37i	2	Q67h	0
Q8pi	1	Q38o	2	Q68pi	0
Q9o	4	Q39a	2	Q69i	1
Q10o	1	Q40s	4	Q70pa	2
Q11h	1	Q41l		Q71d	4
Q12s	3	Q42s	4	Q72a	3
Q13pa	4	Q43pi	2	Q73l	0
Q14d	4	Q44	4	Q74h	0
Q15d	3	Q45o	3	Q75pa	2
Q16p	0	Q46o	4	Q76pi	2
Q17a	4	Q47pa	0	Q77p	2
Q18pi	1	Q48s	2	Q78a	4
Q19	4	Q49s	2	Q79d	4
Q20d	4	Q50pa	2	Q80a	0
Q21i	1	Q51o	3	Q81h	0
Q22d	3	Q52s	3	Q82pa	0
Q23a	3	Q53s	3	Q83pi	3
Q24h	0	Q54d	4	Q84p	4
Q25pa	2	Q55o	3	Q85p	4
Q26d	4	Q56s	3	Q86a	4
Q27s	4	Q57a	3	Q87p	0
Q28o	4	Q58s	3	Q88p	2
Q29d	4	Q59	3	Q89	4
Q30d	4	Q60	4	Q90p	0
	28		28		19

Dimension	Total	No. questions	Raw score	T score
Somatization (12)	38	12	3.17	73S
Obsessive- compulsive (10)	28	10	2.80	63OC
Interpersonal sensitivity (9)	13	8	1.63	53IS
Depression (13)	48	13	3.69	74D
Anxiety (10)	31	10	3.10	65A
Hostility (6)	1	6	0.17	39H
Phobic Anxiety (7)	12	7	1.71	60PA
Paranoid ideation (6)	9	6	1.50	54PI
Psychoticism (10)	20	10	2.00	63P
Additional items (7)	26	7		
Total		89		

		T score
Grand total (GT)	226	
GSI (GT/total)	2.54	67
PSDI (GT/PST)	3.01	63
PST	75	63

FIG 3-4 Symptom Checklist 90 Revised (SCL-90-R): Oral Health Related Quality of Life (OHRQoL). (Form reproduced from Derogatis 1992, with permission.)

the Consortium Network and Orofacial Pain Special Interest Group (Schiffman et al. 2014) to monitor the effect of psychological factors on clinical treatment.

Figure 3-4 is an example of an SCL-90-R (Derogatis et al. 1992) analyzed to indicate the psychological features of a particular patient. The SCL-90-R questionnaire has 90 questions relating to nine behavioral domains in random order, which address somatization, anxiety, depression, interpersonal sensitivity, hostility, paranoid ideation, and psychoticism. The analysis of a psychological profile is presented on Fig. 3-4, and it includes graphical representation of one patient's particular details, which indicate elevated somatization, depression, and anxiety (values at 65 or above warrant further investigation). The value

of this information to the clinician in understanding a patient's psychological status is significant, and such data are desirable as a component of the patient-specific information generally collected to assist in patient management.

The RDC/TMD and the DC/TMD are validated, standardized clinical assessment tools for assessment of subtypes of TMD (jaw muscles and jaw joints) to determine (1) presence of evoked pain, limited mobility, and dysfunction of the physical features (Axis 1) and (2) the psychological status (Axis 2) in relation to signs and symptoms. In addition, this protocol was a means for standardized documentation for clinical research and comparison across clinics involved in TMD and orofacial-pain diagnosis and management.

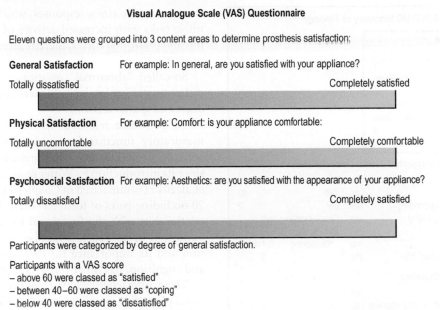

FIG 3-5 Visual Analogue Scale (VAS) Questionnaire. (Reproduced from Feine & Lund 2006, with permission.)

THE NEW PARADIGM

Recognition of the importance of occlusion and mastication as a core element in prosthodontic rehabilitation to maintain or enhance cognitive skills is clearly a new paradigm in clinical management.

Thomas Kuhn (1962) proposed, "science progressed in paradigms": a set of procedures that are shared by the group of proponents of the field, who work within a particular set of guidelines (Greenhalgh 2011). This could apply also to prosthodontic rehabilitation.

The reappraisal of thinking may be a result of interaction with other disciplines. Cross-disciplinary interaction is to be encouraged for innovation and new concept development.

This *new paradigm* in prosthodontics will be explored further in the following section.

CONTINUING CREATIVITY

Continuing creativity is sustainable well into old age, contrary to earlier understandings. Myelination of nerves commences in the newborn as brain circuits develop and expand in childhood and into young adulthood when the breadth of sensorimotor skills and executive functions of the prefrontal cortex are being established.

Importantly, the identification through contemporary imaging (such as fMRI) shows that myelination of nerves continues into advanced age, especially in the temporal cortex, the area of interpretation of executive functions of visual memory, language, meaning, and emotions.

The driver of continual advance of myelination and high-level executive reasoning is the continual reinforcing of activity, which serves to preserve physical and cerebral function.

OCCLUSION AND COGNITIVE HEALTH

The Role of Mastication

Animal and human studies have introduced a new dimension to oral health. Mastication has been reported to be linked with cognitive function through the hippocampus and its role in individual learning and memory (see reviews by Weijenberg et al. 2010, Ono et al. 2010, and Ohkubo et al. 2013).

Decreased mastication has been shown to be an epidemiological risk factor for dementia, decreased spatial memory, and decreased hippocampus neurons. The question of whether this is reversible is of particular importance.

Data indicate that increased mastication influences changes in memory processes by decreased endocrine

RDC/TMD Summary of Findings

Patient	
Date	19/03/2013
Patient ID	7
Clinician	Dr Smith
Age	30
Gender	Female
Race	Australian
Educational level	4
Income	4

Self-reported patient characteristics

Click	yes		
Grating/grinding	yes	CPI	60
Nocturnal clenching/grinding	yes	DP	2
Diurnal clenching/grinding	yes	Graded chronic pain	2
AM stiffness	yes	Mandibular	
Ringing in ears	no	functioning	0.416667
Uncomfortable/unusual bite	yes		

Group 1 Muscle disorders

Myofascial pain	yes
Myofascial pain with limited opening	yes
No group 1	no

Group 2 Disk displacements

Right joint

Disk displacement with reduction	no
Disk displacement without reduction with limited movement	no
Disk displacement without reduction without limited movement	no
No right joint group 2	yes

Left joint

Disk displacement with reduction	no
Disk displacement without reduction with limited movement	no
Disk displacement without reduction without limited movement	no
No right joint group 2	yes

Group 3 Other joint conditions

Right joint

Arthralgia	yes
Osteoarthritis of TMJ	no
Osteoarthritis of TMJ	no
No right joint group 3	no

Left joint

Arthralgia	no
Osteoarthritis of TMJ	no
Osteoarthritis of TMJ	no
No right joint group 3	yes

FIG 3-6 Research Diagnostic Criteria for Temporomandibular Disorders (RDC/TMD). (Form reproduced from Dworkin & Le Resche 1992, with permission.)

and autonomic stress responses, which improve cognitive tasks with increased activity of the hippocampus and prefrontal cortex, thereby increasing cognitive processing.

So-called "abnormal" mastication (e.g., occlusal disharmony in animals) influences chronic stress and decreases spatial learning.

Of particular relevance in this need to preserve masticatory function is the shortened dental arch concept, which has been comprehensively evaluated since its introduction by Witter et al. 2001, Reissmann et al. 2015 (summarized in Chapter 7). Having at least 20 occluding pairs of teeth has been shown to have a relationship with the functional implications of the occlusion. Moreover, this number of teeth in occlusion and its importance for diet, nutrition, obesity, and cognition, has other important implications.

These interrelationships have been explored in a series of studies revealing an additional dimension to the concept of the shortened dental arch. A selection of these data is summarized below.

Morita et al. (2006), in an elderly Japanese population (more than 80 years of age), reported on the recognized scenario, that the progressive loss of teeth affected diet and nutrition and thereby influenced daily activities and mental health (oral examinations were based on WHO criteria, and Kaplan-Meier analysis was used to calculate survival). Of significance was that elderly males with less than 20 occluding pairs of teeth had statistically significantly shorter survival; however, this was not the case with females, where the presence of 20 or more teeth did not influence their survival.

In a similar context, Osterberg et al. (2007) reported associations from a population study of the Nordic countries (Denmark, Finland, and Sweden) between periodontal disease and cardiovascular and cerebrovascular disease. A previous study by Ragnarsson et al. (2004) had suggested that there was a significantly increased prevalence of death from cardiovascular disease correlated with (1) the number of teeth present, (2) edentulism, and (3) the number of years of edentulism. However, when these data were adjusted for confounders, a Cox regression analysis indicated that there was no significance.

Osterberg et al. (2007) analyzed further associations with a population of 75 year olds over a 7-year period. Data identified significant associations between cognitive and cardiovascular function, muscle strength, hearing, and visual ability with number of teeth, although the association varied with the risk factor. There was a lower mortality for both genders with 20 or more teeth, with a relatively lower mortality in women than in men.

In a later follow-up cross-sectional study Osterberg et al. (2008) further investigated the strength of association between four age cohorts and tooth number (greater than or equal to 20 occluding pairs) in 70-year-old subjects over a 7-year period. The 7-year outcomes indicated that there were statistically significant data confirming that the number of teeth was (1) an independent predictor of mortality and (2), importantly, was independent of general health factors, socioeconomic status, and lifestyle. The data also suggested a direct correlation of a 4% decrease in mortality for each remaining tooth above 20 occluding pairs.

In addition to these significant associations, a further study by this group (Osterberg et al. 2010) confirmed significant statistical association (based on logistic regression and adjusted for confounding variables of general health, socioeconomics, and lifestyle), with increased obesity associated with edentulism, particularly in women of 55-75 years of age. In men, the association was weaker.

Some animal studies have investigated diet-induced obesity in mice, which was found to correlate with a decrease in the immune response and an increase in severity of periodontal disease (Amar et al. 2007). Notwithstanding the limitations of correlation of animal and human data, it appears that there are complex changes in the immune responses with diet and obesity.

GLOBAL ORAL AWARENESS

This general feature of individual-specific oral awareness may be investigated and assessed by the following:

- *Aesthetics*—provides satisfaction and enhanced psychosocial well-being and self-confidence
- *Occlusal stability and jaw support*—key elements for optimizing function
- *Function*—includes many features but is primarily mastication and swallowing with improved functional efficiency and comfort as a primary goal of rehabilitation; additionally, phonetics for confi-

dent communication and social interaction engenders self-confidence, and jaw mobility is linked with this

- *Psychophysical*—tactile perception to detect and appreciate food texture and volume; it is also integrated with taste
- *Occlusal vigilance*—the regular behavioral response, whereas occlusal hypervigilance is an amplified behavioral response occurring in the absence of cognitive modulation

HYPOTHESIS

A negative correlation has been identified between mastication and corticosteroid level. This led Ono and colleagues to suggest the hypothesis (1) suppression of the hypothalamic-pituitary-adrenal (HPA) axis occurs by mastication-induced stimulation, and (2) this is a significant component of preservation of cognitive function.

Mastication may induce changes in defective cognitive function and operate through the HPA axis and hippocampal neuronal processes. Data have indicated that mastication preceding cognitive-task acquisition leads to enhanced blood-oxygen level in the prefrontal cortex and hippocampus, as well as increased learning and memory. These findings have led to the hypothesis that mastication appears to provide "medication-free" protection against the development of senile dementia and stress-related disorders (Ono et al. 2010).

REFERENCES

Amar S, Zhou Q, Shaik-Dasthagirisaheb Y, et al: Diet-induced obesity in mice causes changes in immune responses and bone loss manifested by bacterial challenge, *PNAS* 104:20466–20471, 2007.

Bull R, Rumsey N: *The social psychology of facial appearance*, New York, 1998, Springer-Verlag.

Clark GT, Minakuchi H: Oral appliances. In Laskin DM, Greene CS, Hylander WL, editors: *Temporomandibular disorders—an evidence-based approach to diagnosis and treatment*, Chicago, 2006, Quitessence.

Dao T: Musculoskeletal disorders and the occlusal interface, *Int J Prosthodont* 18:295–296, 2005.

Derogatis LR: *SCL-90-R: Administration, Scoring and Procedures Manual—II*, ed 2, Baltimore, 1992, Clinical Psychometric Research.

Dworkin S, Le Resche L: Research diagnostic criteria for temporomandibular disorders: review, criteria, examination and specifications, critique, *J Craniomandib Disord* 6:301–355, 1992.

Feine JS, Lund JP: Measuring chewing ability in randomised controlled trials with edentulous populations wearing implant prostheses, *J Oral Rehabil* 33:301–308, 2006.

Greene CS: Managing the core of patients with temporomandibular disorders: a new guideline for care, *J Am Dent Assoc* 141:1086–1088, 2010.

Greene CS: Relationship between occlusion and temporomandibular disorders: implications for the orthodontist, *Am J Orthod Dentofacial Orthop* 139:11–15, 2011.

Greenhalgh T: Why do we always end up here? Evidence-based Medicine's conceptual cul-de-sacs and some of-road alternative routes. Guest Editorial, *Int J Prosthodont* 26:11–15, 2013.

Klineberg I, Murray G, Trulsson M: Occlusion on implants—is there a problem? *J Oral Rehabil* 39:522–537, 2012.

Kuhn TS: *The structure of scientific revolutions*, Chicago, 1962, University of Chicago Press. (50th anniversary edition 2012).

Lai A, Korgaonkar M, Gomes L, et al: f MRI study on human subjects with sudden occlusal vertical dimension increase, *Jacobs J Dent Res* 2:20–28, 2015.

Lavie L: Oxidative stress in obstructive sleep apnoea and intermittent hypoxia—Revisited—The bad ugly and good: implications to the heart and brain, *Sleep Med Rev* 20:27–45, 2014.

Luraschi J, Korgaonkar M, Whittle T, et al: Neuroplasticity in the adaptation to prosthodontic treatment, *J Orofac Pain* 27:206–216, 2013.

Maner JK, Kenrick DT, Becker DV, et al: Sexually selective cognition: Beauty captures the mind of the beholder, *J Personality Soc Psychol* 85:1107–1120, 2003.

Markland S, Wanman A: Risk factors associated with incidence and persistence of signs and symptoms of temporomandibular disorders, *Acta Odontol Scand* 68:289–299, 2010.

Michelotti A, Farella M, Gallo LM, et al: Effect of occlusal interferences on habitual activity of human masseter, *J Dent Res* 84:644–648, 2005.

Morita I, Nakagaki H, Kato K, et al: Relationship between survival rates and numbers of natural teeth in an elderly Japanese population, *Gerontol Assoc* 23: 214–218, 2006.

Ohkubo C, Morokuma M, Yoneyama Y, et al: Interactions between occlusion and human brain function activities, *J Oral Rehabil* 40(2):119–129, 2013.

Ono Y, Yamamoto T, Kubo YA, et al: Occlusion and brain function: mastication as a prevention of cognitive dysfunction, *J Oral Rehabil* 37(8):624–640, 2010.

Osterberg T, Carlsson GE, Sundh V, et al: Number of teeth—a predictor of mortality in the elderly? A population study in three Nordic localities, *Acta Odontol Scand* 65:335–340, 2007.

Osterberg T, Carlsson GE, Sundh V, et al: Number of teeth—predictor of mortality in 70-year old subjects, *Comm Dent Oral Epidemiol* 36:258–268, 2008.

Osterberg T, Dey DK, Sundh V, et al: Edentulism associated with obesity: a study of four national surveys of 16,416 Swedes aged 55-84 years, *Acta Odontol Scand* 68(6):360–367, 2010.

Patzer GL: *The power and paradox of physical attractiveness*, Boca Raton, Fla, 2008, Brown Walker Press.

Penfield W, Rasmussen T: *The Cerebral Cortex of Man*, New York, 1950, Macmillan.

Ragnarsson E, Eliasson ST, Gudnarson V: Loss of teeth and coronary heart disease, *Intern J Prosthodont* 17:441–446, 2004.

Reissmann DR, Heydeke G, Schierz O, et al: The randomised shortened dental arch study: temporomandibular pain, *Clin Oral Invest* 1:1–11, 2014.

Schiffman E, Ohrbach R, Truelove E, et al: Diagnostic criteria for temporomandibular disorders (DC/TMD) for clinical research applications: Recommendations of the INternation PDC/TMD Consortium network* and orofacial pain special interest group, *J Oral Facial Pain Headache* 28:6–27, 2014.

Sessle BJ: Biological adaptation and normative values, *Int J Prosthodont* 18:280–282, 2005.

Stohler CS: Taking stock: from chasing occlusal contacts to vulnerability alleles, *Orthod Craniofac Res* 7: 157–160, 2004.

Turp JC, Schindler H: The dental occlusion as a suspected cause for TMDs: epidemiological and etiological considerations, *J Oral Rehabil* 39:502–512, 2012.

Weijenberg RAF, Scherder EJA, Lobbezoo F: Mastication for the mind: the relationship between mastication and cognition in aging and dementia neuroscience, *Neurosci Biobehav Rev* 35:483–497, 2010.

Witter DJ, Creugers NH, Kreulin CM, et al: Occlusal stability in shortened dental arches, *J Dent Res* 80:432–436, 2001.

CHAPTER 4

Occlusion and Adaptation to Change: Neuroplasticity and Its Implications for Cognition

Sandro Palla and Iven Klineberg

SYNOPSIS

Occlusion should no longer be considered simply as the occlusal scheme determining the static or dynamic relationship between the dental arches or the jaw position. Rather, it should be regarded within a broader framework that considers the modulation of the somatosensory input from the periodontal, dental, and mucosal mechanoreceptors by the central nervous system, as well as sensorimotor neuroplasticity. These mechanisms, rather than the type of occlusion, ultimately determine whether an individual adapts to the oral perception changes inherent to all dental treatment. Central in this process is likely the patient's degree of vigilance to the somatosensory stimulus because attention increases perception, as well as how this somatosensory input is centrally processed. Notably, it is enough to attend to a stimulus to decrease the discrimination threshold. Thus patients who are hypervigilant to the oral environment are likely more sensitive to abnormal stimuli and therefore more at risk of not adapting even to minute oral or occlusal changes. Nevertheless, hypervigilance is likely to be a necessary but not comprehensive cause of maladaptation, as in the case of occlusal dysesthesia, which requires an imbalance between perceptual and cognitive processes, together with a negative affective response and abnormal illness behavior.

Sensorimotor neuroplasticity is essential to adjust jaw movements to an altered occlusal and/or oral condition after changing jaw position or inserting new reconstructions, with altering tongue space. In some cases, however, this may lead also to maladaptive oral behaviors. Recognition that sensorimotor neuroplasticity does not always lead to a context-specific adaptation of motor behavior prevents performing incorrect and potentially harmful therapies.

CHAPTER POINTS

- Satisfaction of search and premature closure
- Occlusal interferences
- Occlusal perception
- Cortical reorganization
- Modulation of somatosensory inputs: attention
- Occlusal hypervigilance
- Occlusal dysesthesia
- Medically unexplained symptoms
- Neuroplasticity of the sensorimotor cortex
- Dystonia

THE NEED TO ENLARGE THE VIEW OF OCCLUSION

Occlusion in dentistry is still a matter of controversy, especially in relation to its etiological association with craniomandibular disorders, bruxism, and implants survival. Many dentists still refuse to accept that occlusion plays at most, a very limited role in the etiology of craniomandibular disorders, although this has been proven in many epidemiological and experimental human and animal studies. The same is true for the association with bruxism, where a direct association with implant failure and bruxism has not been determined because it has never been measured objectively in such patients.

The term *malocclusion* certainly concurs, at least at a subconscious level, with regard to these erroneous interpretations. The term implies that there are occlusal forms that are detrimental (e.g., "bad" for the masticatory system or the subject's health) and that therefore lead to pathological alterations. Further, the term implies the existence of a "good" or "ideal" occlusion. In reality, such occlusions are not merely the exception; they are a theoretical construct based on a misconception of physiological principles. The "good" or "ideal" occlusion is created by dentists to simplify the technical aspects of the prosthodontic treatment. Further, the term *ideal occlusion* is not synonymous with physiologically "correct" occlusion. Individuals adapt well to various occlusal forms and severely compromised dental arches, or to an Angle Class III, which is the occlusal form most distant from an "ideal" one.

The opinion that occlusion is related to craniomandibular disorders is also due to a misinterpretation of clinical success on which etiological hypotheses are often based. Clinical success should only generate hypotheses to be validated scientifically. In this line of thought, there is also a propensity to rely on experts' opinions rather than scientific proof and to give the results of one's own clinical experience external validity (e.g., to generalize them to other situations and other patients). In addition, there is a tendency to consider that, if an intervention leads to clinical success, it is because it eliminated the cause. For instance, the observation that an occlusal adjustment or the insertion of an occlusal appliance relieves muscle pain or bruxism is still considered by many dentists as proof that "occlusal interferences" are etiologically related to these conditions, as their removal eliminates the symptoms. This thinking trap can be subsumed under the concept of "satisfaction of search" or "premature closure," terms that are normally used to define cognitive errors in the decision-making process (Croskerry 2003, Nendaz & Perrier 2012, Palla 2013, Stiegler et al. 2012). These terms define the condition in which one is satisfied with the first explanation or finding, and as a result, fails to look for alternative ones. This cognitive trap prevents the dentist from understanding that the intervention "occlusal adjustment" or "insertion of an occlusal appliance" is not merely a "mechanical" intervention aiming to eliminate premature contacts or to change the occlusion and restore centric relation. Rather, these therapeutic procedures are likely to be accompanied by additional actions that contribute to symptom remission, such as the clinician speaking positively about treatments, providing encouragement, and developing trust, reassurance, and a supportive relationship. As the beliefs and expectations associated with a therapeutic procedure can mimic, enhance, and mask the beneficial responses to pharmacological agents (Benedetti & Amanzio 2011), it is likely that they have similar effects with nonpharmacological therapies.

Further, the complexity of a biological response is often underestimated, and the masticatory system is considered unique, disregarding the fact that the physiological and pathophysiological mechanisms are the same for the complete musculoskeletal system. Moreover, there is a lack of understanding of the facts that (1) the somatosensory input is continuously modulated by the central nervous system by means of descending mechanisms (see Chapter 1), (2) the sensorimotor system is not hard wired but plastic (e.g., that it has the capacity to adapt to the functional demand), and (3) cognitive, affective, and emotional factors often determine if and how a patient adjusts to dental treatment. Lack of this understanding very often leads to treatment failures, with patients involved in "doctor shopping" and a series of unsuccessful therapies.

These introductory remarks should not be interpreted as a permit to perform less-than-optimum occlusal treatment when restoring a dentition, because, as discussed in the following, there are individual variations in the adaptation or vulnerability to occlusal changes. It simply underlines the need to enlarge the view of occlusion by integrating perceptual modulation and cognitive processes.

The aim of this chapter is to elucidate using two clinical cases of how individuals react to experimental occlusal changes, how the sensory input from tactile receptors is centrally modulated, and how the sensorimotor cortex undergoes neuroplastic changes relevant for understanding adaptation and maladaptation to reconstructive work.

CASE PRESENTATION 4.1

A 48-year-old female received two CAD/CAM-manufactured (Cerec) ceramic inlays on tooth 14 and 15. At insertion, she complained that she felt that tooth 15 was too high. The occlusal check revealed that the occlusal contact was indeed slightly too heavy so it was relieved. Thereafter, the contact between the tooth 14 and 44 was adjusted because the contact also bothered her. However, the occlusal adjustment did not result in a comfortable occlusion; the patient still felt that the "new" occlusion was uncomfortable. However, she was dismissed with the advice that she "would adjust" in "a matter of a few days." The patient returned 1 week later complaining that the occlusion was still uncomfortable. An occlusal check revealed a slight interference between the tooth 14 and 44, which was then removed. About 10 days later, the patient requested an emergency appointment because the occlusion was becoming increasingly uncomfortable. The direct occlusal analysis with manipulation of the mandible in centric relation did not show an interference in the right premolar area but rather the interference was found on the opposite side between the tooth 24 and 34. Because of lack of time and the fact that the Cerec inlays were no longer interfering, the patient was dismissed without therapy and scheduled for a new appointment 1 week later to recheck the occlusion. At the new appointment the patient complained again that the occlusion was uncomfortable and that right facial pain had started a few days before. The pain was strongest on awakening and decreased during the morning. Therefore the dentist decided to perform a new occlusal adjustment and to remove the balancing interference between the tooth 17 and 37. However, this procedure did not lead to a better occlusal perception; therefore it was decided to insert an occlusal appliance (Michigan type) also because, in the meantime, the facial pain had increased, lasting almost during the whole day, and it was exacerbated with chewing. Following this appointment, the patient visited several other dentists who continued to adjust the occlusal appliance, make new ones, and perform further occlusal adjustments without providing a comfortable occlusion or pain relief.

Four points of this history must be emphasized. First, the patient became aware of her occlusion. Second, the uncomfortable bite awareness persisted after the elimination of the interferences, leading the dentist to perform an occlusal adjustment even on teeth that had not been restored. Third, the occlusal awareness did not diminish. On the contrary, it increased the more occlusal therapies were performed. Fourth, the patient began experiencing facial pain.

To understand why this happened, it is necessary to review the literature on the effect of occlusal interferences, on how the occlusal sense is centrally modulated, and on the role of occlusal hypervigilance in the development of an occlusal dysesthesia such as the one the patient was suffering from.

EFFECTS OF THE INSERTION OF EXPERIMENTAL OCCLUSAL INTERFERENCES

Several studies have investigated the effect of the introduction of experimental occlusal interferences in healthy subjects. The earlier studies indicated that an experimental interference might cause symptoms typical of craniomandibular disorders, tooth ache, and altered chewing movements (Karlsson et al. 1992, Magnusson 1985, Randow et al. 1976, Riise &

Sheikholeslam 1982, Rugh et al. 1984, Shiau & Syu 1995, Yashiro et al. 2010). However, these symptoms occurred only in a minority of subjects and lasted only a few days. Interestingly, those investigations reported that the experimental interference lead in several patients to a decrease in bruxing activity during sleep (Randow et al. 1976, Riise & Sheikholeslam 1982, Rugh et al. 1984, Shiau & Syu 1995). Nevertheless, clinicians did not give much credit to this observation and continued viewing occlusal interferences as a cause of bruxism.

The results of these studies have been confirmed by newer investigations performed with a more rigorous study design. Michelotti et al. (2005) performed double blind studies in 11 healthy females without craniomandibular disorders, bruxism, or headache. Each female subject received an active occlusal interference over a period of 7 days and a dummy or placebo interference in a crossover design. The interference effect was monitored by recording the electromyographic activity of the masseter muscle during waking hours (8 hours) in the natural environment by means of portable recorders. The active occlusal interference caused a significant reduction in the number of muscle contractions. The reduction was more pronounced for the high- than for the low-intensity contractions. The active interference did not lead to craniomandibular symptoms but rather to dental discomfort that decreased during the study period. In addition, the masseter muscle pain pressure threshold did not change after insertion of the active interference (Michelotti et al. 2006). The decrease in the number of contraction episodes was interpreted as adaptation to the dental discomfort. In a successive study, the same group of investigators analyzed the effect of an active occlusal interference using a similar design in subjects with parafunction while awake (Michelotti et al. 2012). Twenty female subjects were divided in two groups, differing by the frequency of bruxism while awake, as assessed by the Oral Behaviors Checklist (Markiewicz et al. 2006). As distinct from the first study, the occlusal interference was higher (0.4 vs. 0.25 mm) and the authors did not measure the frequency of masseter muscle contractions but the frequency of tooth contacts while awake, using an ecological momentary assessment (Chen et al. 2007). Results showed that the frequency of tooth contacts while awake decreased in both groups,

the decrease being significantly less in the group with high-frequency parafunction.

In this context, Le Bell et al. (2002) inserted dummy and active interferences in four groups of female subjects. One group consisted of patients with and the other without a history of craniomandibular disorders. Each group was then randomly divided into two groups, one receiving an active and the other the dummy interference during two weeks. The females without a TMD history showed good adaptation to the interference, but the subjects with a TMD history and true interference showed a significant increase in clinical signs compared with the other groups. In addition, these females also reported stronger symptoms that did not decline during the observation time, as was the case for the symptoms in the females without a history of craniomandibular disorders (Le Bell et al. 2006). Support for this finding comes from another study performed by the Michelotti group, showing that the introduction of an occlusal interference in female patients with masticatory muscle pain did not lead to a reduction in the frequency of masseter muscle contraction as observed in healthy females, even though the females with muscle pain also developed tooth ache (Cioffi et al. in press). Thus there appeared to be individual differences in vulnerability to occlusal interferences.

Considering that subjects with craniomandibular disorders, in particular with masticatory muscle pain, have the teeth in contact far more often than healthy subjects do (Chen et al. 2007, Fujisawa et al. 2013, Funato et al. 2014, Glaros et al. 2005a,b, Huang et al. 2002, Kino et al. 2005, Sato et al. 2006) and that the reduction in the frequency of tooth contacts is less pronounced in patients with a high frequency of parafunction, it may be hypothesized that the habit of holding the teeth in contact while awake is the common denominator that makes these subjects more vulnerable to experimental and, by analogy, to iatrogenic occlusal interferences.

To summarize, the results of the studies on placement of experimental occlusal interferences allow two conclusions. First, there are individual differences in vulnerability to occlusal interferences. Second, acute occlusal interferences may cause different symptoms, which in healthy individuals disappear within 1 to 2 weeks at most. It is therefore correct to tell patients "they will adjust" to the new reconstruction. However, longer lasting symptoms are a sign that either the reconstruction is incorrect or the dentist is managing a patient with poor adaptability (e.g., a patient at risk to develop an occlusal dysesthesia). Thus one could hypothesize that the introduction of an occlusal interference could be a test to check the degree of adaptability of a patient. This is a provocative statement, but it underlines the need for a paradigm shift in how dentists must look at the occlusion.

OCCLUSAL PERCEPTION

Determination of the interocclusal tactility threshold (ITT) is a technique used to measure occlusal perception. Foils of different thickness are placed between the teeth, taking care that they do not touch the soft tissues, and the subject is requested to close gently into maximum intercuspation and to report if he or she feels the foil. The smallest ITT is recorded between healthy teeth, and it varies interindividually between 8 μ and 60 μ. The threshold increases when the tooth has an artificial crown or is nonvital, indicating that not only periodontal mechanoreceptors but also pulpal receptors contribute to the ITT. The threshold increases by a factor of 5 (range 2.5× to 8×) during chewing, the range varying between 100 μ and 250 μ (Herren 1988).

The following data on the modulation of the tactile input from skin mechanoreceptors will be used to explain these variations in the ITT. Tactile modulation is used because of the scarcity of data on the modulation of the input from the periodontal mechanoreceptors by higher centers. Moreover, several lines of evidence indicate that the input from the skin and periodontal mechanoreceptors is regulated in the same manner.

Changes in exteroception and proprioception are due to two phenomena: top-down modulation of the incoming signal by higher brain centers and brain neuroplasticity (e.g., its capability to change and adapt to new demands).

One of the clinically relevant mechanisms by which sensitivity to a stimulus is modulated is provided by attention to and distraction from a stimulus: attention leads to an increase and distraction to a decrease in sensitivity. For instance, experiments using functional magnetic resonance imaging showed that the primary somatosensory cortex, the posterior

parietal cortex, and the anterior insula cortex (e.g., areas involved in tactile perception) were significantly more activated when the subject attended to a vibratory stimulus than when the same stimulus was presented in a passive manner (Albanese et al. 2009; see Johansen-Berg & Lloyd 2000 for details). Importantly, attention regulates neuronal excitability both in its presence and in its absence (e.g., during expectation of the stimulus) (Fiorio et al. 2012, Gazzaley & Nobre 2012) or when an individual is required to attend to the spontaneous sensations of a body part in the absence of external stimuli (Bauer et al. 2014), which indicates that those cortical areas are already activated before stimulus presentation.

Attention is necessary because at any time, the individual is subjected to far more perceptual information than he or she can effectively process. In other words, attentional mechanisms evolved out of necessity to focus efficiently on the information relevant to ongoing goals and behaviors. For example, in hearing, auditory environments typically present many competing sounds, and one selects what is most relevant, such as a speaker's voice during a lecture.

The perception of exteroceptive stimuli depends on not only cognitive mechanisms but also the frequency and duration of the incoming peripheral input. Indeed, the brain maintains the capacity to undergo cortical reorganization throughout life (e.g., to alter neural connections, connection strengths, and the cortical representation area of the body following extensive use, practice, and training). For instance, the cortical representation of the fingers of the left hand of professional string players is increased in comparison to that of nonviolin players, and the expansion is related to the years of play (details in Pantev et al. 2001). Therefore it is not surprising that tactile acuity and discrimination increases after repetitive sensory stimulation of a finger (Kowalewski et al. 2012, Schlieper & Dinse 2012). This increase parallels an enlargement of the cortical areas representing the stimulated body part (Hodzic et al. 2004, Hoffken et al. 2007, Pleger et al. 2001). A lowering of the tactile discrimination threshold is obtained also after high-frequency repetitive transcranial stimulation of the primary somatosensory cortex, an effect that outlasts the stimulation time (Ragert et al. 2008), which also parallels an increase in the cortical representation area (Tegenthoff et al. 2005).

Only interindividual variations in the degree of tactility during chewing can be ascribed to different attentional degrees. The marked decrease of occlusal tactility during chewing compared to the nonchewing situation is likely caused by top-down inhibition of the exteroceptive input. It is well known that during movements, perception of tactile stimuli is decreased, as the transmission of somatosensory signals to the primary somatosensory cortex are diminished (sensory gating). This is due to descending inhibition from the primary somatosensory and motor cortex. Involvement of the latter is proved by the fact that the inhibition starts before movement onset. This gating is interpreted as a mechanism that allows enhanced detection of unexpected stimuli (see Chapman & Beauchamp 2006, Seki et al. 2003).

To summarize, different degrees of attention most likely explain interindividual variations in occlusal perception when patients consciously close on a metal foil, whereas descending inhibition concurs, together with the intrusion-related adaptation of the periodontal receptors (Morimoto et al. 2013), to the reduction of the occlusal perception during chewing.

OCCLUSAL HYPERVIGILANCE AND OCCLUSAL DYSESTHESIA

Occlusal dysesthesia, the disorder from which the patient described initially was suffering, is "a persistent complaint of uncomfortable bite sensation for more than 6 months, which does not correspond to any physical alteration related to the occlusion, dental pulp, periodontium, jaw muscles, or the temporomandibular joints" (Hara et al. 2012). Several etiological hypotheses have been proposed to explain occlusal dysesthesia: psychiatric disorders, phantom phenomenon, and alteration in oral proprioceptive input transmission (Hara et al. 2012), none of which by itself can explain the disorder that has a multifactorial etiology.

According to the definition, occlusal dysesthesia can be included in the group of "medically unexplained symptoms" (MUS). Several hypotheses have been proposed to explain these symptoms (see Rief & Broadbent 2007). Most etiological theories consider that persons with MUS have amplified perceptual experiences. Accordingly, the central process is a perceptual one: people need to perceive sensations to describe physical complaints (Rief & Broadbent 2007). Under normal conditions context-irrelevant propio- and exteroceptive inputs are filtered out so that they are not perceived (e.g., they do not reach conscious awareness). For instance, we are not aware of our occlusion, of wearing clothes, of our own weight, or of the heartbeat unless we concentrate on them. However, a down regulation of the filtering mechanisms, such as lack of distraction or increased selective attention (hypervigilance), allows the exteroceptive input to gain consciousness (e.g., to be perceived). Nevertheless, increased perception is not by itself a sufficient cause for developing MUS. This requires a disbalance between perceptual and cognitive processes (attention, expectation, or anticipation of negative effects, catastrophizing, worry, and attribution of sensations to noxious rather than benign causes) along with negative affectivity such as anxiety and abnormal illness behavior (Rief & Barsky 2005, Rief & Broadbent 2007).

Heightened attention to the body (i.e., bodily hypervigilance) and a selective focus on detected sensations, increase the perception of somatic sensations. Clinical experience shows that patients with an occlusal dysesthesia are occlusally hypervigilant (e.g., they continuously check their occlusion). This together with the role that hypervigilance has in the etiology of MUS supports the hypothesis that occlusal hypervigilance is necessary but not sufficient for the development of an occlusal dysesthesia. Occlusal hypervigilance is therefore presumably not simply a by-product of the emotional state of patients with occlusal dysesthesia, but plays together with cognitive, behavioral and affective negativity a major role in symptom causation and maintenance (Fig. 4-1).

It has been discussed that differences in occlusal perception depend upon different degrees of attention. Accordingly, occlusal hypervigilant patients should have an increased occlusal perception. However, although the tactile threshold seems to be significantly lower in somatoform disorder sufferers than in healthy subjects (Katzer et al. 2012), this does not appear to be the case for the degree of occlusal perception in patients with oral dysesthesia (Baba et al. 2005). The median interdental thickness discrimination ability of the 31 healthy subjects was 14 μ, and that of the eight dysesthesia patients was

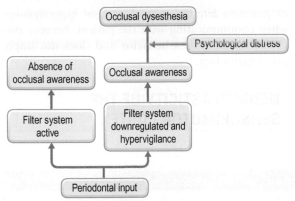

FIG 4-1 Hypothetical Model of Occlusal Dysesthesia

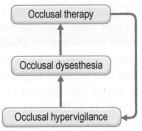

FIG 4-2 The Vicious Cycle of Occlusal Dysesthesia Amplification

8 μ. However, the difference was not statistically significant. Nevertheless, the thoughts and emotions accompanying the sense of an altered occlusion are likely to be more important than the degree of occlusal perception is for the development of the disorder.

A temporal association between the beginning of an occlusal sensation and a psychosocially loaded situation, such as distress, negative emotions, worries, depression, a history of unexplained medical symptoms, or absence of distraction, may increase the abnormal occlusal sensation with the patient focusing increasingly on the occlusion. The lack of recognition by the dentist that the disorder does not have a somatic occlusal etiology, together with the continuation of occlusal therapies, will reinforce the patient's conviction that the occlusion is incorrect, and engender greater occlusal vigilance. Typically, after each occlusal therapy the patient is asked how the occlusion feels. These risks enhance the vicious cycle of occlusal hypervigilance and negative thoughts that worsen the disorder (Fig. 4-2).

MANAGEMENT OF OCCLUSAL DYSESTHESIA

The central role that perception modulation and cognitive, affective, emotional, and behavioral processes play in the etiology of occlusal dysesthesia implies that this disorder cannot be treated by occlusal means. On the contrary, it is necessary to understand not only that occlusal interventions are harmful, as they may initiate the disorder, but also that they encourage its perpetuation. Especially in chronic cases, the management needs to be multidisciplinary, with the most important elements being: (1) establishment of a good therapeutic environment through an empathetic doctor-patient communication and an effective doctor-patient relationship, (2) generic interventions such as motivational interviewing, giving tangible explanations and reassurance, and (3) specific interventions such as cognitive approaches and eventually pharmacotherapy (Heijmans et al. 2011).

Establishment of a positive relationship with the patient based on the dentist's recognition of the somatic complaints and of the patient's suffering is fundamental, as it assures the patient that the care provider is taking him/her seriously (Heijmans et al. 2011, Heinrich 2004, Richardson & Engel Jr. 2004). Confrontation is not helpful. A thorough exploration of patients' beliefs, concerns, and the consequences of these symptoms on patients' daily activities, social environment, and illness behavior not only allows reaching a better understanding of the patients' symptoms and problems but often also provides a starting point to explain the need for the psychological management of the disorder. As the patient comes with a conviction of a somatic, occlusal complaint, he/she does not easily accept that the disorder has a nonsomatic component. Thus, in the management, the dentist plays a central role not only in recognizing the disorder and in assuring the patient that based on the clinical examination there is no serious occlusal problem but especially in finding an efficient manner to refer the patient to a specialist for the treatment of the cognitive, emotional, and affective disorder components.

This referral process is often very difficult, and dentists are generally unprepared and thus feel incompetent. Explaining to the patient about the causative role that occlusal hypervigilance has in the etiology of the disorder, and that occlusal vigilance is a behavior that with appropriate therapy can be reversed, may facilitate a referral. It is therefore suggested not to use the terms *occlusal dysesthesia*, *occlusal neurosis*, or *phantom bite* but that of *occlusal hypervigilance* when communicating with the patient, because this last term refers to a behavior and does not imply psychopathology.

NEUROPLASTICITY OF THE SENSORIMOTOR CORTEX

CASE PRESENTATION 4.2

A 35-year-old female patient received a crown on tooth 46. Immediately after she felt that the crown was too "big" and that "something was wrong with her teeth." She began clenching and developed a headache. The patient described herself as very nervous. When she arrived for the first visit, she stated that the occlusion bothered her and that she could no longer find a comfortable jaw position. The occlusal inspection showed that the patient was biting in an anterior position (Fig. 4-3, *A* and *B*), as if the crown would hinder closing in maximum intercuspation. However, when asked to clench the teeth forcefully, the jaw slid dorsally to close in maximum intercuspation (Fig. 4-3, *C* and *D*), indicating that the crown did not hinder closing into habitual intercuspation. However, the patient stated that this jaw position was very uncomfortable and that the only less-uncomfortable position was an anterior one.

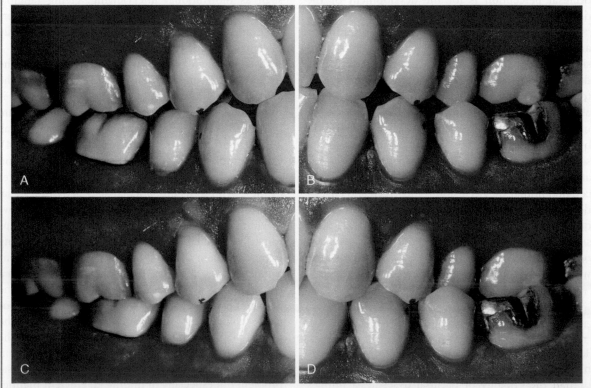

FIG 4-3 A and **B** show the jaw position into which the patient began closing after the insertion of the fixed prosthesis on tooth 46. **C** and **D** show that the fixed prosthesis did not hinder closing into the habitual intercuspation.

SENSORIMOTOR CORTEX

The primary motor cortex receives sensory inputs directly through the thalamus and indirectly through the somatosensory cortex. This somatosensory information is used by the motor cortex to control motor functions. The oral somatosensory cortex is therefore involved not only in somatosensation but also in the modulation of oral motor function, in particular in learning new motor skills, as well as adapting orofacial behavior to alterations in the oral environment, such as after tooth extractions, occlusal alterations, or the insertion of removable reconstructions with tongue space alteration (Sessle et al. 2005).

Several lines of evidence suggest that afferent intraoral inputs are important in modifying oral motor behavior, and dental changes lead to neuroplastic changes within the sensorimotor cortex. For instance, animal studies have shown a change in the representation of the digastric and genioglossus muscles in the motor cortex after extraction or trimming of a rat's lower incisor. These neuroplastic changes were explained by the sensory loss after tooth extraction and/or the alteration of the oral behavior caused by the tooth loss (see Chapter 1; Avivi-Arber et al. 2011, Sessle et al. 2007, Sessle 2011). In humans, neuroplastic changes in the sensorimotor cortex have been documented after the insertion of an implant-supported prosthesis in edentulous patients (Kimoto et al. 2011, Luraschi et al. 2013, Yan et al. 2008).

These neuroplastic changes may be structural or functional, may have a fast or short onset, and may be short lived or long lasting (Citri & Malenka 2008). Fast-onset and short-term changes result from changes in synaptic efficacy or unmasking of existing synaptic connections (see Avivi-Arber et al. 2011). In the vast majority of cases, these neuroplastic changes result in positive adaptation. An example is the almost instantaneous modification of jaw movements to meet a new occlusion and/or a new jaw position that represents a fast-onset motor change. However, in some cases, these neuroplastic changes may lead to a maladaptive behavior, as likely happened in the presented case: disturbing the sensory input, probably together with negative thoughts, altered the motor output to drive jaw closure in a position that the patient felt as being less uncomfortable. This occurred even though the inserted crown actually did not alter the habitual occlusion.

Movement disorders, as in cases of dystonia, are another example of sensorimotor maladaptation. Indeed, increasing evidence suggests that these disorders are caused not only by a dysfunction of the basal ganglia-motor cortex circuits but also by abnormalities in the somatosensory inputs and/or their central processing that interfere with the implementation of motor programs and are thus involved in the pathophysiology of these disorders (Abbruzzese & Berardelli 2003, Patel et al. 2014, Tinazzi et al. 2003).

REFERENCES

Abbruzzese G, Berardelli A: Sensorimotor integration in movement disorders, *Mov Disord* 18:231–240, 2003.

Albanese MC, Duerden EG, Bohotin V, et al: Differential effects of cognitive demand on human cortical activation associated with vibrotactile stimulation, *J Neurophysiol* 102:1623–1631, 2009.

Avivi-Arber L, Martin R, Lee JC, et al: Face sensorimotor cortex and its neuroplasticity related to orofacial sensorimotor functions, *Arch Oral Biol* 56:1440–1465, 2011.

Baba K, Aridome K, Haketa T, et al: Sensory perceptive and discriminative abilities of patients with occlusal dysesthesia, *Nihon Hotetsu Shika Gakkai Zasshi* 49:599–607, 2005.

Bauer CC, Diaz JL, Concha L, et al: Sustained attention to spontaneous thumb sensations activates brain somatosensory and other proprioceptive areas, *Brain Cogn* 87:86–96, 2014.

Benedetti F, Amanzio M: The placebo response: how words and rituals change the patient's brain, *Patient Educ Couns* 84:413–419, 2011.

Chapman CE, Beauchamp E: Differential controls over tactile detection in humans by motor commands and peripheral reafference, *J Neurophysiol* 96:1664–1675, 2006.

Chen CY, Palla S, Erni S, et al: Nonfunctional tooth contact in healthy controls and patients with myogenous facial pain, *J Orofac Pain* 21:185–193, 2007.

Cioffi I, Farella M, Festa P, et al: Short-term sensorimotor effects of experimental occlusal interferences on the wake-time masseter muscle activity of females with masticatory muscle pain, *J Oral Facial Pain Headache* (in press).

Citri A, Malenka RC: Synaptic plasticity: multiple forms, functions, and mechanisms, *Neuropsychopharmacology* 33:18–41, 2008.

Croskerry P: The importance of cognitive errors in diagnosis and strategies to minimize them, *Acad Med* 78:775–780, 2003.

Fiorio M, Recchia S, Corra F, et al: Enhancing non-noxious perception: behavioural and neurophysiological correlates of a placebo-like manipulation, *Neuroscience* 217:96–104, 2012.

Fujisawa M, Kanemura K, Tanabe N, et al: Determination of daytime clenching events in subjects with and without self-reported clenching, *J Oral Rehabil* 40:731–736, 2013.

Funato M, Ono Y, Baba K, et al: Evaluation of the non-functional tooth contact in patients with temporomandibular disorders by using newly developed electronic system, *J Oral Rehabil* 41:170–176, 2014.

Gazzaley A, Nobre AC: Top-down modulation: bridging selective attention and working memory, *Trends Cogn Sci* 16:129–135, 2012.

Glaros AG, Williams K, Lausten L: The role of parafunctions, emotions and stress in predicting facial pain, *J Am Dent Assoc* 136:451–458, 2005a.

Glaros AG, Williams K, Lausten L, et al: Tooth contact in patients with temporomandibular disorders, *Cranio* 23:188–193, 2005b.

Hara ES, Matsuka Y, Minakuchi H, et al: Occlusal dysesthesia: a qualitative systematic review of the epidemiology, aetiology and management, *J Oral Rehabil* 39:630–638, 2012.

Heijmans M, Olde Hartman TC, van Weel-Baumgarten E, et al: Experts' opinions on the management of medically unexplained symptoms in primary care. A qualitative analysis of narrative reviews and scientific editorials, *Fam Pract* 28:444–455, 2011.

Heinrich TW: Medically unexplained symptoms and the concept of somatization, *WMJ* 103:83–87, 2004.

Herren P: *Okklusale Taktilität beim bewussten Zusammenbeissen und beim Kauen (Occlusal Tactility During Conscious Biting and During Chewing)*, Thesis. Zurich, 1988, University of Zurich.

Hodzic A, Veit R, Karim AA, et al: Improvement and decline in tactile discrimination behavior after cortical plasticity induced by passive tactile coactivation, *J Neurosci* 24:442–446, 2004.

Hoffken O, Veit M, Knossalla F, et al: Sustained increase of somatosensory cortex excitability by tactile coactivation studied by paired median nerve stimulation in humans correlates with perceptual gain, *J Physiol* 584:463–471, 2007.

Huang GJ, LeResche L, Critchlow CW, et al: Risk factors for diagnostic subgroups of painful temporomandibular disorders (TMD), *J Dent Res* 81:284–288, 2002.

Johansen-Berg H, Lloyd DM: The physiology and psychology of selective attention to touch, *Front Biosci* 5:D894–D904, 2000.

Karlsson S, Cho SA, Carlsson GE: Changes in mandibular masticatory movements after insertion of nonworking-side interference, *J Craniomandib Disord* 6:177–183, 1992.

Katzer A, Oberfeld D, Hiller W, et al: Tactile perceptual processes and their relationship to somatoform disorders, *J Abnorm Psychol* 121:530–543, 2012.

Kimoto K, Ono Y, Tachibana A, et al: Chewing-induced regional brain activity in edentulous patients who received mandibular implant-supported overdentures: a preliminary report, *J Prosthodont Res* 55:89–97, 2011.

Kino K, Sugisaki M, Haketa T, et al: The comparison between pains, difficulties in function, and associating factors of patients in subtypes of temporomandibular disorders, *J Oral Rehabil* 32:315–325, 2005.

Kowalewski R, Kattenstroth JC, Kalisch T, et al: Improved acuity and dexterity but unchanged touch and pain thresholds following repetitive sensory stimulation of the fingers, *Neural Plast* 2012:974504, 2012.

Le Bell Y, Jämsä T, Korri S, et al: Effect of artificial occlusal interferences depends on previous experience of temporomandibular disorders, *Acta Odontol Scand* 60:219–222, 2002.

Le Bell Y, Niemi PM, Jämsä T, et al: Subjective reactions to intervention with artificial interferences in subjects with and without a history of temporomandibular disorders, *Acta Odontol Scand* 64:59–63, 2006.

Luraschi J, Korgaonkar MS, Whittle T, et al: Neuroplasticity in the adaptation to prosthodontic treatment, *J Orofac Pain* 27:206–216, 2013.

Magnusson T: Signs and symptoms of mandibular dysfunction in complete denture wearers five years after receiving new dentures, *J Craniomandib Pract* 3:267–272, 1985.

Markiewicz MR, Ohrbach R, McCall WD Jr: Oral behaviors checklist: reliability of performance in targeted waking-state behaviors, *J Orofac Pain* 20:306–316, 2006.

Michelotti A, Cioffi I, Landino D, et al: Effects of experimental occlusal interferences in individuals reporting different levels of wake-time parafunctions, *J Orofac Pain* 26:168–175, 2012.

Michelotti A, Farella M, Gallo LM, et al: Effect of occlusal interferences on habitual activity of human masseter, *J Dent Res* 84:644–648, 2005.

Michelotti A, Farella M, Steenks MH, et al: No effect of experimental occlusal interferences on pressure pain thresholds of the masseter and temporalis muscles in healthy women, *Eur J Oral Sci* 114:167–170, 2006.

Morimoto Y, Oki K, Iida S, et al: Effect of transient occlusal loading on the threshold of tooth tactile sensation perception for tapping like the impulsive stimulation, *Odontology* 101:199–203, 2013.

Nendaz M, Perrier A: Diagnostic errors and flaws in clinical reasoning: mechanisms and prevention in practice, *Swiss Med Wkly* 142:w13706, 2012.

Palla S: Cognitive diagnostic errors, *J Orofac Pain* 27:289–290, 2013.

Pantev C, Engelien A, Candia V, et al: Representational cortex in musicians. Plastic alterations in response to musical practice, *Ann N Y Acad Sci* 930:300–314, 2001.

Patel N, Jankovic J, Hallett M: Sensory aspects of movement disorders, *Lancet Neurol* 13:100–112, 2014.

Pleger B, Dinse HR, Ragert P, et al: Shifts in cortical representations predict human discrimination improvement, *Proc Natl Acad Sci U S A* 98: 12255–12260, 2001.

Ragert P, Franzkowiak S, Schwenkreis P, et al: Improvement of tactile perception and enhancement of cortical excitability through intermittent theta burst rTMS over human primary somatosensory cortex, *Exp Brain Res* 184:1–11, 2008.

Randow K, Carlsson K, Edlund J, et al: The effect of an occlusal interference on the masticatory system. An experimental investigation, *Odontol Revy* 27:245–256, 1976.

Richardson RD, Engel CC Jr: Evaluation and management of medically unexplained physical symptoms, *Neurologist* 10:18–30, 2004.

Rief W, Barsky AJ: Psychobiological perspectives on somatoform disorders, *Psychoneuroendocrinology* 30:996–1002, 2005.

Rief W, Broadbent E: Explaining medically unexplained symptoms—models and mechanisms, *Clin Psychol Rev* 27:821–841, 2007.

Riise C, Sheikholeslam A: The influence of experimental interfering occlusal contacts on the postural activity of the anterior temporal and masseter muscles in young adults, *J Oral Rehabil* 9:419–425, 1982.

Rugh JD, Barghi N, Drago CJ: Experimental occlusal discrepancies and nocturnal bruxism, *J Prosthet Dent* 51:548–553, 1984

Sato F, Kino K, Sugisaki M, et al: Teeth contacting habit as a contributing factor to chronic pain in patients with temporomandibular disorders, *J Med Dent Sci* 53:103–109, 2006.

Schlieper S, Dinse HR: Perceptual improvement following repetitive sensory stimulation depends monotonically on stimulation intensity, *Brain Stimul* 5:647–651, 2012.

Seki K, Perlmutter SI, Fetz EE: Sensory input to primate spinal cord is presynaptically inhibited during voluntary movement, *Nat Neurosci* 6:1309–1316, 2003.

Sessle BJ: Face sensorimotor cortex: its role and neuroplasticity in the control of orofacial movements, *Prog Brain Res* 188:71–82, 2011.

Sessle BJ, Adachi K, Avivi-Arber L, et al: Neuroplasticity of face primary motor cortex control of orofacial movements, *Arch Oral Biol* 52:334–337, 2007.

Sessle BJ, Yao D, Nishiura H, et al: Properties and plasticity of the primate somatosensory and motor cortex related to orofacial sensorimotor function, *Clin Exp Pharmacol Physiol* 32:109–114, 2005.

Shiau YY, Syu JZ: Effect of working side interferences on mandibular movement in bruxers and non-bruxers, *J Oral Rehabil* 22:145–151, 1995.

Stiegler MP, Neelankavil JP, Canales C, et al: Cognitive errors detected in anaesthesiology: a literature review and pilot study, *Br J Anaesth* 108:229–235, 2012.

Tegenthoff M, Ragert P, Pleger B, et al: Improvement of tactile discrimination performance and enlargement of cortical somatosensory maps after 5 Hz rTMS, *PLoS Biol* 3:e362, 2005.

Tinazzi M, Rosso T, Fiaschi A: Role of the somatosensory system in primary dystonia, *Mov Disord* 18:605–622, 2003.

Yan C, Ye L, Zhen J, et al: Neuroplasticity of edentulous patients with implant-supported full dentures, *Eur J Oral Sci* 116:387–393, 2008.

Yashiro K, Fukuda T, Takada K: Masticatory jaw movement optimization after introduction of occlusal interference, *J Oral Rehabil* 37:163–170, 2010.

Jaw Movement and Its Control

Greg M. Murray

SYNOPSIS

The jaw muscles move the jaw in a complex three-dimensional manner during jaw movements. There are three jaw-closing muscles (masseter, temporalis, and medial pterygoid) and two jaw-opening muscles (lateral pterygoid and digastric). The basic functional unit of muscle is the motor unit. The internal architecture of the jaw muscles is complex, with many exhibiting a complex pennate (feather-like) internal architecture. Within each of the jaw muscles, the central nervous system (CNS) appears capable of activating separate compartments with specific directions of muscle fibers. This means that each jaw muscle is capable of generating a range of force vectors (magnitude and direction) required for a particular jaw movement. In the generation of any desired movement, the CNS activates motor units in different muscles. Movements are classified into voluntary, reflex, and rhythmical. Many parts of the CNS participate in the generation of jaw movements. The face motor cortex is the final output pathway from the cerebral cortex for the generation of voluntary movements, such as opening, closing, protrusive, and lateral jaw movements. Reflexes demonstrate pathways that aid in the refinement of a movement and can be used by the higher motor centers for the generation of more complex movements. Mastication or chewing is a rhythmical movement that is controlled by a central pattern generator in the brainstem. The central pattern generator can be modified by sensory information from the food bolus and by voluntary commands from higher centers.

At any instant in time during jaw movements, the jaw can be described as rotating around an instantaneous center of rotation. Many devices have been constructed to describe jaw movements, but only six-degrees-of-freedom devices can accurately describe the complexity of movement. Devices for tracking jaw movement have no place in the diagnosis and management of patients, as they lack the required sensitivity and specificity. Masticatory movements are complex, consisting of jaw, face, and tongue movements that are driven by jaw, face, and tongue muscles. Changes to the occlusion appear capable of having significant effects on the activity of the jaw muscles and the movement of the jaw joint.

CHAPTER POINTS

- The jaw muscles move the jaw in a complex three-dimensional manner.
- There are three main jaw-closing muscles (masseter, temporalis, and medial pterygoid) and two main jaw-opening muscles (lateral pterygoid and digastric).
- The functional unit of a muscle is the motor unit.
- The internal architecture of the jaw muscles is highly complex.
- Jaw muscles generate a range of force vectors (magnitude and direction) required for a particular jaw movement.
- In generating a desired movement, the central nervous system (CNS) selects motor units to be activated in different muscles.
- Jaw movements are classified into voluntary, reflex, and rhythmical jaw movements.
- Many parts of the CNS participate in the generation of jaw movements.
- Reflexes demonstrate a pathway that can be used by the higher motor centers for the refinement and generation of more complex movements.
- Mastication is controlled by a central pattern generator in the brainstem.
- At any instant in time, the jaw can be described as rotating around an instantaneous center of rotation.
- The use of devices that provide single point tracings (e.g., pantographs) may provide misleading information if used for diagnostic purposes or in the evaluation of treatment outcomes.
- Changes to the occlusion appear capable of having significant effects on the

activity of the jaw muscles and the movement of the jaw joint.

JAW MUSCLES: THE MOTORS FOR JAW MOVEMENT

An understanding of jaw movement provides background for Chapter 8 on jaw muscle disorders, which describes changes in jaw movement patterns (for review, see Hannam & McMillan 1994, van Eijden & Turkawski 2001).

There are three jaw-closing muscles (masseter, temporalis, and medial pterygoid) and two jaw-opening muscles (digastric and lateral pterygoid).

The contractile element of a muscle is the motor unit. Each motor unit consists of an alpha-motoneuron and all of the muscle fibers (approximately 600 to 1000) innervated by (i.e., connected to and activated by) that motoneuron. Jaw muscle motoneurons are mostly located in the trigeminal motor nucleus in the brainstem.

Three physiological types of motor units contribute to variations in the magnitude of force that different motor units can generate. Type S motor units are slow. They generate low forces and are fatigue resistant. Type FF motor units are fast. They generate the highest forces but fatigue rapidly. Type FR motor units have intermediate speed, force generating capabilities, and fatigue resistance. Type S motor units are recruited first in a muscle contraction. With larger forces, type FR and then type FF motor units are recruited.

Further complexity exists because each face, jaw, or tongue muscle has a complex internal architecture in terms of the arrangement of the muscle fibers within each muscle. Muscle fibers within the masseter and medial pterygoid muscles, for example, are not long fibers running from origin to insertion, but rather, each of these muscles contains groups of short muscle fibers arranged in a pennate manner (i.e., a feather-like arrangement). Figure 5-1 illustrates this pennate arrangement for the medial pterygoid muscle. The figure shows groups of short muscle fibers (shaded red lines in the insert on the left of the figure and shaded red regions on right) being enclosed by aponeurotic sheaths (thick gray lines in figure). The inset on the left of the figure shows an expanded view of

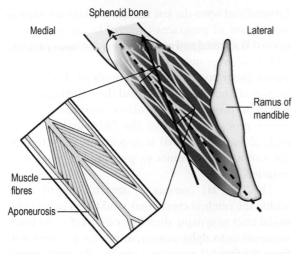

FIG 5-1 Coronal View Through the Medial Ptery-goid Muscle, Base of Skull (sphenoid bone), and Ramus of Mandible Some of the aponeuroses that divide the medial pterygoid have been outlined and are shown in expanded form as thick gray lines in the inset on the left. The feather-like (pennate) arrangement of the muscle fibers is indicated by these gray lines. The solid arrow demonstrates the direction of pull if the muscle fibers on the left side of the inset were to selectively contract. The dashed arrow indicates the direction of pull if the muscle fibers hypothetically passed directly from the base of the skull to the mandible.

part of the muscle, and it illustrates the pennate arrangement of muscle fibers. When motor units on one side of an aponeurosis contract, they direct forces at an angle (the pennation angle) to the long axis of the muscle and generate a force vector (i.e., magnitude and direction of force) at an angle to the force vector that would be generated if muscle fibers passed directly from the base of the skull to the ramus without pennation (dashed arrow). The black solid arrow in Figure 5-1 shows the direction of force generated if only the muscle fibers on the left side of the inset were activated. The masseter muscle also has a similar complex internal architecture. These complexities of muscle-fiber architecture within the jaw muscles provide a wide range of directions with which forces can be applied to the jaw. The brain

can selectively activate these regions, or subcompartments, independently of other regions of the muscle.

When generating a particular movement of the jaw, the sensorimotor cortical regions that drive voluntary movements (see the following discussion) are not organized in terms of specific muscles to activate. Rather, they send command signals to the various motor nuclei to activate those motor units, in whatever muscles are available, that are biomechanically best suited to generate the force vector required for that particular jaw movement. Thus, for example, a grinding movement of the jaw to the right side with the teeth together might be best achieved by activation of some motor units in the inferior head of the left lateral pterygoid, some motor units in the right posterior temporalis to prevent the right side of the jaw moving forward, and some units in the right masseter and anterior temporalis to help pull the jaw to the right side and to keep the teeth together while doing so (Miller 1991). The activation of these motor units will produce a force on the jaw that moves the jaw to the right side.

CENTRAL NERVOUS SYSTEM COMPONENTS IN THE GENERATION AND CONTROL OF JAW MOVEMENTS (FIG. 5-2)

- Motor cortex and descending pathways through pyramidal tract to alpha-motoneurons (drives motor units)
- Cerebellum (refinement and coordination of the movement)
- Basal ganglia (selects and initiates motor programs)
- Supplementary motor area (SMA), premotor cortex (area 6) (contains programs for movements)
- Central pattern generators for mastication and swallowing (programs for generating mastication and swallowing)
- Alpha-motoneurons within brainstem motor nuclei
- Motor units within muscles
- Somatosensory system that conveys and processes somatosensory information about the movement

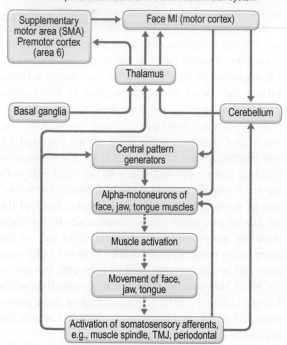

Some important connections of the orofacial motor system

FIG 5-2 Some Important Connections of the Orofacial Motor System Arrows indicate some of the complex linkages in the sequence leading to a motor event. Solid arrows indicate direction of action potentials conveying information. Dotted arrows indicate the result of activation of motoneurons. See Figure 1-2 for a more detailed outline of connections of the orofacial sensorimotor system.

CLASSIFICATION OF JAW MOVEMENTS

- Voluntary movements: for example, playing the piano, speaking, taking an alginate impression, moving the jaw forward
- Reflex movements: for example, knee-jerk reflex, jaw-jerk reflex, and jaw-opening reflex
- Rhythmical movements: for example, chewing, walking, running, and breathing

Voluntary Movements

Voluntary movements are driven by the primary motor cortex (termed MI) and higher motor cortical areas (SMA and premotor cortex; for review, see Hannam & Sessle 1994). The face MI is responsible for driving voluntary movements of the face, jaw, and tongue. When patients are asked to move the tongue

forward and open the jaw (as when taking an impression), a set of programs (much like computer programs) is selected and activated (via the basal ganglia), and these programs send signals to the face MI. The motor programs contain the details of those motor units that must be activated and the sequence of activation, to produce a particular movement. The programs probably reside in the SMA and premotor cortical regions. The MI is responsible for activating the various motor units to produce the movement required.

The face MI consists of specific output zones within the cerebral cortex that send fibers in the pyramidal tract to synapse directly or indirectly (via interneurons) onto alpha-motoneurons. Each output zone from the face MI activates a specific elemental movement: for example, movement of the tongue forward or movement of the tongue to the side, or elevation of the corner of the mouth, or jaw opening or jaw movement to the side. The same movement can be produced at a number of different sites throughout the face MI.

The face MI can be considered the "keys of a piano" that the higher motor centers "play" to allow the generation of the required voluntary movement. Combinations of output zones allow the generation of more complex movements (equivalent to the generation of more complex sounds, as when playing chords on a piano).

The cerebellum continuously coordinates movements by controlling the sensory inputs to the motor areas. Corrections to each movement can also occur via shorter pathways that involve fewer neurons, and many of these pathways are located entirely at the brainstem level. These pathways can be demonstrated clinically by evoking reflexes.

Reflex Movements

Reflex movements are largely organized at the brainstem or spinal cord level (for review, see Hannam & Sessle 1994). They are stereotyped movements that are involuntary and are little modified by voluntary will.

The classic reflex is the knee-jerk reflex, where a sharp tap to the knee evokes contraction in the thigh muscles and a brief lifting of the lower leg. In the jaw motor system, reflexes include the jaw-closing or jaw-jerk reflex, and the jaw-opening reflex.

The jaw-closing reflex occurs when the jaw-closing muscles are suddenly stretched by a rapid downward tap on the chin. This tap causes stretching of specialized sensory receptors called muscle spindles that are stretch sensitive. They are present within all the jaw-closing muscles. When spindles are stretched, a burst of action potentials travels along the group Ia primary afferent nerve fibers coming from the primary endings within the spindles. The primary afferents synapse directly onto and cause activation of the alpha-motoneurons of the same jaw-closing muscle. Thus a stretch of a jaw-closing muscle leads to a fast contraction of the same jaw-closing muscle. This reflex assists in preventing the jaw from flopping up and down during running.

Reflexes demonstrate a pathway that can be used by the higher motor centers for the generation of more complex movements. They also allow fast feedback that adjusts a movement to overcome small, unpredicted irregularities in the ongoing movement and adds smoothness to a movement. Thus, for example, unexpected changes in food bolus consistency during chewing can modulate muscle spindle afferent discharge, and this altered discharge can change alpha-motoneuron activity to help overcome the change in food bolus consistency.

The jaw-opening reflex can be evoked by a variety of types of orofacial afferents. Activity in orofacial afferents, for example, from mucosal mechanoreceptors, passes along primary afferent nerve fibers to contact inhibitory interneurons that then synapse on jaw-closing alpha-motoneurons. The inhibitory interneurons reduce the activity of the jaw-closing motoneurons. At the same time, primary afferents activate other interneurons that are excitatory to jaw-opening muscles, such as the digastric. The overall effect is an opening of the jaw.

Rhythmical Movements

These movements share features of both voluntary and reflex movements (for review, see Lund 1991, Hannam & Sessle 1994). The reflex features of rhythmical movements arise because we do not have to think about these movements for them to occur. For example, we can chew, breathe, swallow, and walk without thinking specifically about the task; however, at any time, we can voluntarily alter the rate and magnitude of these movements.

Rhythmical movements are generated and controlled by collections of neurons in the brainstem or spinal cord. Each collection is called a central pattern generator. The central pattern generator for mastication is located in the pontine-medullary reticular formation. Figure 5-2 shows some relations of the central pattern generators in the brainstem. Swallowing is also controlled by a central pattern generator located in the medulla oblongata.

A central pattern generator is essentially equivalent to a computer program. When activated, the central pattern generator for mastication, for example, sends out appropriately timed impulses of the appropriate magnitude to the various jaw, face, and tongue muscle motoneurons so that the rhythmical movement of mastication can occur. We do not have to think about which motor units in which muscles to activate and the relative timing of activation of the motor units to carry out mastication. This is done by the central pattern generator. We can, however, voluntarily start, stop, and change the rate, magnitude, and shape of the chewing movements, and these modifications are done through descending commands to the central pattern generators from the motor cortical regions.

Figure 5-3, *A*, shows electromyographic (EMG) data from a number of jaw muscles during the right-sided chewing of gum. The associated movement of the midincisor point is shown in the lower panel. Note the regular bursting pattern of EMG activity that occurs in association with each cycle of movement. Note also, in the expanded version in Figure 5-3, *B*, that the EMG activity from the inferior head of the lateral pterygoid muscle and the submandibular group of muscles is out of phase with the jaw-closing muscles. All muscles are controlled by the central pattern generator, and many other jaw, face, and tongue muscles, not recorded here, are being activated similarly.

Sensory feedback is provided by mechanoreceptors located within orofacial tissues: for example, periodontal mechanoreceptors signal the magnitude and direction of tooth contact; mucosal mechanoreceptors signal food contact with mucosa; muscle spindles signal muscle length and rate of change of muscle length as the jaw closes; Golgi tendon organs signal forces generated within muscles; and temporomandibular (TM) joint mechanoreceptors signal jaw position.

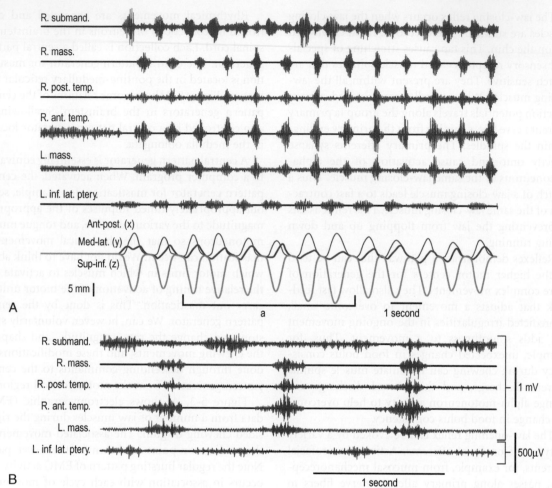

FIG 5-3 Right-Sided Gum Chewing A, EMG data from six jaw muscles (top-six traces) and jaw movement data (bottom-three traces) during 13 cycles of chewing of gum. The EMG activity was recorded from the submandibular group of muscles (*R. submand.*; principally the anterior belly of the digastric muscle), the right and left masseter (*R. mass.*, *L. mass.*), the right posterior temporalis (*R. post. temp.*), the right anterior temporalis (*R. ant. temp.*), and the left inferior head of the lateral pterygoid (*L. inf. lat. ptery.*) muscles. The movement traces display the movement of the midincisor point of the mandible in anteroposterior (*Ant-post.*), mediolateral (*Med-lat.*), and superoinferior (*Sup-inf.*) axes. Thus, for example, the latter shows the amount of vertical displacement of the midincisor point during the opening phase of each chewing cycle. **B,** Expanded form of the EMG data only from the section labeled "a" in **A**.

The muscle spindle is a very complicated sensory receptor. Muscle spindle sensitivity is optimized for all lengths of a muscle. During a muscle contraction, both alpha- and gamma-motoneurons are activated. The alpha-motoneurons cause contraction of the main (extrafusal) muscle fibers and are responsible for the force produced by muscles (Fig. 5-4). The gamma-motoneurons are activated at the same time,

but they cause contraction of the intrafusal muscle fibers within the muscle spindle and thus maintain the sensitivity of the spindles as the muscle and spindles shorten (Fig. 5-4, *C*). The spindle is therefore always able to detect small changes in muscle length, irrespective of the length of the muscle.

Sensory information plays a crucial role in adjusting the chewing cycle to accommodate for changes in

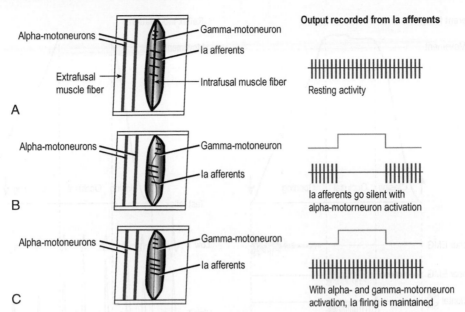

FIG 5-4 Stylized Muscle Showing Extrafusal Muscle Fibers (Thick Red Lines) and Intrafusal Muscle Fibers Within the Muscle Spindle under Three Conditions **A,** The resting condition, where, in this hypothetical muscle, there is a resting tension on the muscle that comes from, for example, the weight of the mandible at postural jaw position. The slight stretch to the muscle from the weight of the mandible results in a slight stretching of the intrafusal muscle fibers and group Ia afferent terminals that results in a continuous barrage of action potentials passing centrally. **B,** In the hypothetical situation where only alpha-motoneurons are firing, muscle fibers contract, and this results in a reduced tension in the muscle spindle and therefore the spindle Ia afferent firing ceases for the duration of the contraction. During this period, the spindle is unable to provide information about unexpected changes in muscle length. **C,** Shows alpha-motoneuron activation accompanied by gamma-motoneuron activation (alpha-gamma coactivation—the usual situation in any voluntary movement) so that the intrafusal muscle fibers contract at the same rate as the extrafusal muscle fibers. This maintains the tension at the terminals of the Ia afferents so that they maintain their firing and are able to respond to, and signal irregularities in, the movement.

food bolus consistency (for review, see Lund & Olsson 1983). Chewing is associated with a barrage of sensory information entering the CNS (Fig. 5-5, *A*). Some of this information travels directly to the cerebral cortex for conscious sensation. Local reflex effects that assist the masticatory process also occur. For example, as food is crushed between the teeth, periodontal mechanoreceptors are activated, and this activity can cause a reflex increase in activity in the jaw-closing muscles to assist in crushing of food.

Many of the orofacial afferents that are activated by food contact during jaw closing can evoke a jaw-opening reflex, as discussed earlier. This would be counterproductive during the closing phase of mastication. Lund & Olsson (1983) have shown that the masticatory central pattern generator depresses the

responsiveness of the jaw-opening reflex during the closing phase of the chewing cycle. The low T (i.e., threshold) test reflex response shown in Figure 5-5, *B*, on the far left is the control jaw-opening reflex response, seen in the digastric muscle, to the activation of orofacial afferents when there is no chewing. During the closing phase of the chewing cycle, the central pattern generator depresses the ability to evoke this reflex. Therefore, in chewing, the excitatory pathway from orofacial afferents to jaw-opening motoneurons is depressed, and this allows the jaw to close unhindered.

An analogous effect occurs during the opening phase of the chewing cycle. During this phase, muscle spindles in jaw-closing muscles will be stretched and will have a tonic excitatory effect on jaw-closing

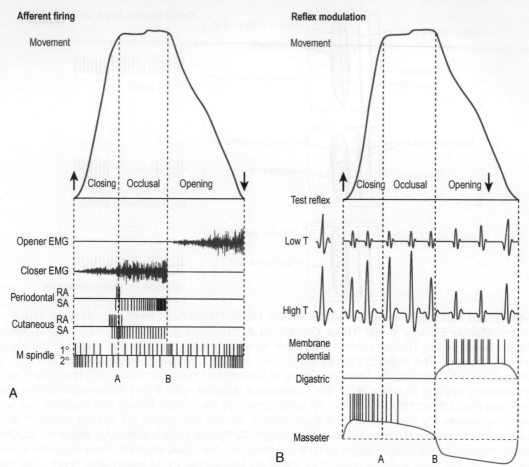

FIG 5-5 A, Some of the patterns of jaw muscle and somatosensory afferent activity during masticatory jaw movements. The movement of the jaw at the midincisor point is at the top. The next two traces show jaw-opener and jaw-closer EMG activity, respectively. Periodontal and cutaneous mechanoreceptive activity is shown next. RA, rapidly adapting, that is, responds only to the dynamic phases of, in this case, a mechanical stimulus; SA, slowly adapting, that is, responds to dynamic and static components of a mechanical stimulus. M spindle 1°, 2°, refers to output from muscle spindle group Ia (provides information on dynamic changes in muscle length), and group II (provides information on new muscle lengths) primary afferents, respectively. Each vertical line in each trace shows the time of occurrence of an action potential that has been recorded in the primary afferent axon. There is a barrage of sensory information that enters the brain during every chewing cycle. **B,** The jaw-opening reflex is modulated during mastication. The left shows the type of reflex response that is recorded from the digastric muscle with the jaw at rest (control). Note that the amplitude of this reflex changes during mastication. When low-threshold afferents are stimulated (*low T,* i.e., nonpainful), the mean amplitude is less, especially during the closing and occlusal phases. In contrast, the response to high-threshold afferents (*high T*) exceeds the control during the late closing and occlusal phases. This pathway is facilitated during the closing phase of the chewing cycle: it is desirable to stop the closing phase of chewing should painful stimuli be encountered during this phase. The lower two traces show that the digastric membrane is at its resting level during these phases, and masseteric motoneurons are hyperpolarized during the opening phase to reduce the possibility of these motoneurons firing, particularly under the influence of group Ia and II muscle spindle afferent barrage arising because muscle spindles are being stretched during the opening phase. (Adapted with permission from Lund & Olsson 1983.)

motor units. This would resist jaw opening. However, the central pattern generator hyperpolarizes (i.e., inhibits) jaw-closing motoneurons during the opening phase of the chewing cycle (Fig. 5-5, B). This hyperpolarization makes jaw-closing motoneurons harder to activate in response to excitatory input from muscle spindles.

BASIC MANDIBULAR MOVEMENTS

The jaw can be viewed as being suspended from the skull by muscles, tendons, ligaments, vessels, and nerves. It is moved in three-dimensional space, with the fixed points being the teeth and the condyles in their respective condylar fossae.

Basic mandibular movements are jaw opening and closing, right-side jaw movement, left-side jaw movement, jaw protrusion, and retrusion. There are a number of anatomical factors playing a role in mandibular movements:

- Condylar guidance—the inclination of the pathway traveled by the condyle during a protrusive or a contralateral jaw movement; the two inclinations in protrusion or contralateral movement will usually be slightly different
- Incisal guidance—the inclination of the pathway traveled by the lower anterior teeth along the palatal surfaces of the upper anterior teeth in a horizontal excursive jaw movement, determined by the magnitude of overbite (vertical overlap) and overjet (horizontal overlap) between the anterior teeth
- Posterior guidance—determined by posterior tooth relationships
- Muscles, vessels, nerves, and ligaments

Movements to and from intercuspal position. Of interest to clinicians are as noted in the following:

- Group function—defined as an occlusion in lateral excursion in which the occlusal load is distributed across at least two pairs of teeth on the working side
- Mutually protected (approximately 10% of natural dentitions; or canine-guided) occlusion—only the anterior (or canine) teeth are in contact in any excursive movement of the jaw

Mastication is not a simple open-close jaw movement because the condyles are able to translate forward, as well as rotate. There are constantly changing combinations of rotation and translation during mastication.

Instantaneous Center of Rotation of the Jaw

At any instant in time, the jaw can be described as rotating around a center of rotation. This center of rotation is constantly shifting because of constantly changing combinations of translation and rotation during most jaw movements.

- A protrusive jaw movement with sliding tooth contact consists largely of translation of the jaw forward, with a slight downward translation. With a steeper incisal than condylar guidance, the jaw will also rotate open slightly. The instantaneous centers of rotation will lie well below and posterior to the jaw.
- For a left-side jaw movement with sliding tooth contact, most of the movement is rotation about a constantly moving center of rotation lying near (usually behind and lateral to) the left condyle. Figure 5-6, A, shows sagittal (upper plots) and horizontal (lower plots) plane views of left condylar movement in a subject performing a working-side mandibular movement (i.e., the jaw moves to the left side). The condyle is represented by a triangle (upper plots in A) for the sagittal view and a quadrilateral (lower plots in A) for the horizontal view. The quadrilaterals are formed by joining the points a, b, c, and d on the actual outline of the condyle in the horizontal plane shown in Fig. 5-6, D. The triangles are formed by joining the points a, e, and c on the condyle; point e is a point 9 mm superior to the other points. A triangle or quadrilateral is plotted each 300 ms from intercuspal position (IP). During this working-side movement in the horizontal plane, the condyle does not rotate about the center of the condyle but rather the center of rotation can be visualized to be behind the condyle.
- At each successive instant in time during chewing, the center of rotation shifts in space. For chewing jaw movements, this center lies between the lower posterior parts of the jaw, toward the midline.

HOW TO DESCRIBE JAW MOVEMENT

For over a century, dentists have had a keen interest in the movement of the jaw and have attempted to describe its movement by graphical devices, such as pantographs, and jaw-tracking devices that are more sophisticated. This interest stems from the need to

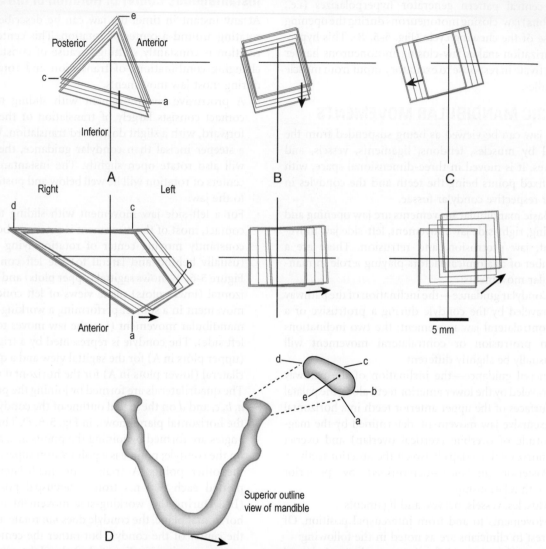

FIG 5-6 Detail of Working-Side Movement of the Left Condyle Sagittal (upper plots) and horizontal (lower plots) plane views of condylar triangles (upper plots in **A**) and quadrilaterals (lower plots in **A**) for the left condyle in a subject performing an ipsilateral working-side mandibular movement, that is, the jaw moves to the left side. A superior view of mandible is shown in **D**, and the condylar points are labeled: a, anterior; b, lateral; c, posterior; d, medial; e, superior (this point was 9.0 mm superior to the other points). The points were determined from computer tomography scans of the subject. **B** shows sagittal (upper) and horizontal (lower) squares generated about the origin of the respective axes in **A**. **C** shows sagittal and horizontal squares generated about an origin that was shifted 30 mm further laterally. A square, triangle, or quadrilateral is plotted each 300 ms, starting at the intercuspal position. In each trace, the outgoing movement only is shown from intercuspal position to maximum lateral excursion, and the approximate direction of movement is indicated by a short arrow. The trajectories of individual condylar points have been omitted for clarity. (Adapted with permission from Peck et al. 1999.)

reduce clinical time required for restorative work for patients.

These systems usually record the movement of the anterior midline of the lower jaw (e.g., see Fig. 5-3) or the terminal hinge axis or the palpated lateral condylar pole in three degrees of freedom (i.e., the movement of a single point along anteroposterior, mediolateral, and superoinferior axes; Fig. 5-3). They do not provide information about the three rotation vectors: pitch, yaw, and roll. This additional information is provided by six-degrees-of-freedom systems.

Considerable error is introduced to the pathway that condylar-point tracings follow simply because of the selection of a different point near the condyle (Peck et al. 1997, 1999). Thus many of the irregularities in condylar-point tracings that have been ascribed diagnostic or prognostic significance could simply have occurred because of the location of the condylar point chosen. Figure 5-6, *B*, shows the movement of points chosen at equal distances about the coordinate center in Figure 5-6, *A*. The resulting squares move in a similar fashion to the quadrilaterals and triangles in *A*. Figure 5-6, *C*, shows the effect on the movement recorded simply by shifting the points 30 mm laterally. The interpretation of the movement of the condyle plotted in *C* would be that the condyle has translated posteriorly and laterally, whereas in fact the condyle has largely translated laterally with some rotation.

Single point tracings may therefore provide misleading information if used for diagnostic purposes or in the evaluation of treatment outcomes. It is also worth quoting the recent American Association for Dental Research policy statement on temporomandibular disorders (TMDs), "the consensus of recent scientific literature about currently available technological diagnostic devices for TMDs is that, except for various imaging modalities, none of them shows the sensitivity and specificity required to separate normal subjects from TMD patients or to distinguish among TMD subgroups" (Greene 2010).

Border movements of the jaw are described in Chapter 1.

MASTICATORY JAW MOVEMENTS

Masticatory jaw movements occur well within border movements, except when the jaw approaches or makes tooth contact toward the end of chewing (Lund 1991).

In the frontal plane, the masticatory cycle is classically described as occurring in a "tear-drop" shape. At the beginning of opening, the midincisor point moves first downward, and at the end of opening, it moves laterally and upward toward the working side (or chewing side). The midincisor point then moves upward and medially, and the food is crushed between the teeth.

The masticatory sequence is highly variable from cycle to cycle in a subject chewing the same or different foods and from subject to subject. Figure 5-3, *A* (lowermost traces), shows that the movement of the midincisor point from cycle to cycle is not identical. Part of this variability relates to the changing consistency of the food bolus from cycle to cycle, as the food breaks down. The movement of the jaw toward the IP is less variable. The jaw muscles must move the jaw precisely toward the teeth at the end of the chewing cycle, so that the teeth glide smoothly along cuspal inclines. Mechanoreceptors (particularly periodontal) provide a continual source of afferent input to the CNS to ensure that the chewing cycle is harmonious with existing tooth guidance (Chapter 1).

Masticatory movements are complex, consisting of jaw, face, and tongue movements that are driven by jaw, face, and tongue muscles. The facial and tongue muscles are involved because the lips, cheeks, and tongue help control the food bolus in the mouth and keep the food contained over the occlusal table for effective comminution.

It is remarkable that the tongue is largely made of the very substance that the teeth commonly break down. The face motor cortex may play an important role here by strongly inhibiting jaw-closing muscle activity during tongue movements that move the food bolus over the occlusal table. The tongue is most active during the opening phase of the chewing cycle when food is required to be collected and repositioned for effective comminution on the occlusal table.

Different phases of masticatory cycles are the following:

- *Preparatory phase*: Jaw, tongue, lips, and cheeks prepare the bolus for effective food comminution
- *Reduction phase*: Period of food comminution associated with salivary flow and mix of food and saliva

- *Preswallowing*: Food is brought together as a bolus with saliva, which commences the chemical breakdown process, and the bolus is prepared for swallowing

The shape and duration of the cycle is influenced by the hardness of food: harder textured foods are associated with wider chewing cycles that have longer duration. Softer foods are associated with more up and down chewing cycles (Gibbs & Lundeen 1982).

CONDYLE AND DISK MOVEMENT

The movement of the condyle and disk during normal jaw movements is complex and not well understood (Scapino 1997). The lateral pterygoid muscle plays an important role because it inserts into the TM joint, with the inferior head inserting exclusively into the condylar neck, and the superior head inserting largely into the condylar neck.

Some fibers of the superior head do insert into the disk-capsule complex of the TM joint, but the long-held view (still held by some) that the superior head inserts exclusively into the disk is completely erroneous! Further, the view that the superior and inferior heads of the lateral pterygoid muscle exhibit reciprocal patterns of activity is also erroneous. Our research group has shown that the superior head and the inferior head of the lateral pterygoid muscle have very similar functions, and the CNS is able to activate different parts independently of each head of the muscle, to provide the appropriate force vector onto the condyle and disk-capsule complex to produce the movement required.

Changes to the occlusion may have an influence on the movement of the jaw and the TM joint and the function of the jaw muscles. Thus restoring teeth in such a way that results in interferences with the normal pathways of a chewing cycle may lead to different levels of firing of orofacial afferents (e.g., periodontal afferents). This information will feed back to the CNS and may cause a change to the central pattern generator controlling mastication. The information can also change activity in higher levels of the CNS: for example, the face motor cortex. These changes in neural activity will change the activity of particular motor units, in particular subcompartments of muscles, so that the appropriate modification to the chewing cycle can occur to accommodate to the change in the occlusion. The new chewing cycle will now avoid this interference unless the interference is too large and beyond the adaptive capacity of the CNS and muscles.

REFERENCES

Gibbs CH, Lundeen HC: Jaw movements and forces during chewing and swallowing and their clinical significance. In Lundeen HC, Gibbs CH, editors: *Advances in Occlusion*, Boston, 1982, Wright, pp 2–32.

Greene CS: Managing the care of patients with temporomandibular disorders: a new guideline for care, *J Am Dent Assoc* 141:1086–1088, 2010.

Hannam AG, McMillan AS: Internal organization in the human jaw muscles, *Crit Rev Oral Biol Med* 5:55–89, 1994.

Hannam AG, Sessle BJ: Temporomandibular neurosensory and neuromuscular physiology. In Zarb GA, Carlsson GE, Sessle BJ, et al, editors: *Temporomandibular Joint and Masticatory Muscle Disorders*, Copenhagen, 1994, Munksgaard, pp 80–100.

Lund JP: Mastication and its control by the brain stem, *Crit Rev Oral Biol Med* 2:33–64, 1991.

Lund JP, Olsson KA: The importance of reflexes and their control during jaw movement, *Trends Neurosci* 6:458–463, 1983.

Miller AJ: *Craniomandibular Muscles: Their Role in Function and Form*, Boca Raton, 1991, CRC Press.

Peck C, Murray GM, Johnson CWL, et al: The variability of condylar point pathways in open-close jaw movements, *J Prosthet Dent* 77:394–404, 1997.

Peck C, Murray GM, Johnson CWL, et al: Trajectories of condylar points during working-side excursive movements of the mandible, *J Prosthet Dent* 81:444–452, 1999.

Scapino RP: Morphology and mechanism of the jaw joint. In McNeill C, editor: *Science and Practice of Occlusion*, Chicago, 1997, Quintessence, pp 23–40.

van Eijden TMGJ, Turkawski SJJ: Morphology and physiology of masticatory muscle motor units, *Crit Rev Oral Biol Med* 12:76–91, 2001.

CHAPTER 6

Anatomy and Pathophysiology of the Temporomandibular Joint

Sandro Palla

SYNOPSIS

The temporomandibular (TM) joint is a freely movable articulation between the mandibular condyle and the glenoid fossa, with the articular disk interposed. Movements occur by a combination of rotation (between condyle and disk) and translation (between the condyle-disk complex and the fossa). This high degree of mobility, in particular of the translatory movement, is reflected in the way in which the disk is attached to the condyle and in the absence of hyaline cartilage.

Condyle and fossa are covered by fibrocartilage, and the disk consists of a dense collagen fiber network oriented in different directions related to functional load.

Condylar movements are complex; during chewing both condyles are loaded, the working less than the nonworking condyle. The TM joint is able to adapt to load changes by remodeling. Once the adaptive capacity is exceeded, TM joint osteoarthritis (OA) develops. In the past this disease was considered noninflammatory and cartilage-centered. However, there is considerable evidence that inflammation is already involved in the pathogenesis at an early stage, and that OA involves all joint structures. Because of its complex etiology, OA is considered the endpoint of numerous disorders with pathological changes sharing a common final pathway that leads to joint destruction. Central to the osteoarthritic process is the imbalance between anabolic and catabolic processes.

This chapter is an overview of the anatomy, histology, and kinematics of the TM joint as well as of the pathophysiology of the two most common conditions encountered in the dental office, that is, disk displacement and joint OA.

CHAPTER POINTS

- Temporomandibular joint anatomy
- Temporal component
- Mandibular condyle
- Articular disk
- Joint capsule
- Disk attachments
- Disk position
- Joint innervation
- Joint lubrication
- Condylar movements
- Rotation versus translation
- Joint loading
- Joint pathophysiology
- Disk displacement
- Joint osteoarthritis

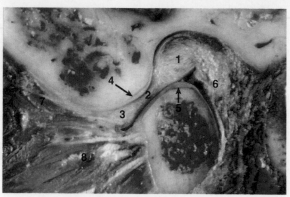

FIG 6-1 Section Through a TM Joint *1*, pars posterior; *2*, pars intermediate; *3*, pars anterior; *4* and *5*, fibrocartilage covering the condyle and fossa; *6*, inferior lamina of the posterior attachment; *7* and *8*, superior and inferior head of the lateral pterygoid muscle. (Courtesy of Dr. Hans Ulrich Luder.)

TEMPOROMANDIBULAR JOINT ANATOMY

The temporomandibular (TM) joint is a freely movable articulation between the mandibular condyle and the glenoid fossa. The condyle articulates against the disk, forming the condyle-disk complex, which articulates with the temporal bone. In comparison with other body articulations, this joint has some unique features. First, functionally the TM joint is a bilateral joint—the right and left joint always function together. Second, movements in the TM joint are characterized by rotation (between condyle and disk) and translation of the condyle-disk assembly. Third, the articular surfaces of condyle and fossa are not covered by hyaline cartilage but by fibrocartilage that is stiffer in tension and softer in compression than hyaline cartilage (Almarza & Athanasiou 2004). Fourth, condylar movements are controlled not only by the shape of the articulating surfaces and the contraction patterns of the muscles but also by the dentition. This determines the end position as well as the movement of the condyle-disk complex when jaw movements are performed under tooth contact, as at the end of chewing or during tooth grinding.

Temporal Component

The temporal component consists of the convex articular tubercle or eminence and the concave glenoid fossa, dorsally limited by the postglenoid tubercle.

This lies immediately anterior to the squamotympanic and petrotympanic fissures (Fig. 6-1).

In the newborn, the glenoid fossa is very shallow (almost flat). The rate of eminence growth does not follow a linear pattern: the eminence develops rapidly during the first years of life and reaches about half its final height by the time the primary dentition is completed. At the age of 5 the growth slows; it stops by the middle to late teens (Nickel et al. 1988, 1997). The early eminence development reflects changes in the direction of joint loading due to condylar growth, transition from suckling to chewing, and variation in the three-dimensional orientation of the musculature caused by growth of the craniofacial complex.

Attempts have been made to correlate the inclination of the posterior slope with occlusal characteristics (e.g., the inclination of the incisal guidance), but no such correlations have been found. However, experimental data support the hypothesis that the steepness of the initial part of the eminence is consistent with the principle of joint-load minimization, thus reducing the risk of cartilage fatigue (Iwasaki et al. 2003, 2010).

The articulating part of the temporal component is covered by a thin layer of fibrocartilage, consisting from the articular surface down to the bone of a fibrous connective tissue zone, a proliferation zone containing undifferentiated mesenchyme cells (not always present), and a cartilage zone. The thickness of this soft tissue varies anteroposteriorly, being thinnest in the roof of the fossa and thickest at the articular eminence (Fig. 6-1—about 0.4 mm at the eminence, 0.2 mm at the slope, and 0.05 mm in the fossa). This reflects the fact that the functionally loaded part of the glenoid fossa is not the roof but the eminence, in particular its posterior slope.

Mandibular Condyle

The condyle normally has an elliptical shape and measures on average 20 mm mediolaterally (range 13 to 25 mm) and 10 mm anteroposteriorly (range 5.5 to 16 mm). The dimension and shape of the condyle present great interindividual variations that may be relevant as far as biomechanical loading. After the age of three, condylar growth occurs mostly in a mediolateral direction, increasing by a factor of 2.5 until adulthood. The growth stops in females in the late teens but may continue into the twenties in males.

The condyles are not aligned in a transverse axis: the condylar long axis (the axes connecting the medial and lateral poles) usually converge in a posterosuperior direction, forming an obtuse angle. The horizontal angle varies between 0° and 30° with a mean of about 15°, whereas the vertical condylar angle varies even more (Fig. 6-2).

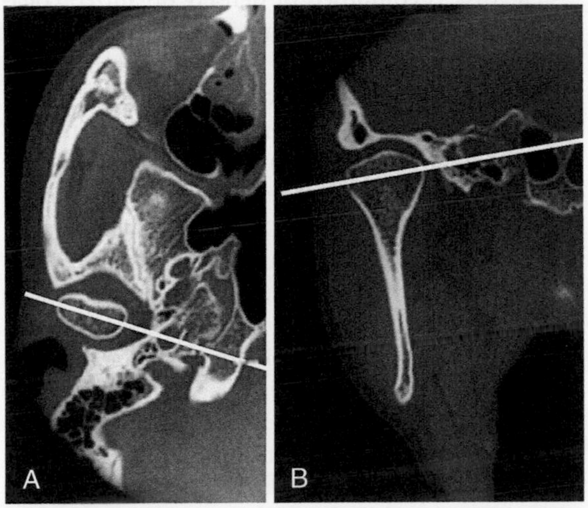

The condyle is covered by a thin layer of fibrocartilage that is thickest superiorly and anteriorly, which are the areas loaded under function and parafunction (Figs. 6-1, 6-3, and 6-4). The condylar cartilage undergoes tissue maturation from the end of condylar growth to adulthood, a process that appears to proceed in two phases. The first phase, between 15 and 30 years of age, is characterized by a progressive cartilaginification of the superficial zone, the disappearance of hypertrophic growth cartilage, the appearance of grid-fibrous fibrocartilage in the deep zone that is accompanied by a decline in endochondral ossification, and formation of a compact, subchondral bone plate. The second phase shows a progressive decrease in cell density and an increase in fibrosis or even cartilage infiltration of the intermediate zone. These last changes appear to reflect adaptive articular remodeling and possibly aging. Both maturational and later age changes seem to depend on articular loading as they do not occur in the nonload-bearing part of the condyle (Luder 1998).

The fibrocartilage differs in many aspects from the hyaline cartilage, including embryonic origin, ontogenetic development, postnatal growth pattern, and histological structures (Shen & Darendeliler 2005). The

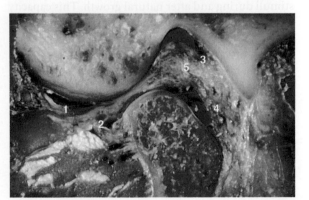

FIG 6-3 Section Through a TM Joint The condyle is in a slightly anterior position. The posterior and anterior attachments and the border between the posterior part of the disk and the bilaminar zone are clearly visible. *1* and *2*, superior and inferior laminae of the anterior attachment; *3* and *4*, superior and inferior laminae of the posterior attachment; *5*, border between posterior band and bilaminar zone. (Courtesy of Dr. Hans Ulrich Luder.)

FIG 6-2 Computed Tomography of the TM Joint (**A**) Horizontal and (**B**) frontal sections indicate the inclination of the condylar long axis in the horizontal and frontal planes.

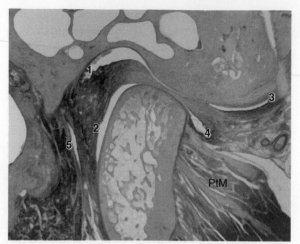

FIG 6-4 Histological section of a TM joint with the condyle in a slightly anterior position Note the different disk attachments and the folds in the superior lamina of the posterior attachment. *1*, posterosuperior attachment; *2*, posteroinferior attachment; *3*, anterosuperior attachment; *4*, antero-inferior attachment; *5*, posterior capsule; *PtM*, lateral pterygoid muscle. (From Luder & Bobst 1991, with permission.)

clinically most important and unique feature of condylar cartilage is its capability to adapt to external stimuli during and after natural growth. This capacity is used by orthodontists to improve mandibular growth in patients with a mandibular deficit. Mandibular forward positioning by functional appliances induces a cascade of reactions that leads to mandibular growth through the releasing of regulatory factors (Owtad et al. 2013, Shen & Darendeliler 2005). It is, however, still unclear if forward mandibular positioning effectively leads to an increase in the total amount of mandibular growth or only enhances the rate at which the genetically predetermined amount of mandibular growth is reached (Owtad et al. 2013).

Joint Capsule

Unlike other joints, the TM joint does not have a circular capsule. A distinct capsule connecting the temporal bone to the mandible exists only laterally; posteriorly, medially, and anteriorly it is absent or so thin that it can hardly be distinguished from the disk attachments. The lateral capsule, into which the disk transverse fibers insert, is stronger in the anterior and

central parts than in the posterior part. This strengthened area forms the lateral ligament (Luder & Bobst 1991, Schmolke 1994). Posteriorly the capsule that is made up mainly of condensed fibrous tissue extends from the anterior slope of the postglenoid tubercle to the condylar neck below the attachment of the lower lamina of the posterior disk attachment (Luder & Bobst 1991).

The lateral part of the capsule is attached to the perimysium of the deep masseter and the temporal muscle by fine fibrous septa (Meyenberg et al. 1986). The fibrous connections allow the capsule to stretch, preventing it from becoming trapped during jaw movements.

The capsule is lined with synovial membrane that continues through a zone of gradual histological transition into the fibrocartilagineous lining of the articular cartilage of condyle, disk, and fossa. The secreted synovial fluid provides nutrition for the cartilage and is involved in joint lubrication and cartilage protection (see the following discussion).

Articular Disk

This fibrocartilaginous avascular and noninnervated structure can be subdivided into an anterior, an intermediate (thinnest), and a posterior part (Fig. 6-1). The anterior and posterior zones are called the anterior and posterior bands.

The disk is composed of densely organized collagen fibers, high-molecular-weight proteoglycans, elastic fibers, and cells that vary from fibrocytes to chondrocytes. The collagen consists mainly of types I and II. Type II collagen is present especially in areas with proteoglycans, which are found predominantly in the posterior band. The collagen fibers have a typical pattern distribution: in the intermediate zone the thick collagen bundles are oriented sagittaly and parallel to the disk surface. The majority of these fibers continue into the anterior and posterior bands to become interlaced or continuous with the transversally and vertically oriented collagen fibers of these bands or pass through the entire bands to continue into the anterior and posterior disk attachments. The vertically and transversely oriented fibers are more pronounced in the anterior and posterior band (Scapino et al. 2006). In the intermediate part there is a weaker crosslinking of the collagen bundles, making this area less resistant to mediolateral shear stresses (see the following discussion). Further details can be found in Scapino 1997, Scapino et al. 2006, and Mills et al. 1994.

Articular Disk Attachments

The attachments allow the disk to rotate around the condyle and to slide anteriorly.

Posterior Attachment

The area of the posterior attachment is normally termed the *bilaminar zone* because it consists of two laminae separated by a loose connective tissue consisting of elastic fibers, blood and lymph vessels, nerves, and fat tissue. The lower lamina inserts into the periosteum of the condyle approximately 8 to 10 mm below the condylar vertex. The lamina consists of thick fibers that originate from almost the entire height of the posterior band and lacks elastic fibers (Figs. 6-3 and 6-4). The lamina is stretched in the closed-mouth position and becomes loose and folded when the condyle rotates, as occurs during jaw opening.

The superior lamina inserts into the periosteum of the fossa in front of the squamotympanic and petrotympanic fissures, is thinner than the lower lamina, and contains thinner collagen fibers. The fibers of both laminae enter the posterior band and become contiguous to or continue into the collagen fibers of the posterior band. Elastic fibers are visible only in the superior lamina and in the posterior capsule. More details can be found in Luder & Bobst (1991).

The collagen fibers of the superior lamina as well as the synovial lining are extensively folded in the closed mouth position and stretch during opening or protrusion, allowing the disk to glide anteriorly (Figs. 6-5 and 6-6). Contrary to previous hypotheses, the stretched elastic fibers do not provide enough force to pull the disk back on closing. The disk position is secured by the lateral and posteroinferior ligaments, a hypothesis supported by the analysis of the tensile stiffness, strength, toughness, and maximum strain of the disk attachments (Murphy et al. 2013).

The loose tissue in the retrocondylar space aprovides compensation for the pressure changes that arise when the retrocondylar space expands during condylar translation. The loose fibroelastic framework allows the blood vessels to expand (Fig. 6-5), and, as a consequence, the posterosuperior lamina is

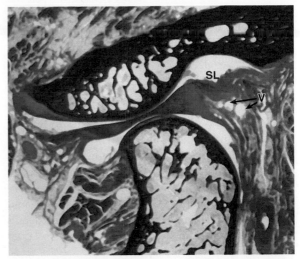

FIG 6-5 Histological Section of a TM Joint with the Condyle in an Anterior Position The superior lamina of the posterior attachment (*SL*) begins to become stretched, and blood vessels (*V*) in the retrodiscal pad dilate. This tissue is pulled anteriorly in the retrocondylar space. The opened joint spaces are artefacts. See Figure 6-6 for comparison in which the posterosuperior lamina is close to the fossa. (Courtesy of Dr. Hans Ulrich Luder.)

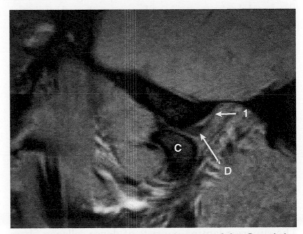

FIG 6-6 Magnetic Resonance Image of the Condyle-Disk Complex at Maximum Mouth Opening The superior lamina of the posterior attachment (*1*) is located close to the fossa and the disk (*D*) lies on top of the posterior part of the condyle (*C*).

pressed against the fossa and the posteroinferior lamina folds upward (Fig. 6-6). The blood vessels are connected with the pterygoid venous plexus located anteromedially to the condyle. Thus on opening the blood is drawn posteriorly and laterally to fill the enlarged space behind the condyle, and on closing it is pushed back into the pterygoid plexus. Pressure compensation is also achieved by the inward bulging of the parotid gland and subcutaneous tissue into the retrocondylar space. The bilaminar zone is thus designed to allow rapid volume changes in the retrocondylar space. Lack of a rapid pressure-compensatory mechanism on opening, closing, or translation would prevent smooth condylar movements. Further details on the posterior attachment may be found in Luder and Bobst (1991) and Scapino (1997).

Lateral and Medial Attachments

There are two types of lateral disk attachment, one inserting into the lateral condylar pole and the other below and behind the lateral pole (Ben Amor et al. 1998). The lateral disk attachment contains, in addition to more or less vertically oriented collagen fibers, fiber bundles that are oriented in an almost concentric fashion. These fibers insert from anterior and posterior directions. With an opening rotation of the condyle the posterior fibers are released while the anterior ones are tightened, and vice-versa during closing. This allows a firm disk-condyle connection preserving condylar rotation (Luder & Bobst 1991).

Medially the disk is attached by its superior lamina to the temporal bone and by its lower lamina to the condyle and the fascia of the lateral pterygoid muscle. The inferior attachment is somewhat thicker than the superior one. The medial attachment inserts below the medial pole and is less firm than the lateral attachment (Fig. 6-7).

Anterior Attachment

The anterior attachment is formed by two laminae. The superior lamina consists of dense collagen fibers and inserts into the periosteum of the infratemporal surface in front of the eminence (temporal attachment) while the inferior lamina inserts into the condyle more superiorly than the posterior attachment (condylar attachment). This lamina is composed of loose wavy fibers, contains sparse elastic fibers, and forms a small recess of the inferior joint

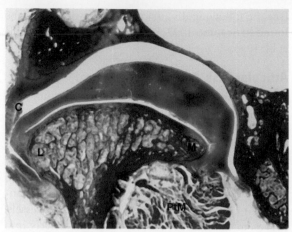

FIG 6-7 Insertion of the Disk to the Lateral (*L*) and Medial (*M*) Pole of the Condyle The medial insertion inserts below the pole. A capsule is only visible laterally (*C*). *PtM*, lateral pterygoid muscle. (From Luder & Bobst 1991, with permission.)

cavity (Figs. 6-3 and 6-4). The temporal attachment is thicker than the condylar attachment. Between these two laminae there are loose connective tissue, fat cells, and a venous plexus similar to that of the retrocondylar area (Luder & Bobst 1991, Schmolke 1994).

Articular Disk and Lateral Pterygoid Muscle

The relation between the disk and the superior head of the lateral pterygoid muscle has been the focus of several investigations because dysfunction of the superior head has been implicated in the etiology of an anterior disk displacement. This hypothesis is not supported by histological and dissection studies. Indeed, except for a couple of studies showing that in a few cases all the fibers of the superior head insert into the disk (Antonopoulou et al. 2013, Naidoo 1996), the majority of the investigations found that all or the vast majority of the fibers insert medially into the pterygoid fovea. In particular, two types of attachments are normally described: one in which all fibers insert into the pterygoid fovea above the insertion of the inferior head and one in which only the most superior fibers of the superior head insert medially into the disk, the remainder of the fibers inserting

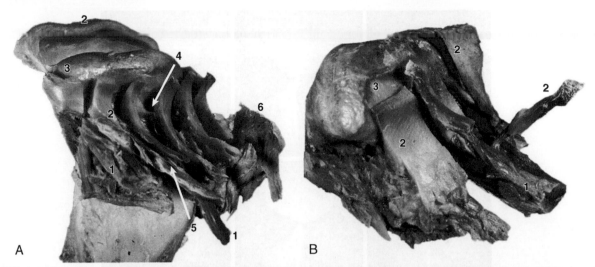

FIG 6-8 Two TM Joint Specimens A, Depicts the insertion of the most superior fibers of the superior head into the pterygoid fovea and the the fibrous septa connecting the inferior disk surface to the muscle fibers. **B,** Shows the most superior fibers of the superior head inserting in the disk, the rest of the fibers inserting in the pterygoid fovea. Notice also the lack of fibrocartilage cranially in the condyle left. *1,* superior head of lateral pterygoid muscle; *2,* disk; *3,* condyle; *4,* anterior disk attachment to the condyle; *5,* septum connecting the disk to the muscle fiber perimysium. (**B,** Reproduced from Meyenberg et al. 1986, with permission).

into the pterygoid fovea (Fig. 6-8; Carpentier et al. 1988, Meyenberg et al. 1986, Wilkinson & Chan 1989; see Antonopoulou et al. 2013 for further references). In the first attachment type the anterior band of the disk is attached to the muscle perimysium by fibrous connections (Meyenberg et al. 1986).

In fresh TM joint tissues, it is impossible to drag the disk anteriorly by pulling the fibers of the superior head. This seems to confirm that an anterior disk displacement cannot be caused by abnormal activity of the superior head. This observation is substantiated by magnetic resonance image (MRI) investigations indicating that disk displacement is not associated with the attachment type (Dergin et al. 2012, Imanimoghaddam et al. 2013).

Articular Disk Position

In maximum intercuspation the posterior band lies above the condyle (Figs. 6-1 and 6-9), and the thin intermediate zone is located between the condyle and the eminence posterior slope (see Fig. 6-1). This disk position is called the "12 o'clock" position on MRIs as the border between the posterior band and

the bilaminar zone of asymptomatic joints often corresponds to the condylar vertex (Fig. 6-9). In reality, there is a range of normalcy, with this border lying within a ±10° angle from a line perpendicular to the Frankfurt plane and crossing the vertex of the condyle (Rammelsberg et al. 1997).

JOINT INNERVATION

The TM joint capsule and the synovia are richly innervated by branches of the trigeminal nerve: the auriculotemporal, masseteric, and deep posterior temporal nerves. Small nerve bundles also innervate the most peripheral parts of the disk, especially the anterior and posterior bands (Asaki et al. 2006, Haeuchi et al. 1999, Morani et al. 1994, Yoshida et al. 1999a). TM joint innervation becomes detectable at the end of the second month of fetal life and increases in density up to the twentieth week (Ramieri et al. 1996). The auriculotemporal nerve provides the main innervation source so that it is sufficient to block this nerve when the TM joint must be anesthetized (e.g., to diagnose whether pain is arthrogeneous or myogeneous).

73

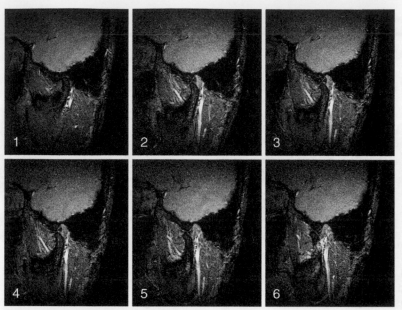

FIG 6-9 Six Positions of the Condyle-Disk Complex During an Opening Movement While the condyle rotates below the disk, the condyle-disk complex glides anteriorly. Note that at maximum opening the disk lies on top of the posterior part of the condylar head.

The TM joint receives inputs from a variety of ganglia, the major contribution being provided by the trigeminal and superior cervical ganglia. Minor contributions come from the sphenopalatine, otic, nodose and cervical dorsal root ganglia at levels C2-C5 (Uddman et al. 1998, Yoshino et al. 1998).

The nerve fibers contain a variety of neuropeptides (substance P, calcitonin gene-related peptide, neuropeptide Y, vasoactive intestinal peptide, pituitary adenylate cyclase-activating peptide) and nitric oxide (Haeuchi et al. 1999, Kido et al. 1993, 2001, Tahmasebi-Sarvestani et al. 1996, Uddman et al. 1998, Yoshida et al. 1999a). Some of the nerve fibers are in close association with blood vessels or synovial cells, or end as free nerves. Thus the TM joint has nociceptive, sympathetic, parasympathetic, and mechanosensitive innervation. As is the case for the other synovial joints, the TM joint capsule also contains mechano-receptors: Ruffini endings, Pacinian-type endings, and Golgi-type endings (Wink et al. 1992) that are part of the peripheral motor control feedback. Innervation of the TM joint is therefore complex, and different sensory and autonomic ganglia are involved.

JOINT LUBRICATION

The frictional coefficient within a joint is very low (Nickel & McLachlan 1994a). Impairment of joint lubrication is a risk factor for TM joint osteoarthritis (OA; see the Osteoarthritis section). The articular cartilage is an efficient, fluid-based tribological system that provides low friction and protects from wear. Optimal lubrication is provided by several mechanisms: fluid film, weeping, and boundary lubrication. Hyaluronic acid (HA) and proteoglycan 4 are two major lubricants involved in boundary lubrication. Proteoglycan 4, also known as lubricin or superficial zone protein, binds to HA to form a cross-linked HA-lubricin complex that is anchored to the cartilage surface by the lubricin itself. As this binding appears to be susceptible to high shear forces, it has been hypothesized that during compression the HA molecules diffusing out of the cartilage into the joint space are mechanically trapped, thus stabilizing the HA-lubricin complex. Details on joint lubrication are provided in Greene et al. (2011) and Tanaka et al. (2008b).

Lubricin, which is expressed by synovial cells and the chondrocytes of the superficial zone of both the fibrocartilage and the articular disk (Leonardi et al. 2012, Ohno et al. 2006, Tanimoto et al. 2011), also has a protective function: it prevents glycosaminoglycan depletion, collagen degradation, and cell loss in the superficial zone (Jay et al. 2010). The expression of this protein is modulated by biomechanical stress as well as cytokines and growth factors: the expression is upregulated by physiological loading and transforming growth factor beta (TGF-β) and downregulated by excessive loading and an increase of interleukin 1 beta (IL-1β) (Kamiya et al. 2010, Ohno et al. 2006).

CONDYLAR MOVEMENTS

Mandibular movements occur by a combination of translation of the condyle-disk assembly and rotation of the condyle beneath the disk (Figs. 6-9 and 6-10). It is likely that the movement between disk and condyle is not always purely rotator, as dynamic MR imaging shows that condylar translation may precede disk translation (see enclosed CD). This is always the case with a displaced disk (Fig. 6-11). Translation between disk and condyle may reflect some laxity of the disk ligaments and could be a first sign of an incipient disk displacement.

Examples of condylar movements are presented in the enclosed CD. Figure 6-12 shows a lateral view of the movement of the condyles during the closing phase of a chewing cycle. The first image represents the position at the beginning of closing. Three features may be appreciated. First, there is a difference in timing between the movements of both condyles: the working condyle reaches its uppermost position before the nonworking condyle. In Figure 6-12, image 4, the working condyle is almost seated in the fossa, while the nonworking condyle is still on the eminence posterior slope. This lead to the hypothesis that the working condyle acts as a stabilizing fulcrum during the so-called power stroke: that is, when force is applied to crush food. Second, during opening, both condyles translate approximately the same amount and are located just behind the eminence. Third, as seen in the compound figure (Fig. 6-12, image 6), the condyle rotates by about 10°, far less than during maximum opening when it rotates on average by 30° (Fig. 6-1 for comparison; Salaorni & Palla 1994.

During so small a rotation, only the superior part of the condyle is loaded, and this is the area where the fibrocartilage is thickest.

Rotation Versus Translation

Condylar rotation and translation of the condyle-disk assembly, in the majority of cases, begin simultaneously. On average, condylar rotation increases or decreases linearly by approximately 2°/mm of anterior or posterior translation during opening or closing, respectively (Salaorni & Palla 1994). However, there is great intraindividual and interindividual variability: three patterns have been described during jaw opening and four during jaw closing. On opening, movements are usually performed by a constant increase in rotation and anterior translation, less often by marked rotation at the beginning of opening, and much less frequently by a marked initial and final rotatory movement. Closing movements show a greater variability between rotation and translation. Further details can be found in Salaorni & Palla (1994).

The amount of condylar rotation does not differ between males and females, a finding which contrasts with the larger maximum interincisal opening of men compared with women due to differences in mandible length (Naeije 2002). Indeed, with the same degree of rotation, the larger the mandible, the larger the mouth opening. Consequently, the degree of interincisal opening cannot be considered as a measure of joint mobility or laxity, unless it is corrected for mandibular size.

JOINT LOADING

A query often raised in dentistry is whether or not the TM joint is loaded during function. The measurement of the minimum condyle-fossa distance by means of dynamic strereometry provides an indirect technique to answer this question. During chewing the minimum condyle-fossa distance was observed to be smaller during the closing than the opening phase, and the decrease was larger on the nonworking than on the working side (Fushima et al. 2003, Palla et al. 1997). This is indirect evidence that the TM joint is loaded during chewing, more on the nonworking than on the working side. These results are in keeping with computer models and recordings in monkeys that consistently predict that the TM joint is loaded

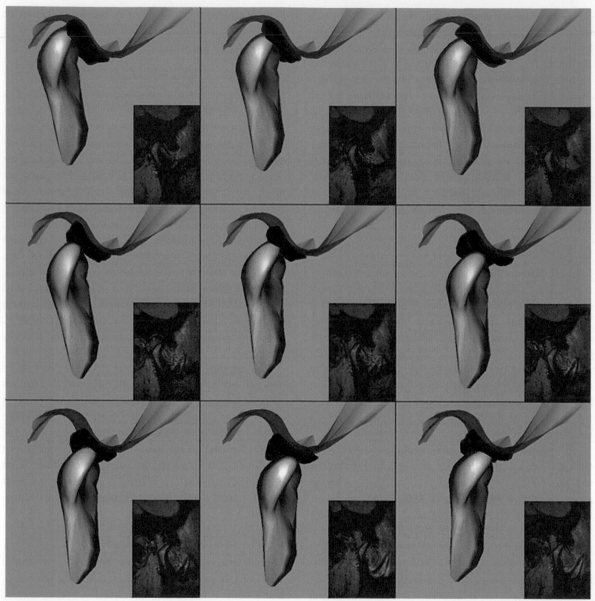

FIG 6-10 Three-dimensional Reconstruction of Nine Positions of the Condyle-Disk Complex During an Opening Movement Note that the condyle-disk complex translates less anteriorly than in the sequence shown in Figure 6-9. As a consequence the degree of rotation of the condyle is less.

during chewing as well as during clenching in eccentric positions. For details see Palla et al. (1997).

Given the incongruence of the articulating surfaces, the stress applied to the TM joint is principally controlled by the disk. Its inherent rheological properties allow its adaptation to the incongruence of the articulating surfaces so that the compressive stress is distributed over a large contact area, reducing the risk of peak loads (Tanaka & van Eijden 2003). The disk compressive module depends on proteoglycan density and therefore varies in different disk regions (Tanaka & van Eijden 2003). Moreover, the disk thickness determines the disk load-bearing capacity: the thinner the disk the more concentrated and intensive the loading of the articular surfaces (Nickel & McLachlan 1994b).

Although thinner than the disk (Hansson & Öberg 1977), the cartilage covering condyle and fossa also contributes to absorbing the compressive stress

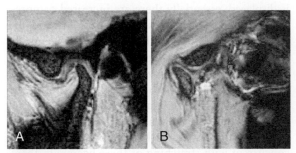

FIG 6-11 Magnetic Resonance Image of Disk Position in Maximum Intercuspation (A) and at Maximum Opening (B) At maximum intercuspation, the condyle lies behind the disk, whereas at maximum opening it is normally positioned below the disk (for comparison, see Fig. 6-9). In order to reach this position the condyle translates below the disk.

(Kuroda et al. 2009, Lu et al. 2009). Interestingly, the cartilage of the apex and posterior slope of the eminence (i.e., of the functional joint parts), can increase in thickness when the disk is anteriorly displaced, likely as an adaptation process to the altered stress (Jonsson et al. 1999).

Mechanical loading during movements is essential for growth, development, and maintenance of the articular tissues because mechanical forces maintain cartilage health by regulating tissue remodeling. Mechanical loading leads to complex changes within the tissue that include matrix and cell deformation, hydrostatic pressure gradients, fluid flow, altered matrix water content, and changes in osmotic pressure and ion concentrations. Chondrocyte mechanoreceptors such as mechanosensitive ion channels and integrins are involved in the recognition of these physical changes (mechanotransduction). For instance, activation of the mechanosensitive ion channels by mechanical stimulation leads to ion influx, in particular calcium ions, and activates intracellular signalling pathways that modulate protein synthesis (Ragan et al. 1999). Chondrocytes respond to mechanical stimuli by activating anabolic or

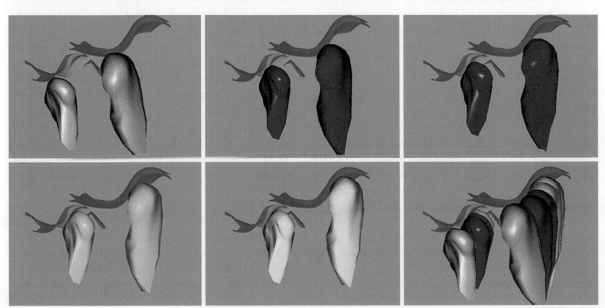

FIG 6-12 Five Positions of the Ipsilateral and Contralateral Condyle During the Closing Phase of a Chewing Cycle The lower right figure is a compound image.

catabolic pathways, and changes from anabolic to catabolic metabolism can lead to OA (see the Osteo-arthritis section). Consequently, cell-matrix interactions are essential for maintaining the integrity of the articular cartilage, and an intact matrix is essential for chondrocyte survival and transmission of mechanical signals. However, not all loading conditions have a positive effect on cartilage metabolism. For instance, while cyclic loading or loading within a physiological range increases proteoglycan synthesis, cartilage over-loading, underloading, and static loading cause pro-teoglycan depletion (Kuroda et al. 2009, Ramage et al. 2009). During parafunction, especially eccentric tooth clenching or grinding, the TM joint is loaded quasi-statically. Static loading, as may happen during para-function, is less favorable for cartilage integrity than dynamic loading (Grodzinsky et al. 2000), as it leads to a decrease in matrix synthesis (Ragan et al. 1999, Torzilli et al. 1997, Wong et al. 1997), increased pro-duction of various metalloproteinases (Fitzgerald et al. 2004), and chondrocyte death in the superficial zone (Lucchinetti et al. 2002).

TEMPOROMANDIBULAR JOINT PATHOPHYSIOLOGY

Articular disk displacement and OA are the two most frequently encountered TM joint problematic conditions in a dental office. Their pathophysiological mechanisms are therefore briefly discussed below.

Disk Displacement

In about one third of subjects without symptoms of TM disorders, the disk is displaced anteromedially or anterolaterally; the prevalence of disk displacement is higher in patients with TM disorders. The etiology of disk displacement is not fully understood. Several risk factors have been suggested: anatomical factors, for example, a large incongruence between condyle and fossa dimensions; a steep and high eminence and a posterior condylar position; biomechanical factors, for example, overloading of the TM joint by para-functional habits; changes in joint lubrication that may lead to a gradual increase of the translator movement between condyle and disk with a gradual stretching of the lateral disk attachments; and disk instability (Naeije 2002). Wake-time parafunction may be a risk factor for the progression of an

intermittently nonreducing to a continuously nonre-ducing disk displacement, and this could be related to joint loading (Kalaykova et al. 2011a, b). However, none of these factors is undisputed. As with all disor-ders and diseases, it is likely that disk displacement is not caused by a single factor but by the interplay of several factors.

The way the disk is loaded changes when the disk is displaced: essentially there are increased compres-sive and tangential stresses in the posterior band, due to the condyle pushing and compressing it against the fossa, and a reduced compressive stress in the inter-mediate and anterior disk zones, the decrease depend-ing on the degree of displacement (partial, total, with or without reduction). In addition the medial, lateral, and anterior disk attachments undergo a higher degree of tensile stress (del Palomar & Doblare 2007) concurrent with stretching of these ligaments, there-fore increasing disk instability.

Inevitably, these load changes cause tissue remod-eling that may continue to disk degeneration. For instance, the posterior attachment that is interposed between the condyle and fossa undergoes fibrotic changes: the collagen fiber bundles become thicker, more rectilinear, and oriented parallel to the attach-ment surface; the elastic fibers thin out; and vascular-ity decreases. In addition, the fibrotic attachment may appear hyalinized and contain cells of cartilage phe-notype and proteoglycans. In the posterior band, the collagen fibers become aligned in all directions and the transverse bundles increase in thickness, probably to resist the increased tensile stress in the mediolateral direction. Rearrangement of the collagen fibers occurs also in the anterior band, and, with a decrease in compressive load, the proteoglycans disappear. In addition, the anterior condylar disk attachment becomes stretched and the disk may flex with a new arrangement of the collagen fibers (see details in Scapino & Mills 1997, Luder 1993).

An anteriorly displaced disk presents histological alterations typical of degeneration that are more pronounced in nonreducing than reducing disks: increase of chondrocyte-like cells and decrease of fibroblast-like cells, hyalinization, alteration of the fiber bundles, clefting, and fraying (Leonardi et al. 2010, Loreto et al. 2011, Natiella et al. 2009). In addition, deformed displaced disks have increased expression of matrix metalloproteinase (MMP) 3 and aggrecanase (Matsumoto et al. 2008, Yoshida et al. 1999b, 2005); beta-defensin 4 (Sicurezza et al. 2013); hyaluronan syntheses (HAS3) that produces low molecular weight HA (Matsumoto et al. 2010); tumor necrosis factor (TNF)-related apoptosis-inducing ligand (TRAIL); and the death receptor DR5 (Leonardi et al. 2010, 2011). Lastly, deformed disks contain a significantly higher number of capsase-positive cells than normal disks (Loreto et al. 2011). TRAIL activates the capsase cascade leading to cell apoptosis.

Osteoarthritis

OA has a complex etiology. The risk factors can be subdivided in three categories: abnormal mechanical loading, genetic factors, and effects of aging. OA is characterized by cartilage degradation, synovial inflammation, and remodeling of the subchondral bone, including sclerosis and osteophyte formation.

Histological and immunohistochemical studies indicate that TM joint OA has a pathophysiological mechanism similar to that of joints with hyaline cartilage. Briefly, in the initial stage there is a proliferation of chondrocytes and increase in metabolic activity. This is interpreted as an attempt by the chondrocytes to repair the initial lesion, an attempt that normally fails because of an imbalance between anabolic and catabolic activity in favor of the latter. In the next stage there is articular swelling due to the disruption of the collagen network and further proliferation of chondrocytes that, under the influence of cytokines, continue producing proteolytic enzymes leading to a steady increase of cartilage damage until there is total cartilage loss (Fig. 6-8). The degradation products may activate synovial cells, producing a secondary synovitis. In turn, cytokines produced by activated synovial cells further activate chondrocytes to overexpress proteolytic enzymes. The final stage is a complete destruction of the cartilage with a thickening of the subchondral bone plate and eventually osteophyte formation (Fig. 6-13). More details can be found in Dijkgraaf et al. (1995) and Luder (1993).

Other findings that underline the similarity are the upregulation of vascular endothelial growth factor (VEGF), osteochondral angiogenesis after subjecting the condyle to mechanical stress (Tanaka et al. 2005, Wong et al. 1997), increased bone turnover during the early stage of OA (Embree et al. 2011), the initiation of OA by abnormal remodeling of subchondral bone (Jiao et al. 2013), and the presence of proinflammatory mediators in the synovial fluid (Tanaka et al. 2008a). The following briefly summarizes actual knowledge on OA pathophysiology in general.

Research in the last decades led to several paradigm shifts. First, while in the past OA was considered noninflammatory, there is today considerable evidence that inflammation is involved: the synovial fluid of OA joints contains inflammatory cytokines, chemokines, and other inflammatory mediators that are produced by chondrocytes and synovial cells in an early phase (Goldring & Otero 2011, Sokolove & Lepus 2013). As a result, the term "osteoarthritis" is used in this chapter instead of "degenerative joint disease" as used in the Diagnostic Criteria for Temporomandibular Disorders (Schiffman et al. 2014). Second, because of its complex etiology, OA is not now considered a single entity but the endpoint of numerous disorders with pathological changes sharing a common final pathway that leads to joint destruction (Sokolove & Lepus 2013). Third, OA is not a cartilage disorder but a disease of the whole joint, including the subchondral bone, the synovial membrane, the ligaments, and the muscles (Brandt et al. 2006). Fourth, changes in the subchondral and periarticular bone may occur early in the course of OA, leading to an imbalance between the higher load adaptive capacity of the bone over that of the cartilage. This imbalance alters the physiological relationship between these tissues, leading to the development of OA (Goldring & Goldring 2010). It is important to underline that there is cross-talk between the cartilage and subchondral bone that is necessary to maintain homeostasis within the subchondral bone-articular cartilage unit (Lories & Luyten 2011). Fifth, the early mechanical cartilage wear theory has been revised to place an imbalance between anabolic and catabolic activity of the chondrocytes at the center of the disease process. The increased catabolic activity leads to breakdown of the extracellular matrix (ECM).

In OA, chondrocytes and cells of the synovial membrane and other joint tissues are activated by several factors, including abnormal mechanical stress, inflammatory cytokines, or ECM degradation products. The activation of stress-induced and inflammation-induced signalling, transcriptional, and posttranscriptional events may cause apoptosis and a phenotypic change of the chondrocytes leading

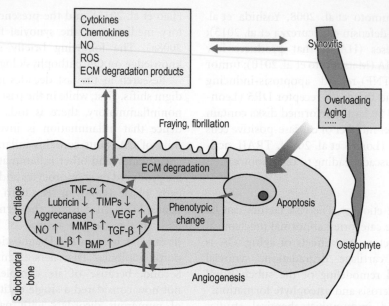

FIG 6-13 Mechanisms Involved in Cartilage Destruction in OA Central is the chondrocytes' phenotypic differentiation that leads to a catabolic metabolism with the upregulation of proteolytic enzymes, chemokines, and other inflammatory mediators. The degradation products cause innate immune responses leading to the upregulation of cytokines, chemokines, and proinflammatory mediators by the synovial cells that further activate the chondrocytes. Chondrocytes can also upregulate the expression of anabolic factors leading to osteophyte formation and blood vessels invasion from the subchondral bone (angiogenesis). *BMP*, Bone morphogenetic proteins; *ECM*, extracellular matrix; *IL-β*, interleukin 1 beta; *MMPs*, matrix metalloproteinases; *NO*, nitric oxide; *ROS*, reactive oxygen species; *TGF-β*, transforming growth factor beta; *TIMPs*, tissue inhibitors of metalloproteinases; *TNF-α*, tumor necrosis factor alpha; *VEGF*, vascular endothelial growth factor.

to an increased expression of proteolytic enzymes such as MMPs, including MMP-13, and aggrecanase. This enhancement is triggered by the release of a number of inflammatory mediators, including interleukin-1-beta (IL-1β), TNF-α, and chemokines by the chondrocytes themselves. The production of proteolytic enzymes, necessary for ECM remodeling, is controlled under physiological conditions by tissue inhibitors of metalloproteinases (TIMPs) that are downregulated in OA (Cawston & Wilson 2006, Leong et al. 2011). In addition, the chondrocytes also upregulate the production of nitric oxide, prostaglandin E, and VEGF and downregulate production of lubricin.

As already pointed out, chondrocytes have receptors that allow monitoring of changes in the ECM. Therefore they respond to abnormal mechanical load by upregulating synthetic activity or by increasing the production of inflammatory cytokines. For instance, unphysiological static compression stimulates the depletion of proteoglycans, damages the collagen network, and decreases the synthesis of cartilage matrix proteins, whereas dynamic cyclic compression increases matrix synthetic activity and inhibits IL-1–induced ECM degradation. Chondrocyte overloading also activates the hypoxia-induced transcription factor1 (HIF-1) resulting in induction of VEGF. This leads, in turn, to enhancement of MMP expression and downregulation of TIMPs (Pufe et al. 2004). Thus chondrocytes may respond to mechanical stress by increases catabolic activity without ongoing inflammation. It is, however, not known whether these are initiating events or serve as feedback to amplify matrix degradation.

There is evidence of an association between cartilage degradation and chondrocyte death through apoptosis and/or a combination of apoptosis and autophagy. For instance, the number of apoptotic chondrocytes increases with OA severity and correlates with mechanical injury, increased production of reactive oxygen species (ROS), disruption of extracellular matrix integrity, and loss of production of growth factor. Chondrocyte apoptosis appears to be an early process in the disease and may be linked with the initiation of cartilage degradation. Support for this hypothesis comes from the fact that chondrocyte numbers decrease while the risk of developing OA increases with aging. However, it is still not clear whether apoptosis is a cause or a result of cartilage degeneration, and a recent study hypothesized that chondrocyte apoptosis is more important for the progression than the initiation of OA (Zamli et al. 2013). Chondrocyte viability depends on maintenance of a proper chondrocyte-matrix interaction; that is, the bond between the pericellular matrix components, such as laminin and fibronectin, and the intracellular cytoskeletal proteins. Thus, degradation of the ECM may lead to loss of the anchorage-viability signals from the surrounding matrix, triggering chondrocyte apoptosis. Indeed, abnormal mechanical loading induces chondrocyte apoptosis. In addition, early cartilage fibrillation may also expose the chondrocyte to catabolic factors such as nitric oxide and cytokines secreted by synovial cells as well as chondrocytes. These mediators, in turn, are likely to induce chondrocyte death by apoptosis. Further details are provided in Zamli & Sharif (2011).

OA affects all joint tissues, including the synovium. The degree of synovitis increases with disease progression. Moreover, synovitis may cause more pronounced cartilage degeneration. Inflammation of the synovia is caused by ECM degradation products, such as fibromodulin, members of the small leucine-rich proteoglycan family, and cartilage oligomeric matrix protein (COMP) that activate innate immune responses. The resulting synovitis leads to the production of proinflammatory mediators and chemokines that diffuse through the cartilage, further activating the chondrocyte catabolic metabolism (Fig. 6-13). Thus synovitis perpetuates cartilage degradation.

Other typical signs of OA are osteophyte formation and invasion of the cartilage at the osteochondral junction by blood vessels from the chondral bone. In OA, chondrocytes upregulate the secretion of TGF-β, bone morphogenetic protein (BMPs), and VEGF. The enhancement of TGF-β and BMP may concur in

osteophyte formation, as recent data showed that in the rat, BMP2 is activated by TGF-β to induce osteophyte formation (Blaney Davidson et al. 2014). The increased expression of VEGF concurs in the angiogenesis process (Lotz 2012). Further details on OA can be found in Berenbaum (2013), Goldring & Goldring (2007, 2010), Goldring & Marcu (2009), Goldring & Otero (2011), Heinegård & Saxne (2011), Kapila (1997), Scanzello & Goldring (2012), and Sellam & Berenbaum (2010).

Once initiated, the osteoarthritic process does not necessarily progress to complete degeneration. It is likely that mechanical factors determine the progression of the disease, as mechanical stress influences the balance between the catabolic and anabolic activity of the chondrocytes. For instance, there is compelling evidence that moderate levels of exercise improve symptoms of OA and even increase proteoglycan content (Leong et al. 2011, Roos & Dahlberg 2005). Thus patients with TM joint OA should be advised to avoid parafunction, as this may overload the joint, and possibly perform a regimen of moderate, still to be designed, functional exercises.

CONCLUSION

Regulation of chondrocyte behavior is a complex process, and cartilage homeostasis is controlled by several interacting factors. Aging, genetic makeup, and local environmental factors, such as inflammation and joint loading, each affect the chondrocyte metabolism. OA is characterized by a phenotypical change in chondrocyte behavior that leads to chondrocyte hypertrophy. These final differentiated chondrocytes upregulate the production of proteolytic enzymes, causing ECM degradation and secondary synovitis. The exact mechanism by which chondrocytes are activated is not fully understood, but may involve several pathways including mechanical stress, oxidative stress, cell-matrix interactions, age-related changes in the ECM, chondrocyte and gene expression, as well as inflammatory mediators and subchondral bone changes.

ACKNOWLEDGMENTS

The author thanks Dr. Hans Ulrich Luder for providing Figures 6-1, 6-3, and 6-5 and for permission to reproduce Figures 6-4 and 6-7 from Luder & Bobst (1991). The author is also grateful to Dr. Konrad Meyenberg for permission to reproduce Figure 6-8, *B*.

REFERENCES

Almarza AJ, Athanasiou KA: Design characteristics for the tissue engineering of cartilaginous tissues, *Ann Biomed Eng* 32:2–17, 2004.

Antonopoulou M, Iatrou I, Paraschos A, et al: Variations of the attachment of the superior head of human lateral pterygoid muscle, *J Craniomaxillofac Surg* 41:e91–e97, 2013.

Asaki S, Sekikawa M, Kim YT: Sensory innervation of temporomandibular joint disk, *J Orthop Surg (Hong Kong)* 14:3–8, 2006.

Ben Amor F, Carpentier P, Foucart JM, et al: Anatomic and mechanical properties of the lateral disc attachment of the temporomandibular joint, *J Oral Maxillofac Surg* 56:1164–1167, 1998.

Berenbaum F: Osteoarthritis as an inflammatory disease (osteoarthritis is not osteoarthrosis!), *Osteoarthritis Cartilage* 21:16–21, 2013.

Blaney Davidson EN, Vitters EL, Blom AB, et al: BMP2 requires TGF-BETA to induce osteophytes during experimental osteoarthritis, *Ann Rheum Dis* 73 (Suppl 1):A70, 2014.

Brandt KD, Radin EL, Dieppe PA, et al: Yet more evidence that osteoarthritis is not a cartilage disease, *Ann Rheum Dis* 65:1261–1264, 2006.

Carpentier P, Yung JP, Marguelles Bonnet R, et al: Insertions of the lateral pterygoid muscle: an anatomic study of the human temporomandibular joint, *J Oral Maxillofac Surg* 46:477–482, 1988.

Cawston TE, Wilson AJ: Understanding the role of tissue degrading enzymes and their inhibitors in development and disease, *Best Pract Res Clin Rheumatol* 20:983–1002, 2006.

del Palomar AP, Doblare M: An accurate simulation model of anteriorly displaced TMJ discs with and without reduction, *Med Eng Phys* 29:216–226, 2007.

Dergin G, Kilic C, Gozneli R, et al: Evaluating the correlation between the lateral pterygoid muscle attachment type and internal derangement of the temporomandibular joint with an emphasis on MR imaging findings, *J Craniomaxillofac Surg* 40:459–463, 2012.

Dijkgraaf LC, de Bont LG, Boering G, et al: The structure, biochemistry, and metabolism of osteoarthritic cartilage: a review of the literature, *J Oral Maxillofac Surg* 53:1182–1192, 1995.

Embree M, Ono M, Kilts T, et al: Role of subchondral bone during early-stage experimental TMJ osteoarthritis, *J Dent Res* 90:1331–1338, 2011.

Fitzgerald JB, Jin M, Dean D, et al: Mechanical compression of cartilage explants induces multiple time-dependent gene expression patterns and involves intracellular calcium and cyclic AMP, *J Biol Chem* 279:19502–19511, 2004.

Fushima K, Gallo LM, Krebs M, et al: Analysis of the TMJ intraarticular space variation: a non-invasive insight during mastication, *Med Eng Phys* 25:181–190, 2003.

Goldring MB, Goldring SR: Osteoarthritis, *J Cell Physiol* 213:626–634, 2007.

Goldring MB, Goldring SR: Articular cartilage and subchondral bone in the pathogenesis of osteoarthritis, *Ann N Y Acad Sci* 1192:230–237, 2010.

Goldring MB, Marcu KB: Cartilage homeostasis in health and rheumatic diseases, *Arthritis Res Ther* 11:224, 2009.

Goldring MB, Otero M: Inflammation in osteoarthritis, *Curr Opin Rheumatol* 23:471–478, 2011.

Greene GW, Banquy X, Lee DW, et al: Adaptive mechanically controlled lubrication mechanism found in articular joints, *Proc Natl Acad Sci U S A* 108: 5255–5259, 2011.

Grodzinsky AJ, Levenston ME, Jin M, et al: Cartilage tissue remodeling in response to mechanical forces, *Annu Rev Biomed Eng* 2:691–713, 2000.

Haeuchi Y, Matsumoto K, Ichikawa H, et al: Immunohistochemical demonstration of neuropeptides in the articular disk of the human temporomandibular joint, *Cells Tissues Organs* 164:205–211, 1999.

Hansson T, Öberg T: Arthrosis and deviation in form in the temporomandibular joint. A macroscopic study on a human autopsy material, *Acta Odontol Scand* 35:167–174, 1977.

Heinegård D, Saxne T: The role of the cartilage matrix in osteoarthritis, *Nat Rev Rheumatol* 7:50–56, 2011.

Imanimoghaddam M, Madani AS, Hashemi EM: The evaluation of lateral pterygoid muscle pathologic changes and insertion patterns in temporomandibular joints with or without disc displacement using magnetic resonance imaging, *Int J Oral Maxillofac Surg* 42:1116–1120, 2013.

Iwasaki LR, Crosby MJ, Marx DB, et al: Human temporomandibular joint eminence shape and load minimization, *J Dent Res* 89:722–727, 2010.

Iwasaki LR, Petsche PE, McCall WD, et al: Neuromuscular objectives of the human masticatory apparatus during static biting, *Arch Oral Biol* 48:767–777, 2003.

Jay GD, Fleming BC, Watkins BA, et al: Prevention of cartilage degeneration and restoration of chondroprotection by lubricin tribosupplementation in the rat following anterior cruciate ligament transection, *Arthritis Rheum* 62:2382–2391, 2010.

Jiao K, Zhang M, Niu L, et al: Overexpressed TGF-beta in subchondral bone leads to mandibular condyle degradation, *J Dent Res* 93:140–147, 2014.

Jonsson G, Eckerdal O, Isberg A: Thickness of the articular soft tissue of the temporal component in temporomandibular joints with and without disk displacement, *Oral Surg Oral Med Oral Pathol Oral Radiol Endod* 87:20–26, 1999.

Kalaykova S, Lobbezoo F, Naeije M: Effect of chewing upon disc reduction in the temporomandibular joint, *J Orofac Pain* 25:49–55, 2011a.

Kalaykova SI, Lobbezoo F, Naeije M: Risk factors for anterior disc displacement with reduction and intermittent locking in adolescents, *J Orofac Pain* 25:153–160, 2011b.

Kamiya T, Tanimoto K, Tanne Y, et al: Effects of mechanical stimuli on the synthesis of superficial zone protein in chondrocytes, *J Biomed Mater Res A* 92:801–805, 2010.

Kapila S: Biology of TMJ degeneration: The role of matrix-degrading enzymes. In McNeill C, editor: *Science and practice of occlusion*, Chicago, 1997, Quintessence, pp 235–258.

Kido MA, Kiyoshima T, Kondo T, et al: Distribution of substance P and calcitonin gene-related peptide-like immunoreactive nerve fibers in the rat temporomandibular joint, *J Dent Res* 72:592–598, 1993.

Kido MA, Zhang JQ, Muroya H, et al: Topography and distribution of sympathetic nerve fibers in the rat temporomandibular joint: immunocytochemistry and ultrastructure, *Anat Embryol (Berl)* 203:357–366, 2001.

Kuroda S, Tanimoto K, Izawa T, et al: Biomechanical and biochemical characteristics of the mandibular condylar cartilage, *Osteoarthritis Cartilage* 17:1408–1415, 2009.

Leonardi R, Almeida LE, Rusu M, et al: Tumor necrosis factor-related apoptosis-inducing ligand expression correlates to temporomandibular joint disk degeneration, *J Craniofac Surg* 22:504–508, 2011.

Leonardi R, Almeida LE, Trevilatto PC, et al: Occurrence and regional distribution of TRAIL and DR5 on temporomandibular joint discs: comparison of disc derangement with and without reduction, *Oral Surg Oral Med Oral Pathol Oral Radiol Endod* 109:244–251, 2010.

Leonardi R, Musumeci G, Sicurezza E, et al: Lubricin in human temporomandibular joint disc: an immunohistochemical study, *Arch Oral Biol* 57:614–619, 2012.

Leong DJ, Hardin JA, Cobelli NJ, et al: Mechanotransduction and cartilage integrity, *Ann N Y Acad Sci* 1240:32–37, 2011.

Loreto C, Almeida LE, Trevilatto P, et al: Apoptosis in displaced temporomandibular joint disc with and without reduction: an immunohistochemical study, *J Oral Pathol Med* 40:103–110, 2011.

Lories RJ, Luyten FP: The bone-cartilage unit in osteoarthritis, *Nat Rev Rheumatol* 7:43–49, 2011.

Lotz M: Osteoarthritis year 2011 in review: biology, *Osteoarthritis Cartilage* 20:192–196, 2012.

Lu XL, Mow VC, Guo XE: Proteoglycans and mechanical behavior of condylar cartilage, *J Dent Res* 88:244–248, 2009.

Lucchinetti E, Adams CS, Horton WE Jr, et al: Cartilage viability after repetitive loading: a preliminary report, *Osteoarthritis Cartilage* 10:71–81, 2002.

Luder HU: Articular degeneration and remodeling in human temporomandibular joints with normal and abnormal disc position, *J Orofac Pain* 7:391–402, 1993.

Luder HU: Age changes in the articular tissue of human mandibular condyles from adolescence to old age: a semiquantitative light microscopic study, *Anat Rec* 251:439–447, 1998.

Luder HU, Bobst P: Wall architecture and disc attachment of the human temporomandibular joint, *Schweiz Monatsschr Zahnmed* 101:557–570, 1991.

Matsumoto T, Inayama M, Tojyo I, et al: Expression of hyaluronan synthase 3 in deformed human temporomandibular joint discs: in vivo and in vitro studies, *Eur J Histochem* 54:e50, 2010.

Matsumoto T, Tojyo I, Kiga N, et al: Expression of ADAMTS-5 in deformed human temporomandibular joint discs, *Histol Histopathol* 23:1485–1493, 2008.

Meyenberg K, Kubik S, Palla S: Relationships of the muscles of mastication to the articular disc of the temporomandibular joint, *Schweiz Monatsschr Zahnmed* 96:815–834, 1986.

Mills DK, Fiandaca DJ, Scapino RP: Morphologic, microscopic, and immunohistochemical investigations into the function of the primate TMJ disc, *J Orofac Pain* 8:136–154, 1994.

Morani V, Previgliano V, Schierano GM, et al: Innervation of the human temporomandibular joint capsule and disc as revealed by immunohistochemistry for neurospecific markers, *J Orofac Pain* 8:36–41, 1994.

Murphy MK, Arzi B, Hu JC, et al: Tensile characterization of porcine temporomandibular joint disc attachments, *J Dent Res* 92:753–758, 2013.

Naeije M: Local kinematic and anthropometric factors related to the maximum mouth opening in healthy individuals, *J Oral Rehabil* 29:534–539, 2002.

Naidoo LC: Lateral pterygoid muscle and its relationship to the meniscus of the temporomandibular joint, *Oral Surg Oral Med Oral Pathol Oral Radiol Endod* 82:4–9, 1996.

Natiella JR, Burch L, Fries KM, et al: Analysis of the collagen I and fibronectin of temporomandibular joint synovial fluid and discs, *J Oral Maxillofac Surg* 67:105–113, 2009.

Nickel JC, Iwasaki LR, McLachlan KR: Effect of the physical environment on the growth of the temporomandibular joint. In McNeill C, editor: *Science and practice of occlusion*, Chicago, 1997, Quintessence, pp 115–124.

Nickel JC, McLachlan KR: In vitro measurement of the frictional properties of the temporomandibular joint disc, *Arch Oral Biol* 39:323–331, 1994a.

Nickel JC, McLachlan KR: In vitro measurement of the stress-distribution properties of the pig temporomandibular joint disc, *Arch Oral Biol* 39:439–448, 1994b.

Nickel JC, McLachlan KR, Smith DM: Eminence development of the postnatal human temporomandibular joint, *J Dent Res* 67:896–902, 1988.

Ohno S, Schmid T, Tanne Y, et al: Expression of superficial zone protein in mandibular condyle cartilage, *Osteoarthritis Cartilage* 14:807–813, 2006.

Owtad P, Park JH, Shen G, et al: The biology of TMJ growth modification: a review, *J Dent Res* 92:315–321, 2013.

Palla S, Krebs M, Gallo LM: Jaw tracking and temporomandibular joint animation. In McNeill C, editor: *Science and Practice of Occlusion*, Chicago, 1997, Quintessence, pp 365–378.

Pufe T, Lemke A, Kurz B, et al: Mechanical overload induces VEGF in cartilage discs via hypoxia-inducible factor, *Am J Pathol* 164:185–192, 2004.

Ragan PM, Badger AM, Cook M, et al: Down-regulation of chondrocyte aggrecan and type-II collagen gene expression correlates with increases in static compression magnitude and duration, *J Orthop Res* 17:836–842, 1999.

Ramage L, Nuki G, Salter DM: Signalling cascades in mechanotransduction: cell-matrix interactions and mechanical loading, *Scand J Med Sci Sports* 19: 457–469, 2009.

Ramieri G, Bonardi G, Morani V, et al: Development of nerve fibres in the temporomandibular joint of the human fetus, *Anat Embryol (Berl)* 194:57–64, 1996.

Rammelsberg P, Pospiech PR, Jager L, et al: Variability of disk position in asymptomatic volunteers and patients with internal derangements of the TMJ, *Oral Surg Oral Med Oral Pathol Oral Radiol Endod* 83:393–399, 1997.

Roos EM, Dahlberg L: Positive effects of moderate exercise on glycosaminoglycan content in knee cartilage: a four-month, randomized, controlled trial in patients at risk of osteoarthritis, *Arthritis Rheum* 52:3507–3514, 2005.

Salaorni C, Palla S: Condylar rotation and anterior translation in healthy human temporomandibular joints, *Schweiz Monatsschr Zahnmed* 104:415–422, 1994.

Scanzello CR, Goldring SR: The role of synovitis in osteoarthritis pathogenesis, *Bone* 51:249–257, 2012.

Scapino RP: Morphology and mechanism of the jaw joint. In McNeill C, editor: *Science and practice of occlusion*, Chicago, 1997, Quintessence, pp 23–40.

Scapino RP, Mills DK: Disc displacement internal derangements. In McNeill C, editor: *Science and practice of occlusion*, Chicago, 1997, Quintessence, pp 220–234.

Scapino RP, Obrez A, Greising D: Organization and function of the collagen fiber system in the human temporomandibular joint disk and its attachments, *Cells Tissues Organs* 182:201–225, 2006.

Schiffman E, Ohrbach R, Truelove E, et al: Diagnostic Criteria for Temporomandibular Disorders (DC/TMD) for Clinical and Research Applications: Recommendations of the International RDC/TMD Consortium Network and Orofacial Pain Special Interest Group, *J Orofac Pain* 28:6–27, 2014.

Schmolke C: The relationship between the temporomandibular joint capsule, articular disc and jaw muscles, *J Anat* 184:335–345, 1994.

Sellam J, Berenbaum F: The role of synovitis in pathophysiology and clinical symptoms of osteoarthritis, *Nat Rev Rheumatol* 6:625–635, 2010.

Shen G, Darendeliler MA: The adaptive remodeling of condylar cartilage—a transition from chondrogenesis to osteogenesis, *J Dent Res* 84:691–699, 2005.

Sicurezza E, Loreto C, Musumeci G, et al: Expression of beta-defensin 4 on temporomandibular joint discs with anterior displacement without reduction, *J Craniomaxillofac Surg* 41:821–825, 2013.

Sokolove J, Lepus CM: Role of inflammation in the pathogenesis of osteoarthritis: latest findings and interpretations, *Ther Adv Musculoskelet Dis* 5:77–94, 2013.

Tahmasebi-Sarvestani A, Tedman RA, Goss A: Neural structures within the sheep temporomandibular joint, *J Orofac Pain* 10:217–231, 1996.

Tanaka E, Aoyama J, Miyauchi M, et al: Vascular endothelial growth factor plays an important autocrine/paracrine role in the progression of osteoarthritis, *Histochem Cell Biol* 123:275–281, 2005.

Tanaka E, Detamore MS, Mercuri LG: Degenerative disorders of the temporomandibular joint: etiology, diagnosis, and treatment, *J Dent Res* 87:296–307, 2008a.

Tanaka E, Detamore MS, Tanimoto K, et al: Lubrication of the temporomandibular joint, *Ann Biomed Eng* 36:14–29, 2008b.

Tanaka E, van Eijden T: Biomechanical behavior of the temporomandibular joint disc, *Crit Rev Oral Biol Med* 14:138–150, 2003.

Tanimoto K, Kamiya T, Tanne Y, et al: Superficial zone protein affects boundary lubrication on the surface of mandibular condylar cartilage, *Cell Tissue Res* 344:333–340, 2011.

Torzilli PA, Grigiene R, Huang C, et al: Characterization of cartilage metabolic response to static and dynamic stress using a mechanical explant test system, *J Biomech* 30:1–9, 1997.

Uddman R, Grunditz T, Kato J, et al: Distribution and origin of nerve fibers in the rat temporomandibular joint capsule, *Anat Embryol (Berl)* 197:273–282, 1998.

Wilkinson T, Chan EK: The anatomic relationship of the insertion of the superior lateral pterygoid muscle to the articular disc in the temporomandibular joint of human cadavers, *Aust Dent J* 34:315–322, 1989.

Wink CS, St Onge M, Zimny ML: Neural elements in the human temporomandibular articular disc, *J Oral Maxillofac Surg* 50:334–337, 1992.

Wong M, Wuethrich P, Buschmann MD, et al: Chondrocyte biosynthesis correlates with local tissue strain in statically compressed adult articular cartilage, *J Orthop Res* 15:189–196, 1997.

Yoshida H, Fujita S, Nishida M, et al: The expression of substance P in human temporomandibular joint samples: an immunohistochemical study, *J Oral Rehabil* 26:338–344, 1999a.

Yoshida H, Yoshida T, Iizuka T, et al: The localization of matrix metalloproteinase-3 and tenascin in synovial membrane of the temporomandibular joint with internal derangement, *Oral Dis* 5:50–54, 1999b.

Yoshida K, Takatsuka S, Tanaka A, et al: Aggrecanase analysis of synovial fluid of temporomandibular joint disorders, *Oral Dis* 11:299–302, 2005.

Yoshino K, Kawagishi S, Amano N: Morphological characteristics of primary sensory and post-synaptic sympathetic neurones supplying the temporomandibular joint in the cat, *Arch Oral Biol* 43:679–686, 1998.

Zamli Z, Adams MA, Tarlton JF, et al: Increased chondrocyte apoptosis is associated with progression of osteoarthritis in spontaneous Guinea pig models of the disease, *Int J Mol Sci* 14:17729–17743, 2013.

Zamli Z, Sharif M: Chondrocyte apoptosis: a cause or consequence of osteoarthritis? *Int J Rheum Dis* 14:159–166, 2011.

SECTION | 2 |

Assessment

Occlusal Form and Clinical Specifics

Iven Klineberg

SYNOPSIS

This chapter reviews relationships of teeth that are important in the clinical management of occlusion. The chapter provides an understanding of tooth contact positions in the natural dentition and the clinical recordings of jaw position for treatment purposes. Occlusal contacts are summarized with recognition given to the prevailing divergent views in defining optimal jaw and tooth contact relationships. The implications of the variations that are described in population studies are considered, and their possible links with jaw muscle pain and temporomandibular disorders (TMDs) reviewed.

A summary statement on occlusal relationships emphasizes the variability of presenting occlusal features in natural dentitions. The border movement diagram is included as an important statement of historical development and as a useful conceptual tool for understanding border positions of the jaw. Anterior and lateral guidance is defined in the light of research evidence, in conjunction with the emerging research data on mediotrusive contacts or interferences. Features of the natural dentition are distinct from guidelines recommended for restoration of occlusions.

Contemporary reports of clinical studies (such as Clark 2006, Stohler 2006, Marklund & Wänman 2010, Greene 2011) systematically clarify previous data, such as that from earlier trials by Pullinger and Seligman (2000) and Seligman and Pullinger (2000). It is also recognized that human physiological studies of jaw and condyle movement; electromyographic (EMG) studies, especially of deep jaw muscles; and microneurographic recordings from periodontal afferents are technically demanding and recruitment of subjects is often difficult. Notwithstanding these challenges, significant progress has been made in the last decade in embracing biology and moving away from our mechanical heritage. Recognition of the biological system and the complexities within which occlusal management is undertaken is of great clinical importance.

CHAPTER POINTS

- Occlusion is the dynamic biological relationship of the components of the masticatory system that determines tooth relationships
- Intercuspal contact (IC) is the contact between the cusps, fossae, and marginal ridges of opposing teeth
- Intercuspal contact position (ICP) is the position of the jaw when the teeth are in IC
- Maximum intercuspation (MI) is the contact of the teeth with maximum clench
- Centric occlusion (CO) is the ICP when the jaw and condyles are in centric relation (CR)
- ICP and CO are not usually the same tooth contact positions; that is, there is usually a slide from CO to ICP
- Median occlusal position (MOP) is a clinically determined tooth-contact jaw position obtained by a "snap" jaw closure from a jaw open position
- Retruded jaw position (RP) is the guided jaw position with the condyles in a physiologically acceptable position for recording transfer records
- Retruded contact position (RCP) is the tooth contact position when the jaw is in RP
- CR is the guided jaw position where the condyles are located anterosuperiorly, in contact with the central bearing surface of the interarticular disk located against the posterior slope of the articular eminence
- Postural jaw position (PJP) is the jaw position determined by the jaw muscles when the subject is standing or sitting upright, with variable space between the teeth
- Occlusal vertical dimension (OVD) is the vertical height of the lower third of the face with the teeth in ICP
- Lateral jaw positions are as noted in the following:
  - Mediotrusive (nonworking) side contact arises when the jaw is moved or guided to the opposite side, and the mediotrusive side moves medially; that is, toward the midline. Tooth contacts on that side are termed mediotrusive (nonworking or balancing) contacts
  - Laterotrusive (working) side contact occurs when the jaw is moved or guided to the side; that is, laterally to the right or left. Tooth contacts on that side are termed laterotrusive (or working) contacts
- Bennett movement is a term that describes lateral movement of the laterotrusive condyle; that is, condyle movement to the laterotrusive (or working) side
- Bennett angle is the angle of the contralateral condyle formed with the sagittal plane on the mediotrusive side as the condyle moves forward downward and medially (mediotrusive condyle movement)
- Protrusive jaw movement describes a forward (straight) jaw movement and protrusive tooth contacts including incisal tooth contact

The term *occlusion* represents a broader concept than just arrangements of teeth. Occlusion refers to the dynamic biological relationships of components of the masticatory system that control tooth contacts during function and dysfunction. It is essentially the integrated action of the jaw muscles, temporomandibular (TM) joints, and teeth.

The essential characteristics of the system morphologically and physiologically are genetically determined (jaw muscle characteristics, jaw shape and size, and tooth eruption sequence), and functional relationships mature during growth and development. However, once established, continual modification of the jaw muscle system occurs with function and parafunction.

Importantly, the influence of parafunction on tooth position and wear may be significant, with ongoing remodeling of jaw bone and jaw muscles allowing adaptation to prevailing circumstances, emphasizing the dynamic nature of this complex biological system.

TOOTH CONTACTS AND JAW POSITIONS

The need to describe jaw and tooth positions accurately for treatment planning, writing of clinical reports, and laboratory prescriptions requires an understanding of the following customarily accepted descriptive terms.

The use of ultrafine occlusal tapes (such as GHM Foil, Gebr. Hansel-Medizinal, Nurtingen, Germany; Ivoclar/Vivadent, Schaan, Liechtenstein) placed between the teeth (teeth need to be air-dried to allow the tape to mark tooth contacts) will allow specific tooth contacts to be identified.

- *Intercuspal contact* (IC) is the contact between the cusps, fossae, and marginal ridges of opposing teeth.
- *Intercuspal contact position* (ICP) is the position of the jaw when the teeth are in IC. Light IC occurs with light tooth contact—in this situation, the number and area of tooth contacts are less than with heavy tooth contact (clenching). ICP is the tooth contact position at the end of the closing phase and the beginning of the opening phase of each chewing cycle of mastication. Most natural occlusions present ICP contacts as a combination of flat and inclined surfaces or inclined planes with supporting cusps contacting opposing tooth fossae or marginal ridges. The greatest number of contacts occurs between molar teeth, and this decreases to 67% contact on first bicuspids and 37% contact on second bicuspids. Light to heavy biting approximately doubles the number of tooth contacts (Riise & Ericsson 1983).
- *Maximum intercuspation* (MI) occurs with clenching (heavy bite force), when the number and area of tooth contacts are greatest. The increase in number and area of tooth contacts occurs as a result of tooth compression within the periodontal space, which for individual teeth may be of the order of 100 μm in healthy periodontal tissues. With periodontal disease and periodontal bone loss, this may be greater.

The distinction between ICP and MI might appear to be of academic rather than clinical interest; however, the recognition of an increase in the number of tooth contacts is relevant when finalizing anatomical tooth form for restorations, to develop the appropriate tooth contact arrangement for function, and to ensure that with clenching the restorations are not too heavily loaded.

- *Centric occlusion* (CO) and ICP may be considered the same for clinical purposes; however, the *Glossary of Prosthodontic Terms* (2005) defines CO as the tooth contact position when the jaw is in centric relation (CR). Thus CO may or may not be the same tooth contact relationship as ICP. CO when the jaw is in CR may be more retruded than at ICP. In an epidemiological study, Posselt (1952) determined that CO and ICP coincided in only approximately 10% of natural tooth and jaw relationships.

In clinical practice, complete denture treatment usually requires working casts to be articulated in CR (see the following discussion). The artificial tooth arrangement and jaw contact position between the denture teeth is then CO by definition.

- *Median occlusal position* (MOP) is a dynamic tooth contact position that may be determined by a "snap" (rapid) jaw closure from a jaw open position (McNamara 1977). Tooth contacts at MOP have been proposed as being equivalent to functional tooth contacts. MOP tooth contacts can only be determined clinically and are useful to indicate functional tooth contacts in clinical occlusal analysis.

It is likely that MOP and ICP (with light tooth contact) are equivalent for clinical assessment purposes.

- *Retruded jaw position* (RP) is the position of the jaw when the condyles are in a physiologically acceptable guided position for the recording of jaw transfer records. This position is a reproducible position for the proposed dental treatment. It is not constant in the long term, as remodeling adaptation of joint components is a feature of biological systems. RP of the jaw is independent of tooth contacts.
- *Retruded contact position* (RCP) is the contact position of the teeth when the jaw is in RP.
- *CR* is the jaw relationship (also termed maxillomandibular relationship) in which the condyles are located in the fossae in an anterorsuperior position in contact with the central bearing surface (the thin avascular part) of the interarticular disk,

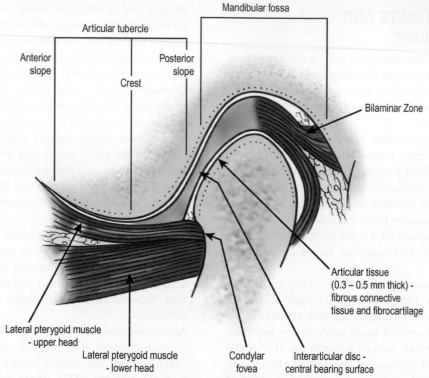

Mandibular fossa

Articular tubercle

Anterior slope

Posterior slope

Crest

Bilaminar Zone

Articular tissue
(0.3 – 0.5 mm thick) -
fibrous connective
tissue and fibrocartilage

Lateral pterygoid muscle
- upper head

Lateral pterygoid muscle
- lower head

Condylar fovea

Interarticular disc -
central bearing surface

FIG 7-1 Mid-Sagittal Section of the Human Temporomandibular Joint (1) The extent of the central bearing surface of the interarticular disk. (2) The thickness of articular tissue varies, being thickest in those areas under greatest functional shear stress and load. This is illustrated in the lower right of the diagram where the surface tissues of the articulation are shown varying in thickness in the condyle, disk, and temporal component. The dark areas represent the relative thicknesses, confirming that function occurs between condyle and articular tubercle rather than between condyle and fossa. (3) The anterior thick band (or foot) of the interarticular disk is bound down on the medial third to the superior surface of the superior lateral pterygoid muscle. Most muscle fibers insert into the condylar fovea. Some muscle fibers insert into a junctional zone between upper and lower head of the lateral pterygoid muscle, which then inserts into the fovea. More laterally, the anterior thick band attaches to the anterior capsular ligament. (Redrawn with permission from Klineberg 1991.)

against the posterior slope of the articular eminence (Figure 7-1). This position is independent of tooth contact. RP and CR describe similar clinical anatomical relationships. It is the condylar position at RP or CR which is used for clinical recording of the jaw (or maxillomandibular) relationship for transfer of casts of the teeth and jaws to an anatomical articulator.

- *Postural jaw position* (PJP) is the position of the jaw in a relaxed and alert individual sitting or standing upright. There is variable space between maxillary and mandibular teeth, termed *free-way* or *speaking* space. The PJP is determined by the

weight of the jaw and the viscoelastic structural elements of the postural jaw muscles, tendons, and ligaments, as well as myotatic reflex contraction of postural muscles. This contraction is brought about by stretching of muscle spindles, which activates alpha-motoneurons innervating the extrafusal muscle fibers of the jaw-closing muscles. PJP is important in the assessment of lower face height (lower third of the face as a proportion of the overall facial proportions) and in determining the occlusal vertical dimension (OVD) in treatment planning for dentate and edentulous patients.

- *OVD* is the vertical height of the lower third of the face when the teeth are in contact in ICP. The lower third of the face is an important component of facial aesthetics and is an essential element of treatment planning in conjunction with PJP. The free-way or speaking space is a variable separation of the teeth between PJP and OVD and is an important determinant with anterior tooth position and orientation of speech clarity and verbal communication. As a result, dental restorations may have a significant influence on speech in both dentate and edentulous treatments.
- *Lateral jaw positions*: The terms "nonworking or balancing" and "working or nonbalancing" are articulator (mechanical) terms. The biological or anatomical terms are "ipsilateral" (working) and "contralateral or mediotrusive" (nonworking).
  - *Mediotrusive* (nonworking or balancing) side refers to the side of the jaw which moves toward the midline (or medially) in lateral jaw movements. The term "balancing" may also be understood in functional terms as the "nonworking" side, that is, the side opposite the chewing side.
  - The term nonworking side is considered in the analysis of casts on an articulator and in the arrangement of the teeth for removable prostheses—complete or partial dentures—in which nonworking or balancing tooth contacts may be a desirable arrangement in prosthesis construction. The term is also used in clinical occlusal analysis to identify the arrangement of teeth and the presence of mediotrusive (balancing or nonworking) tooth contacts or interferences.
  - *Laterotrusive* (or working) side refers to the side of the jaw that moves laterally away from the midline in jaw movement. This may also be termed the "working" or chewing side in function; that is, the side where chewing occurs.
  - A particular aspect of laterotrusive jaw movement is the number and arrangement of the teeth that are in contact in lateral jaw movement or laterotrusion. This may also be termed *disclusion*. Disclusion may involve the anterior teeth only—if the canine tooth only, it is termed *canine disclusion*; when it involves incisor and canine teeth it is termed *anterior disclusion*. It may involve posterior teeth only—bicuspid and/or molar teeth, which is termed *posterior disclusion*, or both anterior and posterior teeth, which is termed *group function*.
- *Bennett movement* and *Bennett angle* are terms originally described by Sir Norman Bennett (British dentist 1870-1947) in 1906. Bennett conducted the first clinical study that identified lateral or sideward movement of the jaw and differentiated the bilateral features of condyle movement with remarkable clarity from movement of a light source in one subject (Bennett himself).
  - *Bennett movement* describes a lateral component of movement of the condyle with laterotrusive jaw movement. Bennett described a lateral horizontal component of movement, which has also been described in relation to the setting of articulator condylar guidance as "immediate side shift" (ISS). The latter is strictly an articulator term. There is some evidence from three-dimensional (six degrees of freedom) clinical recordings (Gibbs & Lundeen 1982) that Bennett movement occurs in function, in some individuals, at the end of the closing path of a chewing movement.
  - *Bennett angle* is the angle formed by movement of the contralateral condyle with the sagittal plane during lateral jaw movement. The contralateral (mediotrusive or balancing) condyle moves downward, forward and medially, forming an angle (Bennett angle) with the sagittal plane when viewed anteriorly (from the front) or superiorly (from above).
  - The articulator term for movement of the contralateral (or balancing) condyle is "progressive side shift" (PSS).

OCCLUSAL RELATIONSHIPS

Occlusion and Temporomandibular Disorders

Confusion remains concerning what defines optimum occlusal relationships; however, evidence is now clear that there is no valid association of occlusal variables and temporomandibular disorder (TMD).

In attempting to define optimum occlusal relationships, it is acknowledged that stable occlusal relationships are the norm in the population, even though there is great variation in craniofacial morphology and functional features. The broad range of structural characteristics matches the general ranges of body size, shape, posture, and gait and is expected across any group or population.

There are no controlled studies on the optimum features of a harmonious natural and/or restored occlusion. Earlier studies (Pullinger & Seligman 2000, Seligman & Pullinger 2000, Tsukiyama et al. 2001) on the relationship between occlusal variables and TMDs provided a clue. However, it needs to be emphasized that there is no relationship between the way the teeth contact or the number of tooth contacts and TMD. Overwhelmingly, contemporary studies refute any such association (Clark et al. 1999, Stohler 2004, DeBoever et al. 2008, Greene 2006, 2011).

The studies by Pullinger and Seligman (2000) and Seligman and Pullinger (2000) investigated 12 independent variables, together with age, and reported a significant overlap of occlusal features between asymptomatic control subjects and patients with TMDs. These data are of interest as they suggested that asymptomatic controls were characterized by:
- A small amount of anterior attrition
- Small or no RCP-ICP slide (<1.75 mm)
- Absence of extreme overjet (<5.25 mm)
- Absence of unilateral posterior crossbite

However, sensitivity (61%) and specificity (51%) in these studies did not reach appropriately high levels (>75% and >90%, respectively) to support undisputed evidence of association. An absence of any identifiable link between changes in the occlusal scheme with dental and or orthodontic treatment and the development of TMDs is the prevailing understanding based on validated data from clinical trials (Marklund & Wänman 2010, Turp & Schindler 2012). In light of these contemporary data, it can be concluded that variations in occlusal morphology or management are not associated with TMDs and are acceptable as optimum for the individual.

Importantly, any association between occlusal variables and TMD signs and symptoms is weak, and statistical associations do not indicate a causal relationship. Furthermore, a number of occlusal variables are likely to have arisen as a result of TMD not as a preceding factor. Such a view was first postulated in the classic publication of Laskin (1969), and has been verified by contemporary studies (Turp & Schindler 2012).

The recognition of an absence of any role for occlusal variables in TMDs is significant and justifiably replaces the emphasis previously given to occlusion and its etiological role in TMD.

Therapeutic Occlusions

In contrast with natural occlusions, therapeutic restoration requires a systematic approach to optimize outcomes. There is now significant clinical research to justify, on evidence-based terms, a specific occlusal design to confidently address each patient's needs according to these powerful clinical guidelines:

- Establish an appropriate OVD at tooth contact for aesthetics (lower face height proportionally) and functions of speech, mastication, and swallowing. It may also be necessary to increase interocclusal distance to provide adequate space for restorations.
- Harmonize tooth contacts (MI) with a stable position of the condyles, ideally in an unstrained condylar position with interarticular disks appropriately aligned, to allow fluent function between condyle and eminence.
- The specific tooth contact pattern requires cusp-fossa and cusp-marginal ridge contacts to provide stable tooth relationships (Wang & Mehta 2013). There is no clinical evidence for more complex tooth contact patterns such as tripodized contacts.
- Data from a laboratory Finite Element Analysis (FEA) analysis on cuspal inclination (Rungsiyakull et al. 2011) indicate differential load concentration at the coronal region of the tooth root or implant with lower loads when low cusp inclination and smaller occlusal table are used (Figure 7-2). These occlusal features are recommended for clinical rehabilitation.
- An increased number of tooth contacts influences bite force. Clinical research (Wang et al. 2010, 2013, Gonzales et al. 2011, Nishigawa et al. 2012) based on an acknowledged protocol has evaluated tooth contacts (stable occlusion) and bite force (at maximum voluntary clench [MVC] and recorded jaw muscle electromyography [EMG]).
  Data indicate that bite force level varies ($P < 0.05$) significantly with the number of tooth

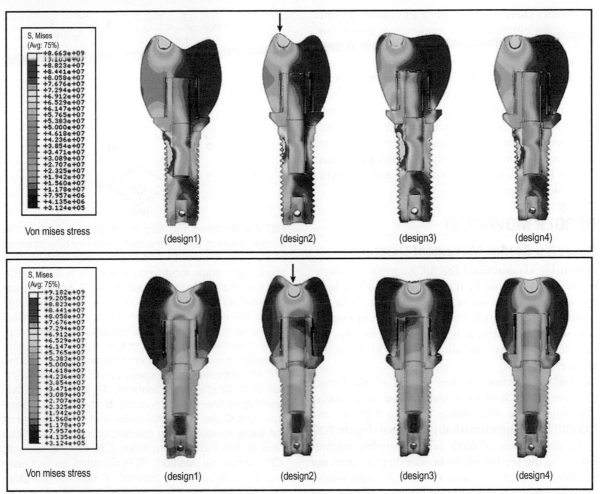

FIG 7-2 Longitudinal Section of a Bicuspid Crown Cemented onto a Single Implant and Subjected to Occlusal Loading Stress distributions (MPa) on the implant and simulated bone with loading of the crown at 2 mm along the cusp incline (upper images) and in the central fossa (lower images). Note stress concentration at the coronal margin in upper images compared with lower.

contacts. With a greater number of tooth contacts that are bilaterally distributed there is:

(a) greater bite force generated.

(b) a reduction in the surface EMG. Specifically, with an increase from 50% MVC to 100% MVC, the number of occlusal contacts increased bilaterally by 50%, but the surface EMG of anterior temporalis and masseter muscles decreased.

It appears that the dominant role of periodontal mechanoreceptor feedback (to jaw muscle motoneurons) is modulated by trigeminal and central neural circuitry through unloading reflexes to protect the joint and periodontal tissues.

In addition, jaw elevator-muscle bite force is reduced preceding peak force as a stable IC is reached.

These new data (Wang et al. 2013) confirm the complexity of bite force–jaw muscle control and the subtle inbuilt protective mechanisms.

- Anterior tooth arrangement (see also the Canine Guidance section) is crucial for aesthetics and speech. There is no evidence to indicate a preference for either anterior guidance or group function (Marklund & Wänman 2000, Yang et al. 2000). However, in a consideration of the biomechanics of lateral tooth contact, anterior guidance resulted in reduced bite force as well as reduction in the reaction force at the condyles (Belser & Hannam 1985). Smooth lateral and protrusive movements support fluent function and are important in optimizing jaw muscle activity. Further, group function is associated with tooth wear and is a feature of older dentition.

BORDER MOVEMENT

Posselt's Border Movement Diagram

Posselt (1952) described the full range of jaw movement in three planes by tracing the path of the lower incisor teeth as the jaw is guided through the border paths. The border path traces the maximum range of jaw movement, which is determined by the jaw muscles, ligaments, limitations of the TM joints, and the teeth.

The teeth define the top section of the border diagram, which is of particular interest in restorative dentistry, as the relationship between ICP (IP) and CO (RCP) is diagrammatically indicated (Figure 7-3).

In the absence of teeth (as in complete edentulism), the top section of the border diagram does not differentiate ICP (IP) and CO (RCP). The border diagram may be displayed in sagittal, frontal, and horizontal planes. The sagittal plane view of the border movement of the jaw in dentate individuals, as defined by the movement of the lower incisor teeth, shows features of particular interest:

- The top of the border path is defined by the position and cuspal inclines of the teeth (Figure 7-3: ICP to RCP, ICP to Pr).
- The retruded path is defined by the anatomy of the TM joints (Figure 7-3: RCP to H; H to O).

ANTERIOR OR LATERAL GUIDANCE

The physical features of tooth guidance vary with tooth arrangement and interarch relationships. Anterior guidance is provided by the vertical (overbite) and horizontal or anteroposterior (overjet) relationships of anterior teeth. Posterior guidance is

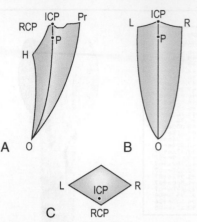

FIG 7-3 A shows the sagittal (or profile) view of the border diagram with the anteroposterior relationships of ICP, RCP, and Pr. This view also shows that the lower incisor tooth movement from ICP to RCP requires the jaw to be guided into RCP. Lower incisor movement from RCP to H follows a curved path indicating the initial rotatory movement of the condyles. This is also described as rotation around the intercondylar or terminal hinge axis, that is, the axis of rotation between the condyles when they are guided around CR. The movement changes from rotation to translation (H to O) after approximately 15 to 20 mm of jaw opening at the lower incisors. **B** shows the frontal view and **C** the horizontal view of the movement of the lower incisors along the border path. The sagittal view is the most informative. *CR*, Centric relation; *ICP*, intercuspal position; *RCP*, retruded contact position; *Pr*, protruded jaw position; *P*, postural jaw position; *O*, maximum jaw opening; *H*, hinge arc of opening. Approximate range of jaw movement in adults: RCP to ICP 0.5 to 2.0 mm; ICP to O 40 to 70 mm; RCP to H 15 to 20 mm; P to ICP 2 to 4 mm; ICP to Pr 5 to 10 mm.

determined by the relationships of supporting cuspal inclines, particularly of opposing molar teeth. Posterior guidance may be increased in the presence of missing teeth, with tilting and drifting of teeth, and by the degree of curvature of the occlusal plane anteroposteriorly (curve of Spee) and laterally (curve of Wilson). As a result of tooth arrangement variability, functional tooth guidance is individually specific and directly influences the approach and departure angle of mandibular to maxillary teeth with each

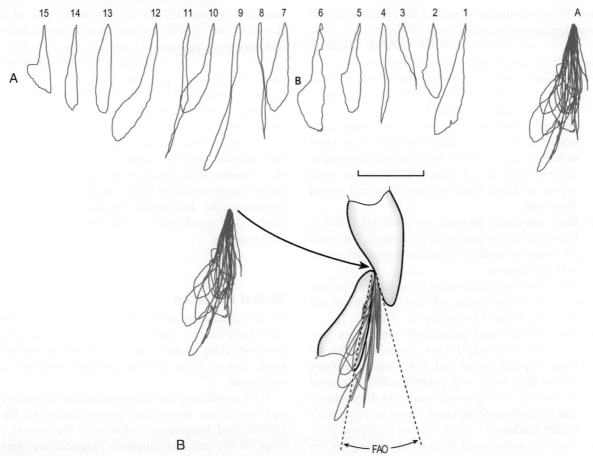

FIG 7-4 A, Tracings 1 to 15 represent individual recordings of human chewing cycles (or envelopes) obtained by monitoring the movements of the lower incisor tooth while chewing gum. The movement of the lower incisor teeth was recorded with a Kinesiograph (K5 Myo-tronics Research Inc., Seattle, Washington), via a magnet cemented at the incisors, and movement of the magnet was recorded with an array of sensors (flux-gate magnetometers) attached to a headframe. Note the individual variations in each chewing cycle. The 15 cycles comprise the functional envelope of movement for this individual. Scale bar = 10 mm. **B,** Tracings of the lower incisor tooth obtained as in **A** while chewing gum. The composite envelope of function is composed of the 15 individual chewing cycles shown in **A.** The relationship of the functional envelope to the incisor teeth is shown and the functional angle of occlusion (FAO) represents the approach and departure of the lower incisors into and from tooth contact.

chewing cycle. This is termed the functional angle of occlusion in chewing. The *chewing cycle* is also termed the *envelope of function*, details of the superior part of which are determined by the tooth guidance (Figure 7-4).

The functional loading of teeth and the associated stimulation of periodontal and associated mechanoreceptors provide a reference point for tooth contact

and establish a beginning and end of jaw movement in mastication and swallowing (Trulsson 2006).

CANINE GUIDANCE

Data reported by Trulsson and colleagues from human microneurographic recordings of periodontal afferents have identified that periodontal mechanoreceptors (located in periodontal tissues supporting tooth roots) provide precise signals of the effects of vertical and horizontal forces on teeth (Trulsson et al. 1992, Trulsson and Johansson 1994, 1996a,b, Trulsson 2006). Such mechanoreceptors are especially sensitive to low forces, and anterior and posterior teeth have different load thresholds, described in terms of dynamic and static sensitivity:

a. Dynamic sensitivity—anterior teeth respond to low forces of <1.0 N and posterior teeth respond to higher forces >4.0 N. Anterior teeth respond to varying loads in all directions; posterior teeth appear to detect loads only on distal and lingual directions.

b. Static sensitivity increases progressively, which is important in the control of increases in bite force on posterior teeth to generate the power stroke with mastication.

The clinical implications of these findings are significant and define specific roles for both anterior and posterior teeth (see Klineberg et al. 2012):

a. Anterior teeth and particularly canines are anatomically designed (robust crown with lingual ridge dividing mesial and distal lingual surfaces, and a long root) and periodontally innervated to respond with greatest sensitivity to anteriorly and anterolaterally directed forces as occurs with canine guidance.

b. Posterior periodontal innervation is designed for the control of vertical (distolingual) and lateral forces and the generation of large bite forces for mastication on posterior teeth.

In addition, the lingual surface of maxillary canine teeth may influence condyle-disk movement. As already indicated, the prominent lingual axial ridge provides mesial or distal guidance, depending on where the opposing tooth makes contact in lateral jaw movements. Lateral guidance on the distal canine surface may direct the ipsilateral (working) jaw distally, while initial tooth contact on the mesial canine incline may direct the jaw mesially. This may influence condyle-disk relationships; evidence of association with this clinically observed influence has been reported by Yang et al. (2000) and is supported by geometrical assessment (Figure 7-5).

Distal Guidance

During function or parafunction (tooth grinding), if anterior tooth guidance restricts the anterior com-

ponent of movement (as is seen in the case of a deep bite), the closing jaw movement follows a more distal approach path to tooth contact. The more distal approach to tooth contact may also arise as a result of distal guidance from the canine that restricts forward translation in jaw closing. The more distally directed movement requires a predominance of condyle rotation.

It is hypothesized that with more rotation, the interarticular disk may more readily rotate beyond the posterior thick band of the disk and become trapped anteromedially. With translation, in contrast to rotation, the disk moves with the condyle, maintaining the condyle-disk relationship against the eminence.

Mesial Guidance

Mesial guidance along the mesial canine incline may allow both rotation and translation. As a result, the jaw closes along a more anterior path and approaches tooth contact from a more anterior direction of movement.

It is hypothesized that this combination of rotation and translation encourages approximation of the condyle and interarticular disk with the posterior slope of the articular eminence, maintaining their contact relationships.

The association between mesial or distal canine guidance in lateral jaw movements and the effect at the condyle is complex and linked with jaw muscle activity and resolution of force vectors, as well as condyle-disk relationships. There is some clinical research evidence correlating distal canine guidance with a more posterior condylar path (Yang et al. 2000). Yang et al. described a correlation between distal canine guidance; that is, a retrusive laterotrusive path and a lateral and posterior movement of the ipsilateral (working) condyle. In contrast, mesial canine guidance resulted in lateral and inferior movement of the ipsilateral condyle.

It is acknowledged that clinical studies to correlate jaw muscle activity with condyle disk relationships and determine the influence of canine guidance are difficult. The sophistication of equipment needed for accurately tracking condyle movement is a limitation, and the solution to the problem of

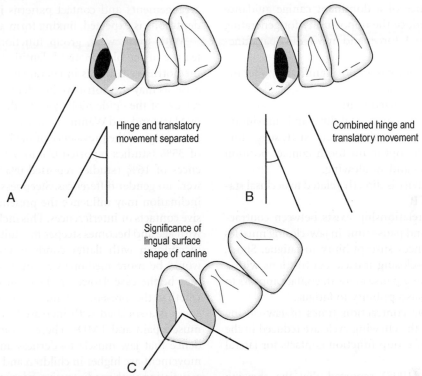

Hinge and translatory
movement separated

Combined hinge and
translatory movement

Significance of
lingual surface
shape of canine

FIG 7-5 Anterior Guidance—Functional Angle of Occlusion A, Anterior guidance on the distal incline of the ipsilateral canine tends to separate the distal hinge and translatory jaw movements, which may direct the condyle and disk along a more distal path and away from the eminence. **B,** Anterior guidance on the mesial incline of the ipsilateral canine tooth tends to provide a combined hinge and translatory movement, which may direct the condyle and disk along a more anterior path toward the eminence. **C,** The lingual contour of the maxillary canine has a longitudinal ridge which divides the lingual surface into distinct mesial and distal fossae. The opposing teeth (ideally the mandibular canine) may contact the distal or mesial fossa, and lateral jaw guidance will be different in each case. The distal fossa will tend to direct the jaw along a more distal (posterior) path and the mesial fossa will tend to direct the jaw along a more mesial path.

identifying an appropriate point within the condyle for three-dimensional measurement has not been standardized (Peck et al. 1999).

Although not necessarily a feature of the natural dentition, with clinical restoration of the dentition it is considered desirable to avoid mediotrusive (non-working) and laterotrusive (working) interferences (Wassell & Steele 1998, Becker et al. 2000). The presence of guidance on canines is also preferred as a restorative convenience, although group function, where several teeth provide simultaneous lateral guidance, may lead less readily to muscle fatigue (Bakke 1993).

A number of clinical physiological studies with EMG and/or jaw tracking have attempted to deter-

mine the features of anterior guidance and have helped in understanding the complexity of the neuromuscular control of mastication, as follows:

- Less muscle force is generated with anterior tooth contact only (Manns et al. 1987), and maximum muscle force is developed with molar tooth contact; guidance from the anterior part of the jaw results in resolution of muscle force vectors to guide the jaw smoothly into IP.
- Belser and Hannam (1985) reported that:
  - There is no scientific evidence to indicate that either canine guidance or group function is more desirable.
  - The steepness of the anterior guidance is not of primary importance.

- The presence of a dominant canine guidance tends to reduce the opportunity for generating high interarch forces and may reduce parafunctional loads.
- Canine guidance does not significantly alter the masticatory stroke.
- Bakke (1993) reported that:
  - Maximum occlusal stability and maximum elevator muscle activity occur at IP, suggesting that it is the optimum tooth contact position for chewing and swallowing.
  - Muscle activity is directly related to occlusal stability in ICP.
  - A critical relationship exists between contraction time and pause time in jaw-closing muscles and influences susceptibility to fatigue. Short, strong jaw-closing muscle contractions with a relatively long pause at tooth contact appears to minimize susceptibility to fatigue.
  - The relative contraction times of jaw-closing muscles in the chewing cycle are reduced in the presence of group function contacts for lateral guidance.
- Ogawa et al. (1998) reported that the chewing cycle is influenced by occlusal guidance and occlusal plane inclination. Their studies used chewing gum and recorded three-dimensional movement of jaw and condyle in relation to tooth guidance and occlusal plane orientation. They concluded that:
  - Both tooth guidance and occlusal plane orientation influence the form of the chewing cycle.
  - Occlusal guidance (overbite and overjet) influences the sagittal and frontal closing paths over the final 0.5 mm of jaw movement into tooth contact.
  - The occlusal plane angle influences the sagittal and frontal closing paths over the final 2.0 to 5.0 mm of jaw movement into tooth contact (Figure 7-4).

MEDIOTRUSIVE (BALANCING) CONTACTS OR INTERFERENCES

Canine or anterior guidance is often present in the natural dentition of young individuals; however, tooth orientation in growth and development may result in posterior guidance. The variation in tooth arrangements and contact patterns in healthy adult dentitions is expected, linking form and function.

With tooth wear, group function develops as a feature of the older natural dentition. In the process, mediotrusive contacts in lateral jaw movements may arise, as may mediotrusive interferences. A systematic review of the epidemiology of mediotrusive contacts by Marklund and Wänman (2000) suggested a median percentage of the prevalence of mediotrusive contacts of 35% (studies reported 0% to 97%) and interferences of 16% (studies reported 0% to 77%). There were no gender differences. Steepness of the condylar inclination may influence the presence of mediotrusive contacts or interferences. This inclination changes with age and becomes steeper in adults. It follows that in children with flatter condylar inclinations there would be more mediotrusive interferences, and this may be the case. However, the clinical significance is whether the presence of these contacts or interferences is associated with increased prevalence of jaw muscle pain and TMDs. There is some reported evidence that jaw muscle tenderness and impaired jaw movement are higher in children and young adults in association with mediotrusive interferences; however, the evidence is weak.

Contemporary evidence indicates that:
- There is no direct cause-and-effect relationship between posterior tooth contact and either jaw muscle pain or TMDs (see reviews by Clark et al. 1999, Clark 2006, Stohler 2006).
- Other factors are involved in the etiology of TMDs (Stohler 2004, Greene 2011).

A biomechanical study of mediotrusive contacts and clenching by Baba et al. (2001) reported that canine guidance caused a small displacement at the ipsilateral molars and the largest displacement at the contralateral molars. A similar effect on condyle position is suggested, leading to limited compression of the ipsilateral joint and larger compression of the contralateral joint. It is possible that TM joint compression arising in this way may alter the biomechanical relationships of jaw muscles, condyle, and disk, but such minor changes would be accommodated by the adaptive capacity of the jaw muscle system.

EMG studies have confirmed specific changes in jaw muscles with mediotrusive and/or laterotrusive contacts, but no direct association with TMDs.

Recent studies on the influence of tooth contact interferences on jaw and joint position and jaw muscles suggest that:

- Specific changes in the occlusal scheme, such as placing mediotrusive (balancing) or laterotrusive (working) interferences and canine guidance, cause predictable changes in jaw orientation (or tilt) with clenching (Minagi et al. 1997, Baba et al. 2001).

- Biomechanical associations may occur as a result. However, interpretations of such changes need to recognize the biology and adaptive capacity of the jaw muscle system instead of a strictly mechanical interpretation.
  - A mediotrusive interference and heavy bite force or clenching establish a lever arm with the interference as the fulcrum, leading to greater elevation of the ipsilateral molars and possible compression of the ipsilateral TM joint with a change in reaction force (Belser & Hannam 1985, Korioth & Hannam 1994, Baba et al. 2001).
  - The presence of canine guidance eliminates mediotrusive interferences and changes the biomechanical effects of bite force and clenching on the TM joint.

- Baba et al. (2001) showed that ipsilateral contact from canine to bicuspids to molars (that is, group function) with clenching leads to contralateral jaw elevation and joint compression. Canine guidance results in minimal joint compression, while ipsilateral molar contact interference with clench leads to greater contralateral joint compression. The implications of such biomechanical changes with clenching are unclear but need to be understood within the adaptive capacity of the system.
  - Balanced occlusion appears to provide a "protective role" for the joints and may not lead to an increase in either ipsilateral or contralateral TM joint compression.
  - In support of this biochemical situation, Minagi et al. (1997) found a positive correlation between the absence of contralateral (mediotrusive) tooth contacts and increased prevalence of joint sounds. The corollary from this study is that mediotrusive contacts may have a protective role for the joint in association with jaw clenching.

- In EMG studies, canine guidance results in increased unilateral anterior and posterior temporal muscle activity. The presence of mediotrusive (balancing side) contacts recruits contralateral jaw muscles and results in bilateral anterior and posterior temporal activity (Belser & Hannam 1985, Baba et al. 2001, Minagi et al. 1997).

SHORTENED DENTAL ARCH

It has been consistently reported that individuals may have satisfactory aesthetics and occlusal function with fewer posterior teeth (Käyser 2000, Wolfart et al. 2005, Walter et al. 2010). These data have led to the so-called shortened dental arch (SDA) concept and the realization that it is not essential to replace missing posterior teeth.

Of particular interest in the management of the occlusion is the recognition of the concept of the SDA as a viable treatment option. This section concerns specific tooth contact relationships and the controversial effects of clenching on the TM joints and describes studies based on the presence of posterior (bicuspid and molar) teeth.

In the absence of the molar and possibly bicuspid teeth, the specific lever arm effects and TM joint reaction forces from loading would be reduced. Whether or not this is advantageous to the jaw muscle system would depend on remaining tooth distribution and their ability to withstand functional and parafunctional loading.

More importantly, the often claimed association between the lack of posterior teeth predisposing to TM joint loading and the possible development of TMD is not supported by clinical studies. Long-term data on the clinical effects of the SDA indicates that the absence of molar teeth does not predispose to TMD or orofacial pain and allows adequate function for long-term health of the jaw muscle system.

The minimum number of teeth needed for function varies with individuals. The goal of maintaining a complete dental arch, although theoretically desirable, may not be attainable or necessary. The SDA data have confirmed through long-term studies that the anterior and premolar segments meet all functional requirements—20 occluding teeth (Käyser 2000). See Chapter 3 for further clarification of the implications of the SDA.

When priorities have to be set, restorative treatment should preserve the most strategic anterior and premolar segments. The need for partial dentures or complex treatment to restore molar segments (implant, bridgework, endodontics, and root and tooth resection) should be questioned and based on individual patient wishes.

REFERENCES

Baba K, Yugami K, Yaka T, et al: Impact of balancing-side tooth contact on clenching-induced mandibular displacement in humans, *J Oral Rehab* 28:721–727, 2001.

Bakke M: Mandibular elevator muscles: physcology, action, and effect of dental occlusion, *J Dental Res* 101:314–331, 1993.

Becker CM, Kaiser DA, Schwalm C: Mandibular centricity: centric relation, *J Prosth Dent* 83:158–160, 2000.

Belser UC, Hannam AG: The influence of altering working-side occlusal guidance on masticatory muscles and related jaw movement, *J Prosth Dent* 53:406–414, 1985.

Clark GT: Treatment of myogenous pain and dysfunction. In Easkin DM, Greene CS, Hylander WL, editors: *TMDs: An Evidence Based Approach to Diagnosis and Treatment*, Chicago, 2006, Quintessence, pp 483–500.

Clark GT, Tsukiyama Y, Baba K, et al: Sixty-eight years of experimental interference studies: what have we learned? *J Prosth Dent* 82:704–713, 1999.

DeBoever JA, Nilner M, Orthlieb JD, et al: Recommendations by the EACD for examination, diagnosis, and management of patients with temporomandibular disorders and orofacial pain by the general dental practitioner, *J Orofacial Pain* 22:268–278, 2008.

Gibbs CH, Lundeen HC: Jaw movements and forces during chewing and swallowing and their clinical significance. In Lundeen HC, Gibbs CH, editors: *Advances in Occlusion*, Boston, 1982, Wright, pp 2–32.

Gonzales Y, Iwasaki LR, McCall WD Jr, et al: Reliability of electromyographic activity vs bite-force from human masticatory muscles, *European J Oral Sci* 119:219–224, 2011.

Greene CS: Concepts of TMD etiology: Effects on diagnosis and treatment. Chapt 14. In Laskin DM, Greene CS, Hylander WL, editors: *Temporomandiular Disorders—An Evidence-based Approach to Diagnosis and Treatment*, Chicago, 2006, Quintessence, pp 219–228.

Greene CS: Relationship between occlusion and temporomandibular disorders: Implications for the orthodontist, *American J Ortho Dent Orth* 139:11–15, 2011.

Käyser AF: Limited treatment goals—shortened dental arches, *Periodont* 4:7–14, 2000.

Klineberg I: *Occlusion Principles and Assessment*, Boston, 1991, Wright-Butterworth-Heinemann Ltd.

Klineberg IJ, Trulsson M, Murray G: Occlusion on implants—is there a problem? *J Oral Rehab* 39:1–16, 2012.

Korioth TW, Hannam AG: Mandibular forces during simulated tooth clenching, *J Orofacial Pain* 8:178–189, 1994.

Laskin DM: Etiology of the pain-dysfunction syndrome, *J Am Dent Assn* 79:147–153, 1969.

Manns A, Chan C, Miralles R: Influence of group function and canine guidance on electromyographic activity of elevator muscles, *J Prosth Dent* 57:494–501, 1987.

Marklund S, Wänman A: A century of controversy regarding the benefit or detriment of occlusal contacts on the mediotrusive side, *J Oral Rehab* 27:553–562, 2000.

Marklund S, Wänman A: Risk factors associated with incidence and persistence of signs and symptoms of temporomandibular disorders, *Acta Odont Scand* 68:289–299, 2010.

McNamara DC: The clinical significance of median occlusal position, *J Oral Rehab* 5:173–186, 1977.

Minagi G, Ohtsuki H, Sato T, et al: Effect of balancing-side occlusion on the ipsilateral TMJ dynamics under clenching, *J Oral Rehab* 24:57–62, 1997.

Nishigawa K, Suzuki Y, Ishikawa T, et al: Effect of occlusal contact stabiliaty on the jaw closing point during tapping movements, *J Prosth Res* 56:130–135, 2012.

Ogawa T, Koyano K, Umemoto G: Inclination of the occlusal plane and occlusal guidance as contributing factors in mastication, *J Dent* 26:641–647, 1998.

Peck CC, Murray GM, Johnson CWL, et al: Trajectories of condylar points during working-side excursive movements of the mandible, *J Prosth Dent* 81:444–452, 1999.

Posselt U: Studies in the mobility of the human mandible, *Acta Odont Scand* 10:1–160, 1952.

Pullinger AG, Seligman DA: Quantification and validation of predictive values of occlusal variables in temporomandibular disorders using a multi-factorial analysis, *J Prosth Dent* 83:66–75, 2000.

Riise C, Ericsson SG: A clinical study of the distribution of occlusal tooth contacts in the intercuspal position in light and hard pressure in adults, *J Oral Rehab* 10:473–480, 1983.

Rungsiyakull P, Rungsiyakull C, Appleyard R, et al: Loading of a single implant in simulated bone, *Int J Prosths* 24:140–143, 2011.

Seligman DA, Pullinger AG: Analysis of occlusal variables, dental attrition, and age for distinguishing healthy controls from female patients with intra capsular temporomandibular disorders, *J Prosth Dent* 83:76–82, 2000.

Stohler CS: Taking stock: from chasing occlusal contacts to vulnerability alleles, *Orth Cran Res* 7:157–160, 2004.

Stohler CS: Management of dental occlusion. In Lasken DM, Greene CS, Hylander WL, editors: *TMDs: An Evidence Based Approach to Diagnosis and Treatment*, Chicago, 2006, Quintessence, pp 403–411.

Trulsson M: Sensory motor function of human periodontal mechanoreceptors, *J Oral Rehab* 33:262–273, 2006.

Trulsson M, Johansson RS: Encoding of amplitude and rate of forces applied to the teeth by human periodontal mechanoreceptive afferents, *J Neurophys* 72:1734–1744, 1994.

Trulsson M, Johansson RS: Encoding of tooth loads by human periodontal afferents and their role in jaw motor control, *Prog Neurobiol* 49:267–284, 1996a.

Trulsson M, Johansson RS: Forces applied by the increases and roles of periodontal afferents during food-holding and biting tasks, *Exp Brain Res* 107:486–496, 1996b.

Trulsson M, Johansson RS, Olsson KA: Directional sensitivity of human periodontal mechanoreceptive afferents to forces applied to the teeth, *J Physiol* 447:373–389, 1992.

Tsukiyama Y, Baba K, Clark GT: An evidence-based assessment of occlusal adjustment as a treatment for temporomandibular disorders, *J Prosth Dent* 86:57–66, 2001.

Turp JC, Schindler H: The dental occlusion as a suspected cause for TMDs: epidemiological and etiological considerations, *J Oral Rehab* 39:502–512, 2012.

Walter MH, Weber A, Marré B, et al: The randomized shortened dental arch study: tooth loss, *J Dent Res* 89:818–822, 2010.

Wang M, Mehta N: A possible biomechanical role of occlusal cusp-fossa contact relationships, *J Oral Rehab* 40:69–79, 2013.

Wang MQ, He JJ, Zhang JH, et al: SEMG activity of jaw-closing muscles during biting with different unilateral occlusal supports, *J Oral Rehab* 37:719–725, 2010.

Wang XR, Zhang Y, Xing N, et al: Stable tooth contacts in intercuspal occlusion makes for utilities of the jaw elevators during maximal voluntary clenching, *J Oral Rehab* 40:319–328, 2013.

Wassell RW, Steele JG: Considerations when planning occlusal rehabilitation: a review of the literature, *Int Dent J* 48:571–581, 1998.

Wolfart S, Heydecke G, Luthardt RG, et al: Effects of prosthetic treatment for shortened dental arches on oral health-related quality of life, self-reports of pain and jaw disability: results from the pilot-phase of a randomized multicentre trial, *J Oral Rehab* 32:815–822, 2005.

Yang Y, Yatabe M, Ai M, et al: The relation of canine guidance with laterotrusive movements at the incisal point and the working-side condyle, *J Oral Rehab* 27:911–917, 2000.

Further Reading

Forssell H, Kalso E, Koskela P, et al: Occlusal treatments in temporomandibular disorders: a qualitative systematic review of randomised controlled trials, *Pain* 83:549–560, 1999.

Kirveskari P, Jamsa T, Alanen P: Occlusal adjustment and the incidence of demand for temporomandibular disorder treatment, *J Prosth Dent* 79:433–438, 1998.

McNamara JA, Seligman DA, Okeson JP: Occlusion, orthodontic treatment and temporomandibular disorders. A review, *J Orofacial Pain* 9:73–90, 1995.

CHAPTER 8

Occlusal Diagnostics for Treatment Planning

Iven Klineberg

SYNOPSIS

In treatment planning, an assessment of the teeth and their relationship with the jaw muscle system is an integral part of diagnosis. A broad distribution of tooth contacts disperses force vectors from function and parafunction over many teeth and reduces force concentration on a limited number of teeth.

Clinical occlusal analysis allows a detailed assessment of tooth contacts in retruded contact position (RCP), intercuspal contact positions (ICP) or its dynamic equivalent median occlusal position (MOP), and lateral and protrusive jaw excursions. Modification of tooth contacts in these jaw positions may be indicated in restorative care. Occlusal adjustment and selective grinding are discussed in Chapter 21.

Indications of parafunctional tooth wear are described and the value of provocation tests linked with bruxofacets is discussed. Provocation tests may indicate an association between the particular tooth-wear pattern with jaw posture and orofacial symptoms. This information may be of importance in restorative treatment planning.

CHAPTER POINTS

- Jaw guidance techniques are described
- Tooth contacts in MOP and RCP are identified with ultrafine plastic tapes, and their relevance is indicated
- Lateral guidance, balancing contacts or interferences, and mediotrusive contacts or interferences are specified
- Bruxofacets are identified as evidence of parafunction with discussion of whether a combination of attrition and erosion is present
- Provocation tests are described to determine whether they evoke clinical symptoms:
  - Temporomandibular (TM) joint provocation test to determine the presence of TM joint pain or discomfort with clenching on a unilateral posterior support
  - Jaw muscle provocation test to determine the effect on jaw muscles of clenching in intercuspal position (ICP)

("centric bruxing") and clenching on opposing bruxofacets

Occlusion represents static and dynamic tooth relationships and the integrated action of the jaw muscles and temporomandibular (TM) joints (see Chapter 7). A comprehensive assessment of occlusion includes:

- Assessment of the positional relationships of the teeth and interarch tooth contacts in "centric" and eccentric jaw positions
- Jaw mobility measurement to determine TM joint function
- Jaw muscle palpation following a defined protocol

The comprehensive protocol for the assessment of TM joints and occlusion was described by Helkimo in 1972 and is known as the Helkimo Dysfunction Index. More recently a validated protocol—the Research Diagnostic Criteria for Temporomandibular Disorders (RCD/TMD) of Dworkin & LeResche (1992)—has been accepted as the international benchmark for temporomandibular dysfunction (TMD) assessment (Truelove et al. 1992). This specific clinical approach became the accepted standard TMD assessment protocol and follows studies on validation of data collection by clinicians calibrated against a gold standard. This development has been an important step in standardizing clinical assessment to justify comparison of clinical studies. The most recent revision of the RCD/TMD approach has been considered by a collaborative group and is now termed Diagnostic Criteria for Temporomandibular Disorder (DC/TMD) (Schiffman et al. 2014).

In addition, the American Association for Dental Research has approved a new "Standard of Care" for management of patients with TMDs (Greene CS, American Association for Dental Research see http://www.aadronline.com/i4a/pages/index.cfm?pageid= 3465 and the Int J Prosthodont 2010;23:190-191).

One of the shortcomings of studies of TMD assessment and management in general has been the lack of a standardized approach to experimental design and clinical assessment (Mohl & Ohrbach 1992, Antczak-Bouckoms 1995), which has prevented valid data comparison. The standardized and validated RCD/TMD protocol has encouraged multicenter studies and the development of large databases for analysis, such as data from Ohrbach et al. (2011) and Visscher et al. (2009). This protocol was designed for clinical research and has been reasonably successful. The revised protocol (Schiffman et al. 2014) is also applicable for routine practice-based application.

This chapter will discuss details of an assessment of jaw and tooth relationships but will not include an assessment of the TM joints and jaw muscles. These topics are separately described in Chapters 13 and 14, respectively.

A detailed assessment of the static and dynamic relationships of teeth is important in clinical assessment for all aspects of dental practice. The information will provide an understanding of specific tooth relationships associated with function and parafunction, upon which treatment will be based. The number of tooth contacts around the arch relates directly to jaw muscle activity (Ferrario et al. 2002). This knowledge is important for prognosis and management of treatment and allows the clinician to more confidently manage the wishes and expectations of patients. It is recognized that, in older patients, loss of posterior teeth may nevertheless allow appropriate jaw function as described by the shortened dental arch (SDA) concept (Witter et al. 2001).

CLINICAL OCCLUSAL ASSESSMENT

Clinical assessment of tooth contact details is valuable in restorative and prosthodontic treatment planning. It requires operator confidence in determining jaw positions with guidance, and the use of high-quality ultrafine marking tapes (e.g., GHM Foil, Gebr. Hansel-Medizinal, Nurtingen, Germany; Ivoclar/Vivadent, Schaan, Liechtenstein) to accurately determine tooth contact and jaw relationships. Ultrafine tapes such as these minimize contact artifacts and clearly indicate tooth contact detail. It is recognized that operator experience is important for consistency of tooth contact markings and that a gold standard approach has not been defined (Millstein & Maya 2001, Harper & Setchell 2002).

A practical approach in clinical assessment is the use of different-colored tapes (GHM Foils) for identifying specific tooth contacts. For convenience, red, black, and green tapes are suggested for comparisons, as described in Box 8.1. (See Chapter 7 for revision of jaw and tooth positions.)

Box 8.2 lists the requirements for clinical occlusal assessment.

Retruded Contact Position

Jaw guidance into retruded contact position (RCP) may be carried out using chin, chin and jaw, or bilateral jaw guidance. Each clinical approach is satisfactory, and each may be applied confidently. However,

practice and experience is required to gain confidence in being able to guide the jaw reproducibly. Clinician confidence is often challenged by the difficulty that most patients have in relaxing the jaw to allow guidance into RCP (Figures 8-1 and 8-2, A-D). The rationale for clinical recordings of RCP is that for a given treatment requiring laboratory and technical support, a reproducible position of the jaw is required for equivalent clinical and laboratory relationships.

Median Occlusal Position

Median occlusal position (MOP) is examined with a different colored tape (red) to assess the distribution of functional contacts and whether this contact distribution is different from RCP. The optimum tooth arrangement provides multiple bilateral simultaneous contacts on many, and often on all, posterior teeth, and if the anterior tooth arrangement allows (depending on degree of overjet), there may be anterior tooth contacts as well (Figure 8-2, D-F).

Lateral Tooth Guidance

The physical features of tooth guidance vary with the intraarch tooth arrangement and the interarch relationships of anterior and posterior teeth and are described in Chapter 7.

Lateral guidance from RCP (gentle operator guidance only) is examined with tape (green), and the presence of mediotrusive and/or laterotrusive contacts or interferences will be identified by tape marks on the teeth concerned (Figure 8-2, G-J).

PARAFUNCTIONAL TOOTH WEAR

Parafunction is a term that has been used to describe those jaw movements not related to function, or more specifically, not related to mastication, swallowing, speech, facial expression, and jaw postures with and without tooth contact.

Functional jaw movements of chewing, swallowing, and speech involve relatively short durations of tooth contacts. However, parafunctional clenching commonly occurs while awake (awake bruxism) and appears to be driven by psychosocial factors generating daytime stress and mood changes (Glaros et al. 2005, Manfredini & Lobbezoo 2010). Episodic daytime clenching is of longer duration than sleep bruxism episodes. When clenching occurs during sleep (sleep bruxism), the cause may be associated with a variety

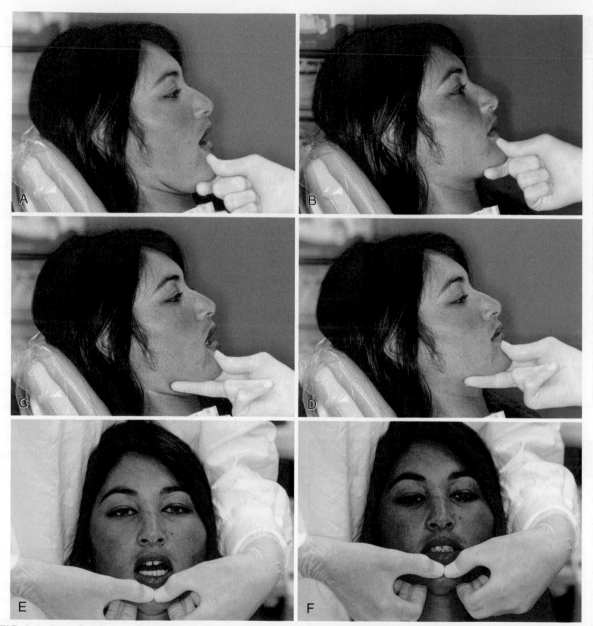

FIG 8-1 Jaw Guidance Techniques Each clinical technique is appropriate for occlusal analysis and clinical recording of jaw position. **A** and **B,** Jaw guidance by supporting the chin point with the thumb and the index finger and middle finger on the lower border of the jaw bilaterally. The jaw is rotated open and closed with the axis of rotation between the condyles. **C** and **D,** Jaw guidance by supporting the chin point with the thumb and index finger. The same procedure is followed in obtaining a centric relation record. **E** and **F,** Bilateral jaw guidance with the patient lying supine. The jaw is guided with each thumb depressing the chin while the fingertips support the lower border of the jaw. The head is stabilized by the operator seated at the 10 or 11 o'clock position with the head between the chest and inner surface of the left arm (for a right-handed operator). Firm bilateral support, with gentle guidance and the presence of the sensitive fingerpads along the lower border of the jaw, allows recording and testing of the retruded jaw position or centric relation.

of factors related to sleep—such as body position, snoring, apnea–hypopnea episodes, breathing difficulty, and hypertension. Sleep bruxism is characterized by rhythmic masticatory muscle activity (i.e., repetitive jaw muscle contractions with or without tooth contact) and is defined as a movement sleep disorder or a parasomnia, as is snoring (Lavigne & Palla 2010). Each trigger appears to be associated with a change in central nervous system drive to jaw muscle motoneurons and an increase in the following:

- Tooth contact time
- Muscle contraction force and duration
- Possible increased loading of articular tissues in tension or compression

A commonly presenting form of tooth contact parafunction from clinical observation appears to be lateroprotrusive parafunction. This may be destructive to teeth, contribute to their wear, and induce remodeling changes in alveolar bone and articular tissues. It may in some instances lead to muscle fatigue and myogenic pain. Sustained jaw muscle contraction has been shown in clinical studies of healthy adults to evoke a dull ache in the face, temple, or forehead, similar to the orofacial pain described by patients (Glaros et al. 2005, Greene 2010). In addition, clenching in an eccentric jaw position, that is, not at intercuspal centric position (ICP) or centric occlusion (CO), may also lead to jaw muscle pain and tenderness on palpation. In eccentric lateroprotrusive or protrusive jaw positions, the jaw muscle system has less resistance to loading, especially when there are no posterior supporting tooth contacts on laterotrusive (working) and mediotrusive (nonworking) sides. In centric bruxism (which appears to occur most commonly when awake), posterior tooth support best resists joint loading. However, TMD jaw muscle pain may occur with centric clenching (see Wänman 1995, for review).

Box 8.3 summarizes tooth contacts and non–tooth-contact parafunction.

As described, parafunction may occur when awake (awake bruxism), or when asleep (sleep bruxism) and may occur without the individual being aware of either of these events. However, many patients who present for treatment with signs of parafunction are aware of their awake habit. Sleep bruxism may be drawn to a person's attention by their room-mate or sleep partner. Sleep bruxism may occur at any age and

---

BOX 8.3 PARAFUNCTION

Tooth contact parafunction includes:

- Jaw clenching (centric bruxism)
- Jaw grinding (bruxism), which occurs in a lateroprotrusive direction
- Tapping of teeth
- Forced postures of the jaw in which teeth may also be inlocked (such as holding the jaw forward in protrusion with the anterior teeth inlocked in a class II relationship) or placed in a lateroprotrusive position

Non-tooth-contact jaw postures include:

- Holding the jaw in a fixed posture without tooth contact, usually with a varying degree of protrusion; may be a deliberate attempt to improve facial aesthetics
- Pipe smoking
- Nail biting, pencil biting
- Thumb or finger sucking, particularly in children

---

is often noticed in children by their parents. Bruxism in children has been reported to have a similar etiology to that occurring in adults.

Clinical studies provide strong evidence that parafunctions, and bruxism especially, are not caused by local dental factors, that is, there is no association between tooth arrangement or tooth contact patterns, such as interferences (from RCP to ICP, mediotrusive or balancing interferences) and the etiology of parafunction (Seligman et al. 1988). There is now strong evidence to indicate that parafunction, especially sleep bruxism, is induced within the central nervous system and is recognized as a sleep disorder or parasomnia (Lavigne 2005, Lavigne & Palla 2010, Manfredini & Lobbezoo 2010). A multicenter study (Lobbezoo et al. 2013) proposed the concept of bruxism presenting with two circadian rhythms, associated with the etiology of awake and sleep bruxism.

Further, a detailed analysis (Raphael et al. 2012, 2013) on sleep bruxism, supported by sleep laboratory data from polysomnography, investigated possible associations between sleep bruxism and muscle-based TMD. Concerns have existed (Marbach et al. 2003) about the widely held clinical view that there is a casual link between sleep bruxism and TMD based on self-reporting of bruxism (self-reporting reliability and consistency is of concern). Of particular

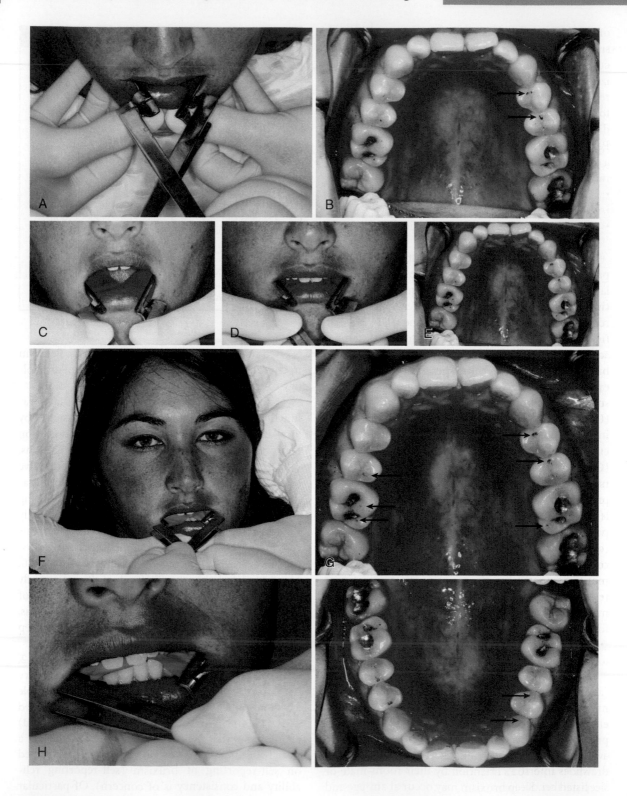

FIG 8-2 Clinical Occlusal Analysis Recording A and **B,** Clinical recording of retruded jaw position (RP) with bilateral jaw guidance. The dental assistant supports Miller holders for right and left quadrant recordings with black tape. RP contacts (black) marked with tape (arrows). Definite RP tooth contacts are seen on teeth 1.5 (buccal incline of lingual cusp), 1.6 (contact on distolingual cusp, lighter on mesiolingual marginal ridge), 2.4 (mesial marginal ridge 2 marks), and 2.5 (mesial marginal ridge and fossa). **C** and **D,** Clinical recording of MOP. The clinician holds Miller holders for right and left quadrant recordings with red foil. MOP contact is obtained by requesting the patient to snap the teeth together (**D**) from a jaw opened position (**C**). The tape marks (*red*) provide a pattern similar to functional tooth contacts. **E, G,** MOP contacts are seen to be similar to RP contacts (**B**). Contacts on the right: 1.4 (buccal incline of lingual cusp—light); 1.6 (buccal incline of mesiolingual cusp, and buccal incline of distolingual cusp). Contacts on the left: 2.4 (mesial marginal ridge); 2.5 (mesial marginal ridge); 2.6 (distolingual cusp). Original RP contacts are arrowed to indicate the differences between RP and MOP. **F, H,** Lateral jaw guidance to the left. **I,** Lateral guidance to the left provided by tooth contacts (*arrowed*) on 2.3 (distal—minor guidance), 2.4 (distolingual—major guidance), and 1.7 (buccal incline of mesiolingual cusp). Lateral guidance to the right provided by anterior teeth (*arrowed*) 2.2 (incisal edge), 1.3 (mesiolingual light contact), and 2.4 (lingual incline of buccal cusp light contact).

importance was the fact that the polysomnographic data together with the sleep-related electromyographic episodes of jaw muscle contractions showed no correlation between sleep bruxism and TMD. These data have for the first time explicitly refuted such an association and require clinicians to review their clinical explanation in patient management (see also Lavigne & Palla 2010).

OCCLUSAL ANALYSIS

An occlusal analysis protocol has been developed for standardized documentation of tooth features and contact details for restorative treatment planning (Figure 8-3). In this protocol, tooth contacts are indicated by circling the appropriate teeth of the odontograms. The details recorded may indicate the need for further assessment and referral for an apparent sleep-related disorder.

- ICP/MOP. For clinical occlusal analysis MOP is recorded (red tape), followed by RCP contacts (black tape).
- A slide from RCP to ICP (in 90% of individuals from Posselt's data) is identified (black tape) by asking the patient to bite on the teeth once the initial RCP contact is determined by clinician guidance. The black tape mark is usually distinct, and the presence of a slide may also be observed through the movement of the lower incisor teeth with biting from initial RCP contact if the jaw slides into ICP. The slide dimensions may also be listed on the form.

- Laterotrusive contacts are identified (green tape), with operator guidance, as the patient moves the jaw from RCP into right and then left laterotrusion. Initial lateral guidance is also indicated on the form.
- Protrusive contacts from RCP to edge-to-edge contacts are identified (green tape).
- Bruxofacets are observed with the use of a dental mirror and light reflection from tooth surfaces that show signs of wear; these surfaces are usually highly reflective with a good light source. Tooth surface loss is graded (see the code at the bottom of Figure 8-3) for both attrition and erosion.
- Vertical dimension is determined in the customary way by observing lower face height proportion and its relationship with facial aesthetics.

Once the occlusal features are listed, the details may be scored by adding the number of tooth contacts, the RCP-ICP slide dimensions, and the score for tooth surface loss.

Score values are an indication of the degree of tooth contact and surface loss and may be used for intraindividual comparison for case maintenance in the long term. A comparison between patients indicates a greater or lesser degree of tooth contact and/or tooth wear.

Clinical Signs

Clinical signs are summarized in Box 8.4. The most common presenting sign is wear on teeth, and attritional wear often presents in conjunction with erosion

OCCLUSAL ANALYSIS

JAW RELATIONSHIP: ant-post: .... vertical: .... transverse: ....

(Angle molar relationship) (incisor relationship) (crossbite)

ICP/MOP (red)

1	2
8 7 6 5 4 3 2 1	1 2 3 4 5 6 7 8
8 7 6 5 4 3 2 1	1 2 3 4 5 6 7 8
4	3

No. of contracts ☐

RCP (black)

1	2
8 7 6 5 4 3 2 1	1 2 3 4 5 6 7 8
8 7 6 5 4 3 2 1	1 2 3 4 5 6 7 8
4	3

No. ☐

SLIDE (black)

RCP – ICP distance ant-post .... mm

vertical .... mm

lateral displacement .... mm

R or L

LATEROTRUSION R (green)

1	2
8 7 6 5 4 3 2 1	1 2 3 4 5 6 7 8
8 7 6 5 4 3 2 1	1 2 3 4 5 6 7 8
4	3

No. of contracts ☐

LATEROTRUSION L (green)

1	2
8 7 6 5 4 3 2 1	1 2 3 4 5 6 7 8
8 7 6 5 4 3 2 1	1 2 3 4 5 6 7 8
4	3

No. ☐

INITIAL LATERAL GUIDANCE:

(tick box) maxillary tooth

	R	L
mesial	☐	☐
distal	☐	☐

PROTRUSION (green)

1	2
8 7 6 5 4 3 2 1	1 2 3 4 5 6 7 8
8 7 6 5 4 3 2 1	1 2 3 4 5 6 7 8
4	3

No. of contracts ☐

BRUXOFACETS

1	2
8 7 6 5 4 3 2 1	1 2 3 4 5 6 7 8
8 7 6 5 4 3 2 1	1 2 3 4 5 6 7 8
4	3

No. ☐

TOOTH SURFACE

	Inc	can	prem	mol
Attrition*	☐	☐	☐	☐
Erosion*	☐	☐	☐	☐

VERTICAL DIMENSION:

(tick box)

optimal	reduced	severely reduced	open bite anterior	lateral
☐	☐	☐	☐	☐

Scoring the form:

No. of contracts RCP........ Lat. R .... Lat. L .... Pro........... **Score** ☐

Slide: Ant-Post: 0; 0 –1.0; 1.0 –1.5; 1.5 –2; **Vert:** 0; 0 –1.0; 1.0 –1.5; 1.5 –2; **Lat:** 0; 0 –1.0; 1.0 –1.5; 1.5 –2; **Score** ☐

Score 0 1 2 3 0 1 2 3 0 1 2 3

Tooth surface loss

Bruxofacets: No. of teeth with attrition................ attrition guide**.................. **Score** ☐

Erosion: erosion................ erosion guide**.................. **Score** ☐

Total ☐

**Tooth surface loss guide:
0 – nil; 1 – only enamel; 2 – dentine; 3 – dentine extensively; 4 – dentine and secondary dentine;

FIG 8-3 Occlusal Analysis Form Clinical occlusal analysis may be standardized by completing an occlusal analysis form.

BOX 8.4 PARAFUNCTION: CLINICAL SIGNS

Teeth
- Wear on teeth and restorations; degree of wear on teeth depends on:
  - Enamel hardness
  - Interocclusal forces generated and their duration
  - Frequency of habit
- Mobility and spreading of teeth
- Fractured cusps and split teeth

Muscles
- Muscle pain
- Muscle hypertrophy, especially masseter
- Elevated masseter EMG

TM joints
- Possible overloading
- Articular sounds (popping, clicking)
- Internal derangement
  - Reciprocal click
  - Closed-lock
- Radiographic changes in condyle contour

and abrasion (Bartlett et al. 1998, Young 2002). The rate of tooth surface loss is usually of the order of 50 μm per year for posterior teeth (Seligman & Pullinger 1995); there is a nonlinear relationship with age and variable enamel mineral content is likely to influence resistance to wear and demineralization (Bartlett et al. 2006, Sierpinska et al. 2013). It has been reported (Seligman & Pullinger 1995, Bartlett & Dugmore 2008) that the degree of attrition does not increase in a linear manner with age, and that canine or laterotrusive attrition occurs to a greater degree and more rapidly than posterior attrition. The laterotrusive component of parafunction initially provides some protection of posterior tooth wear. Once reduced anterior guidance develops, the rate of posterior attritional wear increases. However, the presence of wear facets (bruxofacets) is evidence of previous or ongoing parafunction. It has been reported that approximately 75% to 80% of tooth wear (attrition) is attributed to parafunction and the remainder to function, including erosion (Seligman & Pullinger 1995). Bruxofacets can usually be matched between opposing tooth surfaces. Figure 8-4 shows bruxofacets of varying severity.

During bruxing (particularly sleep bruxism) and centric clenching, the customary controls of jaw movement appear to be absent. Variable isometric jaw muscle contraction occurs with varied motor unit contributions, leading to rhythmical contractions and generation of bite forces that appear to be less than those occurring during mastication. Sustained and repeated tooth contact results in the development of bruxofacets with progressive wear of tooth structure and restorations.

The loss of permanent tooth structure on contact surfaces of opposing teeth is usually clearly evident in adults, and early signs of tooth wear may also be seen in teenagers and young adults, indicative of a parafunctional habit. Because parafunctional clenching and grinding usually occur with the jaw in eccentric positions, bruxofacets are readily seen on the contact surfaces of the teeth providing lateral guidance; usually, the incisor and canine teeth. The loss of tooth structure varies widely in different individuals and is a function of:
- Duration of tooth contact episodes
- Frequency of parafunctional episodes
- Bite force developed
- Whether there is static clenching or dynamic grinding of tooth surfaces
- Abrasion resistance and mineral content of enamel

PROVOCATION TESTS

Provocation tests are a useful component of occlusal assessment. They are used to provoke a response in teeth, jaw muscles, or TM joints, which may match symptoms or concerns that a patient has been experiencing and may or may not have reported.

Jaw movement as part of TM joint assessment, such as jaw opening or lateral and protrusive jaw movements, could be regarded as a provocation test. In addition, those tests described below are generated by bite force for assessment of the teeth, TM joints, and jaw muscles.

Temporomandibular Joint Provocation Test
- The patient is asked to bite on a unilateral posterior contact or pivot (e.g., cotton roll or wooden spatula 2 mm thick) placed in the first molar region, on one side at a time, for 30 seconds.
  - Pain or discomfort may be experienced in the contralateral joint or joint area from the effects of loading by compression or tension of the

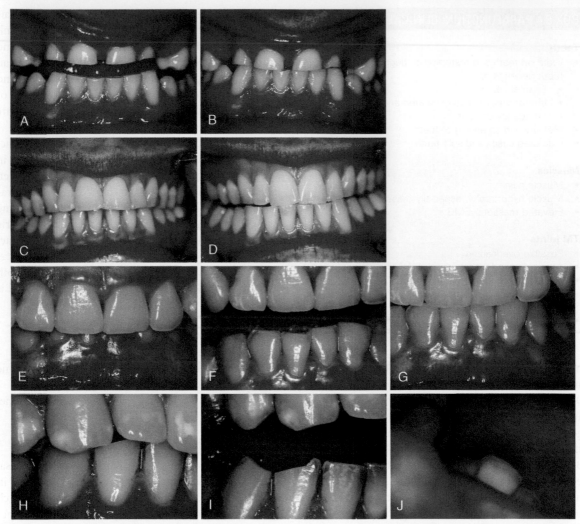

FIG 8-4 Tooth Wear **A, B,** and **C,** Tooth wear involving the anterior teeth. In **B** a protrusive jaw position is required for these tooth contacts to occur in tooth clenching. Wear is obvious in **C,** which shows incisal edge wear of tooth 1.1 and that the tooth is in a labial position outside the maxillary arch contour; this is likely to have developed from protrusive clenching. **D, E,** and **F,** Early signs of tooth wear involving the anterior teeth. The flattening of the incisal edges is apparent. Note the deep overbite in **D** and the protrusive jaw position in **E** for tooth clenching. The incisal wear is more apparent on mandibular teeth in **F.** Such wear is unrelated to function, and the protrusive posturing of the jaw to gain tooth contact allows loading on teeth, TM joints, and muscles. The patient is an 18-year-old student. **G** and **H,** Tooth wear indicated by flattening of incisal edges of anterior teeth at a more advanced stage than in **A-F.** This patient is a 25-year-old dental postgraduate. **I** and **J,** Tooth surface loss of an advanced nature in a 43-year-old male showing marked destruction of tooth structure. Such wear is unrelated to function, and there may also be components of erosion and abrasion. The wear on anterior teeth has been accelerated by loss of some posterior teeth, and the wear pattern is characteristic of attrition with awake bruxism.

joint. The ipsilateral joint may be under tension with possible distraction of the condyle.

- This occurs as the jaw rotates around the ipsilateral posterior support, which acts as a fulcrum. Provoked discomfort may be linked with a patient's symptoms and concerns and assists diagnosis and management.
- Alternatively, the provocation test may not provoke any symptoms or concerns.

Jaw Muscle Provocation Test

- The patient is asked to bite in ICP (CO)—so-called centric clenching for 30 seconds.
  - Pain, discomfort, or muscle fatigue (weakness or tiredness) may be provoked and may be similar to symptoms that the patient has experienced in the head, face, and/or jaws. This suggests that a clenching habit may be related to such symptoms.
  - Alternatively, this test may not provoke any symptoms or concerns.
- Bruxofacets: Where there is evidence of tooth wear, clenching on opposing bruxofacets (on maxillary mandibular teeth) for 30 seconds is likely to reproduce the habit.
  - Bruxofacets on anterior teeth can usually be matched with the jaw in a protrusive or lateroprotrusive position.
  - The patient is often unaware of this jaw posture habit and may be surprised at the forced and often uncomfortable nature of the jaw position.
  - Matching of the bruxofacets in these jaw positions should be carefully explained to the patient: the use of a face mirror is helpful to visually indicate the jaw postures that have unconsciously developed.
  - A careful explanation of the clenching habit is an important step in patient education. As part of the explanation, emphasis is given to the fact that these specific jaw positions, which contribute to tooth wear, are not associated with chewing, swallowing, or talking.
  - This is an important aspect of the conservative management of tooth clenching and its many effects.

A focus on patient education is important in the management of patient-specific needs. The use of a tailored self-care program for management of TMD was reported in a randomized controlled trial by Dworkin et al. (2002) and shown to be equally as effective as other treatments in managing TMD. The data indicated reduced TMD pain, reduced jaw muscle tenderness, and an enhanced ability to cope with any residual TMD. This emphasis is now recognized as the Standard of Care by the American Association of Dental Research, as indicated in the Introduction to this chapter.

REFERENCES

Antczak-Bouckoms AA: Epidemiology of research for temporomandibular disorders, *J Orofac Pain* 9: 226–234, 1995.

Bartlett DW, Coward PY, Nikkah C, et al: The prevalence of tooth wear in a cluster sample of adolescent school children and its relationship with potential explanatory factors, *B Dent Jour* 184:125–129, 1998.

Bartlett D, Dugmore C: Pathalogical or physiological erosion—is there a relationship with age? *Clin Oral Invest* 12(Suppl 1):27–31, 2008.

Bartlett JD, Lee Z, Eright JT, et al: A developmental comparison of matrix metalloproteinase-20 and amelogenin null mouse enamel, *Europ J Oral Sci* 114(Suppl s1):18–23, 2006.

Dworkin SF, Huggins KH, Wilson L, et al: A randomised clinical trial using research diagnostic criteria for temporomandibular disorders—axis II to target clinical cases for a tailored self-care TMD treatment program, *J Orofac Pain* 16:48–63, 2002.

Dworkin SF, LeResche L: Research diagnostic criteria for temporomandibular disorders: review, criteria, examinations and specifications, critique, *J Cranio Dis Fac Oral Pain* 6:301–355, 1992.

Ferrario VF, Serrao G, Dellavia C, et al: Relationship between number of occlusal contacts and masticatory muscle activity in healthy young adults, *J Craniomandibular Practice* 20:91–98, 2002.

Glaros AG, Williams K, Lauten L: The role of parafunctions, emotions and stress in predicting facial pain, *J Am Dent Assoc* 136:451–458, 2005.

Greene CS: Managing the core of patients with temporomandibular disorders: a new guideline for care, *J Am Dent Assoc* 141:1086–1088, 2010.

Harper KA, Setchell DJ: The use of shimstock to access occlusal contacts: a laboratory study, *Int J Prosthodont* 15:347–352, 2002.

Lavigne G: Sleep related bruxism. In Sateia MJ, editor: *The International Classification of Sleep Disorders:*

Diagnostic and Coding Manual, ed 2, Westchester, 2005, American Academy of Sleep Medicine, pp 189–192.

Lavigne G, Palla S: Transient morning headache recognizing the role of sleep bruxism and sleep-disordered breathing, *J Am Dent Assoc* 141:297–299, 2010.

Lobbezoo F, Ahlberg J, Glaros AG, et al: Bruxism defined and graded: an international consensus, *J Oral Rehab* 40:2–4, 2013.

Manfredini D, Lobbezoo F: Relationship between bruxism and temporomandibular disorders: a systematic review of the literature from 1998 to 2008, *Oral Surg Oral Med Oral Path Oral Radiol Endod* 109:e26–e50, 2010.

Marbach JJ, Raphael KG, Janal MN, et al: Reliability of clinician judgements of bruxism, *J Oral Rehabil* 30:113–118, 2003.

Millstein P, Maya A: An evaluation of occlusal contact marking indicators. A descriptive quantitative method, *J Am Dent Assoc* 132:1280–1286, 2001.

Mohl ND, Ohrbach R: The dilemma of scientific knowledge versus clinical management of temporomandibular disorders, *J Prosth Dent* 67:113–120, 1992.

Ohrbach R, Fillingim RB, Mulkey F, et al: Clinical findings and pain symptoms as potential risk factors for chronic TMD: Descriptive data and empirically identified domains from the OPPERA case-control study, *J Pain* 12(Suppl 3):T27–T45, 2011.

Raphael KG, Sirois DA, Janal MN, Wigren PE, Dubrovsky B, Nemelivsky LV, Klausner JJ, Krieger AC, Lavigne GJ: Sleep bruxism and myofascial temporomandibular disorders: a laboratory-based polysomnographic investigation, *J Am Dent Assoc* 143:1223–1231, 2012.

Schiffman E, Ohrbach R, Truelove E, et al: Diagnostic criteria for temporomandibular disorders (DC/TMD) for clinical research applications: recommendations of the International RDC/TMD Consortium network* and orofacial pain special interest group, *J Oral Facial Pain Headache* 28:6–27, 2014.

Seligman DA, Pullinger AG: The degree to which dental attrition in modern society is a function of age and of canine guidance, *J Orofac Pain* 9:266–275, 1995.

Seligman DA, Pullinger A, Solberg WK: The prevalence of dental attrition and its association with factors of age, gender, occlusion and TMJ symptomatology, *J Dent Res* 67:1323–1333, 1988.

Sierpinska T, Oryway K, Kuc J, et al: Enamel mineral content in patients with severe tooth wear, *J Prosth* 26:423–428, 2013.

Truelove EL, Sommers EE, LeResche L, et al: Clinical diagnostic criteria for TMD: new classification permits multiple diagnoses, *J Am Dent Assoc* 123:47–54, 1992.

Visscher CM, Naeije M, De Laat A, et al: Diagnostic accuracy of temporomandibular disorder pain tests: a multicenter study, *J Orofac Pain* 23:108–114, 2009.

Wänman A: The relationship between muscle tenderness and craniomandibular disorders. A study of 35-year-olds from the general population, *J Orofac Pain* 9:235–243, 1995.

Witter DJ, Creugers NH, Kreulen CM, et al: Occlusal stability in shortened dental arches, *J Dent Res* 80:432–436, 2001.

Young WG: The oral medicine of tooth wear, *Aust Dent J* 46:236–250, 2002.

CHAPTER 9

Articulators, Transfer Records, and Study Casts

Rob Jagger and Iven Klineberg

SYNOPSIS

New technologies are transforming clinical practice from clinical data capture and analysis to a virtual clinical environment for case planning. The progression of computer-aided design and computer-aided manufacture (CAD/CAM) is creating the "plasterless laboratory."

Nevertheless, during this progressive transition, articulators will remain a relevant component of restorative dentistry. In the traditional context, casts of a patient's dental arches are placed on an articulator to assess the dental occlusion and to allow construction of dental prostheses and indirect restorations.

There are many designs of articulator and each to a greater or lesser extent reproduces the relationship of a patient's maxilla to mandible at least as a static relationship.

This chapter describes the different types of articulators and how they are used.

CHAPTER POINTS

- Articulators are described under the following headings:
  - Simple hinge
  - Average value
  - Semiadjustable
  - Fully adjustable
- Facebows and their application are described.
- Occlusal records are an associated component of restorative dentistry. Their relevance to articulator systems is indicated.
  - Retruded jaw position (RP) or centric relation (CR)
  - Intercuspal contact position (ICP) or centric occlusion
  - Lateral and protrusive records
  - Dynamic records
  - Wireless motion sensors
  - Selecting an articulator

ARTICULATORS

An articulator is a mechanical device wth upper and lower components to which maxillary and mandibular casts are attached and which is intended to reproduce the static relationship of a patient's maxilla to mandible (in intercuspal or retruded contact positions [RCPs]) and may provide to a limited extent for lateral and protrusive movements.

Articulators are used for the following:

- Study individual teeth and full dental arches for diagnosis and treatment planning
- Allow adjustment of fixed and removable prostheses and indirect dental restorations

Articulators have been the cornerstone requirement of prosthodontics and restorative dentistry. However, their key role is changing with the progressive incorporation of technological advances. The development of digital records and virtual articulators is transforming all aspects of dental practice; as the most far-reaching and definitive change for case management and education, it is an exciting transformation.

Nevertheless, this is a progressive change, and the use of articulators by dental clinicians will continue into the foreseeable future.

There are many designs of articulators, but in general there are four different types:

- Simple hinge
- Average value (plane-line)
- Semiadjustable
- Fully adjustable

Simple hinge articulators provide a single hinge movement without lateral movements (Fig. 9-1, *A*). The distance of the maxillary arch to the intercondylar axis is much less than in the patient, and therefore intercuspal position recordings are an approximation. They have a limited application.

Average value articulators have their condylar angle fixed at 30°. There is no provision for an adjustment for condylar side shift but they may have an adjustable incisal guidance (Fig. 9-1, *B*).

Semiadjustable articulators allow adjustment of condylar inclination and side shift (Bennett angle or progressive side shift) and in some designs for Bennett

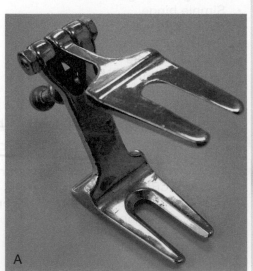

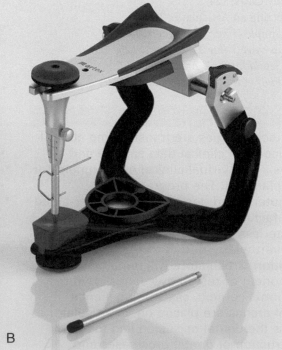

FIG 9-1 A, Hinge articulator. **B,** Average value articulator (Artex CN).

movement or immediate side shift. Intercondylar width is usually fixed at 110 mm, but some articulators allow different intercondylar width settings.

These articulators may be either arcon or nonarcon in design (Fig. 9-2, *A-C*). The description "arcon" is an acronym for "articulator-condyle."

Arcon design describes articulators in which the condylar elements are designed with the fossa box in the upper member of the articulator and the condylar sphere in the lower member, which is similar to the anatomical arrangement of the temporomandibular (TM) joints. The arrangement allows distraction of the condyles, which may occur in function or dysfunction.

Nonarcon articulators have a ball-and-slot mechanism in which the condylar ball is attached to the upper member and the slot mechanism to the lower member.

Condylar and Bennett angles are obtained from protrusive and lateral occlusal records (see below) or are set at average values.

Incisal guidance, the anterior guiding component of the articulation, is produced on the articulator by alteration of the angle of inclination of the incisal guidance. The setting may be made by reference to the overbite and overjet relationship of the anterior teeth. If there is no existing guidance (where anterior teeth are absent), an average value can be set. Custom-made incisal guidance tables may be set from an existing incisal scheme or, where this is not appropriate, from a diagnostic preparation as the plan for the final restoration.

The position of the occlusal plane of the maxillary teeth may be placed in an average position relative to the intercondylar axis as in the average value articulator. Alternatively a facebow may be used in conjuction with most semiadjustable articulators.

Fully adjustable articulators are more complex in their mechanical design and mechanism of data transfer from a patient and are believed to allow closer reproduction of condylar movements. These articulators are designed to duplicate TM joint features by a series of condylar adjustments and also allow curved condylar translation paths (Fig. 9-2, *D-H*). The condylar settings may be determined by pantographic tracings and stereographic records.

However, the accuracy has always been questioned, and no controlled studies have verified the purported accuracy. Nevertheless, it would be assumed that repeated use by experienced clinicians would inevitably provide greater accuracy.

Virtual articulators are used in CAD/CAM production of indirect dental prostheses and has been used to study mandibular movement.

A digital camera is used to obtain images of the dental arches, and data may be captured by computer software which stores and processes the data for CAD/CAM production and on-screen visualization.

Increased use of CAD/CAM technology is transforming the recording of clinical records, and the application of three-dimensional (3D) computer imaging is creating a virtual environment for case planning (Maestre-Ferrín et al. 2012, Farias-Neto et al. 2013).

TRANSFER RECORDS

Facebows

A *facebow* is an instrument that records the relationship of the maxilla to the hinge axis of rotation of the mandible. It allows a maxillary cast to be placed in an equivalent relationship on the articulator (Fig. 9-3).

To identify the hinge axis, it is necessary to use a *hinge axis locator* and *hinge axis facebow*.

More commonly, average value recordings are accepted as adequate. Arbitrary axis facebows may be used with an arbitrary hinge axis that is located at a point 12 mm along a line drawn from the upper aspect of the superior border of the tragus of the ear to the outer canthus of the eye. This point bilaterally is used to position the condylar locator of the facebow. Alternatively and now more commonly the external ear canal is used as the reference point with an ear facebow, which provides an arbitrary point of reference for each TM joint (Denar Slidematic facebow system). The geometric relationship of the ear canal to the TM joint is accommodated in the design of the facebow.

Facebows also allow transfer of intercondylar distance, which can be adjusted on some articulators.

In dentate patients the facebow fork is used to locate the occlusal and incisal surfaces of the maxillary teeth. Wax or impression compound attached to the fork must locate the tooth cusps positively but not extend into undercuts to avoid distortion. In partially dentate or edentulous patients the fork may be attached to a maxillary occlusal rim.

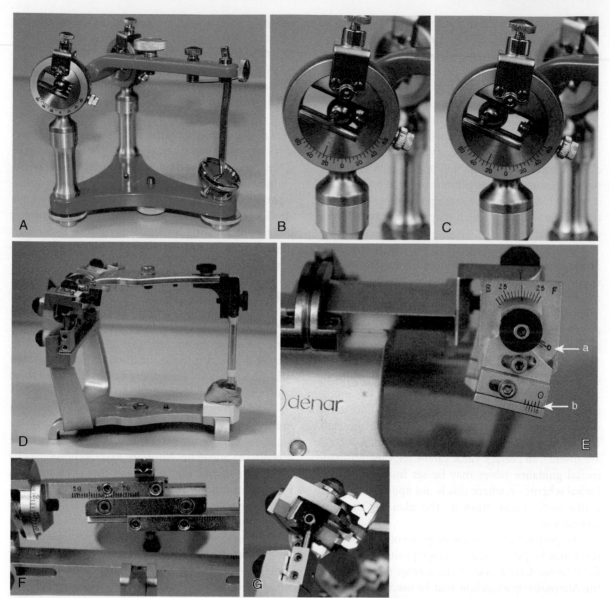

FIG 9-2 A, Dentatus semiadjustable articulator. **B, C,** Magnified views of condylar element "ball-and-slot" mechanism. In **B,** the zero position, the condylar sphere (*arrowed*) contacts the anterior stop. In **C,** with a right lateral movement of the articulator, the sphere moves distally along the slot (*arrowed*). This is a "nonarcon" or "condylar" articulator in which the condylar sphere is attached to the upper member. **D-G,** A Denar D5A fully adjustable articulator. The condylar elements (*arrowed*) are different from those in **A.** This is an "arcon" articulator in which the condylar sphere is attached to the lower member, similar to the anatomical arrangement in the skull. The magnified view (**E**) shows the superior aspect of the right condylar element and identifies where adjustments to the fossa box are made; the progressive side shift (medial wall) (*arrow a*) and the immediate side shift (*arrow b*). The magnified view (**F**) shows the intercondylar width adjustment. The magnified view (**G**) shows the fossa box of the D5A articulator containing the condylar sphere in the zero position.

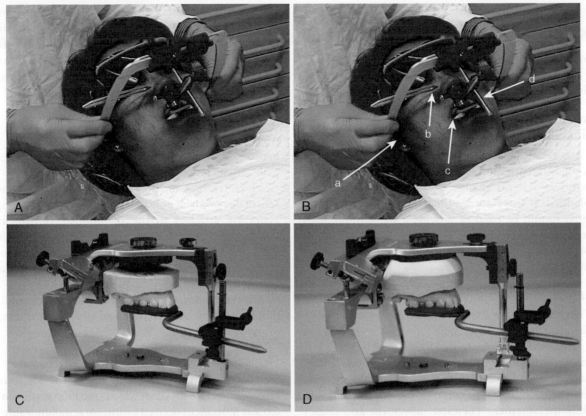

FIG 9-3 A, B, Facebow transfer with Slidematic facebow, fork, and connecting jig in position. Ear rod locator (*a*) for facebow in position in the patient's right external ear. The third point of reference marker (*b*) attached to a Slidematic facebow aligned with a mark placed on the side of the nose 43 mm above the incisal edge of tooth 1.1 or 2.1. Facebow fork in position supported by cotton rolls (*c*) against the mandibular teeth. The rod linking the facebow fork with the facebow is shown in (*d*). This is also used to attach the mounting block to the articulator as seen in **C** and **D. C,** Facebow fork, jig, and mounting block assembled on a Denar (MkII) articulator. **D,** Maxillary cast attached to upper bow of articulator with mounting stone.

Occlusal Records

Retruded Contact Position or Centric Relation Record

This record is used to articulate casts for diagnosis and treatment planning. The CR is recorded with the teeth slightly apart in order to avoid any deflection by tooth contacts. RCP or CR is also used for complex or multiple restorations to restore an occlusal scheme and for complete denture construction.

Recording Centric Relation

- Trim a metal mesh to fit the palatal aspect of the maxillary arch.

- Adapt the mesh with hard wax to the palatal surfaces.
- Add two layers of a hard wax (e.g., Integra Miltex wax [formerly Moyco wax]).
- Soften the wax on the mesh in hot water and place on the upper arch, and then guide the mandible around the hinge axis so that the mandibular teeth indent but do not penetrate the wafer.
- Remove the wax wafer, cool in cold water, and add a small amount of registration material (e.g., zinc oxide–eugenol paste).
- Replace the mesh and wafer in the mouth. Guide the mandible into the hinge position, and allow the paste to set.

- Remove the record, and verify by placing each cast in turn into its correct position.

Details of a technique that can be recommended for articulate casts using a CR record are given in Fig. 9-4, and Fig. 9-5 indicates a verification procedure once casts are articulated.

Intercuspal Contact Position or Centric Occlusion Record

Casts are articulated in this relationship of maximum tooth intercuspation for study and case planning purposes and if no change to the occlusal scheme is planned. If there are insufficient teeth, wax occlusal rims should be used to provide a stable intercuspal record for articulation. Handheld casts have some preliminary application for limited treatment planning needs.

Lateral and Protrusive Records

These records are used to set the condylar angles of the articulator.

Recordings similar to that for CR may be taken but in required lateral or protrusive jaw positions. Alternatively one of a number of graphical analysis systems may be used to record condylar inclination, and side shift measurement (Bennett movement and angle) may be used. These systems require an upper and lower clutch attached to the upper and lower teeth to support and attach an upper and lower bow. The upper bow holds a grid on which the condylar movement details are marked, and the lower bow contains the measuring and marking rods. Once the system is attached the hinge axis may be determined and condylar inclination on jaw opening and immediate and progressive side shift (Bennett movement and angle) recorded during lateral border movements with gentle jaw guidance.

Dynamic Records
Single Plane

Dynamic recordings of mandibular movements in a single plane can be made with tracing plates or acrylic molding devices attached to intraoral clutches, which are attached to the teeth. The acrylic clutches are thin plastic plates or clutches that engage tooth undercuts, or clasp retention may be needed. The mandibular clutch has a tracing plate attached which, during jaw movements, contacts a tracing pin attached to the center of the maxillary clutch. The tracing made on the plate when the patient moves the jaw forward and back from the retruded to protruded positions then from retruded to lateral border positions makes an arrowhead form known as a "Gothic arch" tracing. The apex of the arch represents the RP or CR.

Pantographic Tracings

A pantograph is a device used in conjunction with a matched, fully adjustable articulator that traces border paths of jaw movement in three planes.

These tracings in three axes are used to set the articulator condylar guidance mechanisms. Six tracing plates are attached to the mandibular clutch. Six tracing pins are attached to the maxillary clutch. When the mandible is guided along the border movements, the individual pins capture both horizontal and vertical tracings on the plates.

The traces allow the determination of CR (in addition to a Gothic arch record) and degree and timing of condylar side shift.

Stereographic Recording

Stereographic recordings are used with the TM joint articulator (Fig. 9-6). They are 3D recordings of mandibular movement derived by intraoral molding autopolymerizing acrylic resin on clutches attached to the maxillary and mandibular arches. The mandibular clutch has a central bearing screw, and the maxillary clutch has four cutting studs. Acrylic resin at the dough stage is placed onto the lower clutch at the location of the studs in the upper clutch. The patient is guided through border movements, which molds the acrylic resin as it sets.

Once the acrylic resin has set, the jaw is again guided through the border movements to now allow the studs to define the moldings and capture a precise record.

The record may then be transferred to the articulator, and the Gothic arch moldings captured by the studs are retraced within each molding to generate customized condylar moldings (also in autopolymerizing resin) within the right and left fossa box of the articulator.

In this way personalized articulator moldings are made that capture the right and left condylar inclination and side shift features bilaterally for each patient.

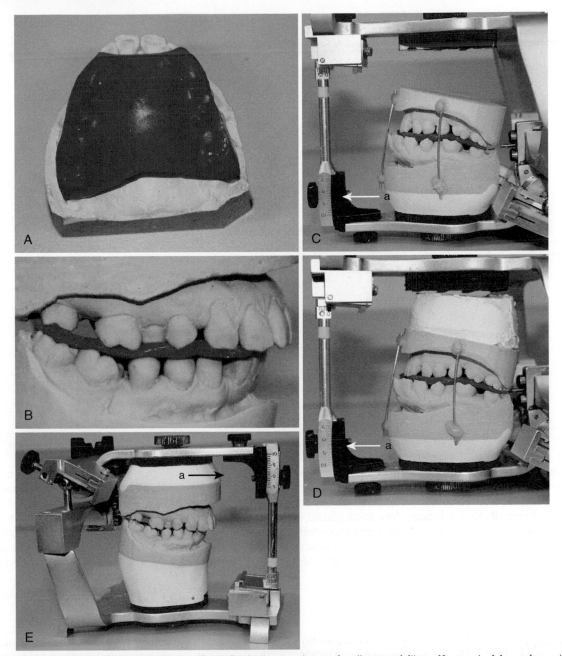

FIG 9-4 Articulating The Mandibular Cast **A,** Jaw record transfer (Integra Miltex [formerly Moyco] wax) on the maxillary cast. **B,** Jaw record transfer in place between maxillary and mandibular casts following trimming of excess wax. **C,** The assembly rigidly supported before mounting stone is added. The arrow (*a*) shows the incisal pin set at +3 mm to account for the thickness of the wax transfer record. **D,** Mounting of mandibular cast by using a two-stage technique: first pour finishes just short of the mounting ring. Note arrow (*a*) as in **C.** **E,** Mounting of mandibular cast completed. Note that the incisal pin is raised 2 or 3 mm in **D** to accommodate the thickness of the Integra Miltex (formerly Moyco) wax record; in **E** the incisal pin has been returned to the zero position (*arrow a*) because the wax record has been removed.

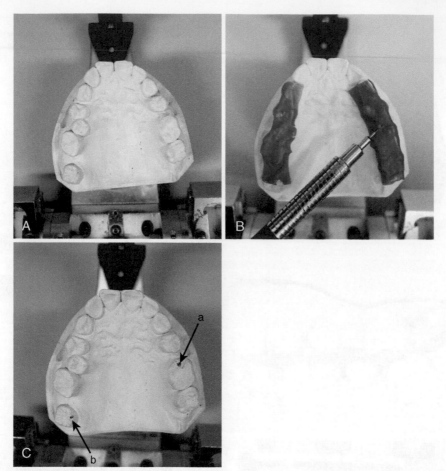

FIG 9-5 Verification of articulator mounting. Verification is desirable to ensure that the articulated dental casts are an accurate representation of the intraoral dental relationships. This is particularly important if occlusal analysis of casts is required and/or a diagnostic wax-up for treatment planning. **A,** Occlusal surface of the articulated maxillary cast. **B,** Kerr Indicator Wax strips placed on the posterior tooth segments of the maxillary cast; the strips have been used intraorally to record the initial tooth contact positions of the jaw in the retruded (guided) position. The first contacts are evident as perforations in the wax and a soft pencil is used to mark the cast through these initial contacts. **C,** Initial contacts indicated on the cast on teeth 1.8 (mesiolingual cusp) and 2.6 (mesial marginal ridge).

Wireless Motion Sensors

Several systems have been developed that use a motion sensor to track mandibular movement (e.g., ARCUS-digma KaVo GmbH, Biberach, Germany). Data are transferred via Bluetooth connection to a computer. Software allows a wide range of parameters to be determined that can be used for the settings for semi-adjustable or fully adjustable articulators or for a virtual articulator.

STUDY CASTS

Casts should be obtained from accurate impressions that record the complete dental arch and ridge and fossa areas to allow reproduction of all tissue contours. Alginate impressions are generally used and if poured promptly produce accurate casts. Bubbles and defects may be removed by trimming the casts. Silicone impressions are accurate, dimensionally stable, and produce superior surface detail.

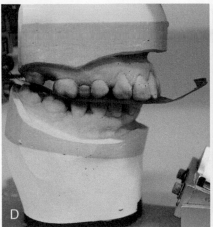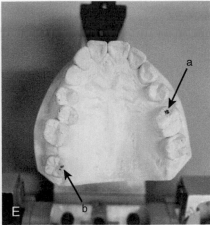

FIG 9-5, cont'd D, The articulator is then closed onto a strip of red plastic articulating ribbon and placed along each posterior segment; the incisal pin is lifted from the incisal guidance plate to allow the initial tooth contacts to imprint the plastic strip. **E,** The occlusal surface of the maxillary cast to indicate the marked contacts (in pencil) and the red contacts (in plastic ribbon). Note the coincidence of tooth 2.6 contacts and the almost coincident marks on 1.8. There is close approximation of the articulated casts compared with the intraoral natural tooth contact in the guided jaw position; this provides verification of the accuracy of the articulation.

It is important to ensure that the articulated casts accurately reproduce the situation in the patient's mouth. There are several causes of errors in cast articulation. Common errors are from an incorrect occlusal record, inaccurate impressions, and casts and articulator mounting errors (see Fig. 9-5 for verification of articulator mounting of casts).

SELECTING AN ARTICULATOR

Simple Hinge Articulators

These articulators are of limited value in restorative dentistry and prosthodontics but allow a preliminary evaluation of static tooth arrangement on study casts and aid discussion with patients. A randomized controlled trial showed that a satisfactory outcome for complete denture provision may be obtained for patients using a hinge type of articulator (Kawai et al. 2005).

Average Value Articulators

These articulators produce an approximation of condylar movements and may be used for construction of simple, indirect restorations and for partial and complete denture construction.

A systematic review (Klineberg et al. 2007) indicated that all occlusal scheme designs provide a satisfactory outcome for most complete denture patients. Clinical experience, however, suggests that some complete denture patients benefit from a balanced articulation. The average value articulator allows a dental technician to produce a balanced occlusion when setting artificial teeth (see Chapter 18).

Semiadjustable Articulators

These articulators are appropriate for most restorative and prosthodontic purposes. Articulating the casts using an RCP (CR) record allows an examination of RCP (CR) features and RCP to ICP differences (see Chapter 7).

The decision whether to use an arcon or nonarcon semiadjustable articulator is largely a matter of operator preference. However, arcon articulators reproduce the anatomical relationship of a patient's maxilla and mandible to the intercondylar axis,

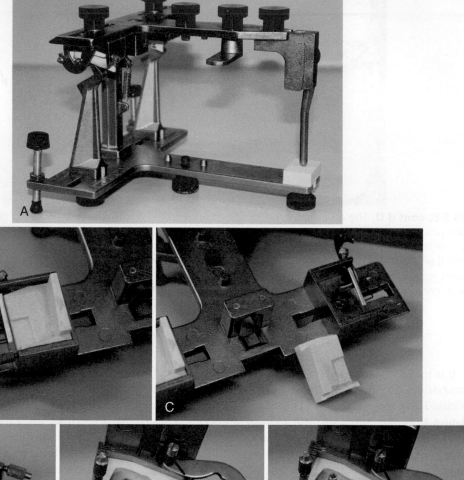

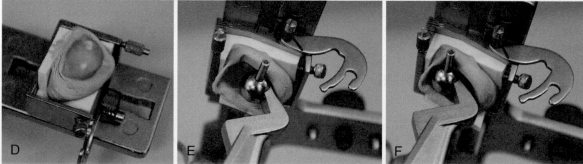

FIG 9-6 Stereographic TM joint system. The stereographic articulator allows customized condylar fossa moldings to be prepared individually for each patient. The moldings incorporate the specific details of condylar movement. **A,** TM joint fully adjustable arcon articulator. **B,** Inferior view of the fossa box (metal) with the plastic insert above. The plastic insert supports the acrylic resin dough while molding of fossa details is in progress. **C,** Inferior view of the fossa box incorporating the plastic insert. **D,** Inferior view of a molded fossa. The condylar element has been removed to show the details of the fossa molding (or condylar analogue). **E,** Inferior view of the condylar element showing movement of the condylar sphere along the molded fossa into a protrusive jaw position. **F,** Inferior view of the condylar element showing the condylar sphere in the centric reference position in the molded fossa analogue.

and both arcon and nonarcon are designed with dimensions that allow realistic approximation of anatomical relationships of teeth and arch form of articulated casts, condyle relationships, and intercondylar distance.

The maxillary cast articulation with a facebow relates the maxillary cast to the arbitrary condylar axis and a closer approximation of the arc of rotation of the jaw in CR. However, any increase of occlusal vertical dimension (OVD) by raising the height of the articulator pin will introduce error, without the use of a hinge axis facebow transfer. Given that a semiadjustable articulator only provides accurate static relationships of tooth contacts on articulated casts or prepared restorations, any required change in OVD needs to be determined clinically and transferred as the maxillomandibular transfer.

A systematic review of the literature has shown that the use of facebows is unnecessary for complete denture construction (Farias-Neto et al. 2013). The review also concluded that the use of facebows is unnecessary for occlusal splint construction. Carlsson (2009) stated that few prosthodontists in Scandinavia use facebows and noted that as long ago as 1991 the Scandinavian Society for Prosthetic Dentistry (SSPD) presented a consensus publication stating that use of a facebow was unnecessary not only for complete denture fabrication but also in other types of prosthodontic treatment. That recommendation was based on the fact that there was no published evidence that the use of a facebow will lead to better clinical end results than when not using a facebows. However, in the absence of evidence, many dentists will remain more comfortable using facebow and other transfer records for fixed prosthodontic restorations. Given that articulators and the transfer of clinical information for laboratory purposes will continue, notwithstanding the introduction of digital intraoral recordings, a realistic reproduction of a patient's jaw relationships relative to the TM joints will remain a goal of occlusal management with a primary aim of reducing the amount of occlusal adjustment at insertion.

Fully Adjustable Articulators

Fully adjustable articulators have the potential to provide the most accurate replication of jaw relationships and lateral and protrusive jaw mandibular movement. However, they are complex instruments and are technique-sensitive, and the complex condylar adjustments for individual patients require pantographic tracings. The reproducibility of the transfer of this condylar information to the articulator is an expectation. Their indication has been principally for extensive fixed prosthodontics and restorative dentistry with the assumption that all aspects of fixed prosthodontic laboratory work can be completed on such articulators and their individualized condylar settings (derived from pantographic tracings), with minimal clinical verification. They are seldom used in clinical practice because semiadjustable articulators with clinical verification and adjustment where indicated has become the acceptable approach.

REFERENCES

Carlsson GE: Critical review of some dogmas in prosthodontics, *J Prosthodont Res* 53:3–10, 2009.

Farias-Neto A, Dias AHM, de Miranda BFS, et al: Face-bow transfer in prosthodontics: a systematic review of the literature, *J Oral Rehabil* 40:686–692, 2013.

Kawai Y, Murakami H, Shariati B, et al: Do traditional techniques produce better conventional complete dentures than simplified techniques? *J Dent* 33: 659–668, 2005.

Klineberg I, Kingston D, Murray G: The bases for using a particular occlusal design in tooth and implant-borne reconstructions and complete dentures, *Clin Oral Implants Res* 18(Suppl 3):151–167, 2007.

Maestre-Ferrín L, Romero-Millán J, Peñarrocha-Oltra D, et al: Virtual articulator for the analysis of dental occlusion: an update, *Med Oral Patol Oral Cir Bucal* 17:160–163, 2012.

Further Reading

Dixon DL: Overview of articulation materials and methods for the prosthodontic patient. Find all citations in this journal (default). Or filter your current search, *J Prosthet Dent* 83:235–247, 2000.

Freilich MA, Altieri JV, Whale JJ: Principles for selecting interocclusal records for articulation of dentate and partially dentate casts, *J Prosthet Dent* 68:361–367, 1992.

Starke EN: The history of articulators: from facebows to the gnathograph, a brief history of early devices developed for recording condylar movement—part II, *J Prosthodont* 11:53–62, 2002.

Starke EN: The history of articulators: a critical history of articulators based on geometric theories of mandibular movement—part I, *J Prosthodont* 11: 134–136, 2002.

Weiner S: Biomechanics of occlusion and the articulator, *Dent Clin North Am* 39:257–284, 1995.

Wilson PHR, Banerjee A: Recording the retruded contact position: a review of clinical techniques, *Br Dent J* 196:395–402, 2004.

SECTION | 3 |

Oral Implant Occlusion

CHAPTER 10

Physiological Considerations of Oral Implant Function

Krister G. Svensson and Mats Trulsson

SYNOPSIS

Normal regulation of oral functions, such as biting and chewing, is dependent on information provided by several sensory organs, including the periodontal mechanoreceptors (PMRs) surrounding natural teeth. The detailed information on the magnitude and spatial aspects of the forces involved in tooth-food contact provided by the PMRs is processed by the central nervous system in a feedback manner (moment-to-moment control) to regulate the level and direction of bite forces. In addition, information provided by these same receptors is used in a feedforward manner to adjust the rate of increase in force to the intrinsic properties (e.g., hardness) of the food, as well as to optimize the direction of the bite force vector.

Absence of information from the PMRs (e.g., as a result of anesthesia or the presence of bimaxillary implant-supported prostheses) disturbs such regulation. Furthermore, the presence of PMRs around teeth connected in a fixed prosthesis does not appear to be beneficial to spatial control during positioning of the food or adaptation to its hardness during mastication. Thus jaw function with a full-arch dental implant prosthesis will be similar to that with a full-arch tooth-supported one. In addition, in the case of the partly edentulous jaw, implants in between free-standing natural teeth may allow preservation of at least some of the rich sensory information provided by the PMRs.

CHAPTER POINTS

A fundamental difference between a natural tooth and a dental implant is that the latter lacks the periodontal ligament and, consequently, also the periodontal mechanoreceptors (PMRs). Intact functioning of PMRs plays important roles in:
- Regulation of bite force, as well as the rate of bite force production when holding and splitting food between the teeth
- Adaptation of the activity of jaw muscles to the hardness of food
- Fine tuning and spatial adjustment of the forces involved in precision biting and positioning for subsequent chewing

Treatment of edentulous individuals with a prosthesis supported by osseointegrated dental implants results in considerable improvement of function and comfort. The reliability of this treatment has, indeed, made it a worldwide success (Brånemark et al. 1977, Adell et al. 1990, Zarb & Schmitt 1990a,b, Lindquist et al. 1996, Lekholm et al. 1999). As part of the minimal invasive approach to dentistry, the use of dental implants that avoid involvement of neighboring teeth in partially edentulous individuals has also increased in recent decades. The efficiency of chewing with an implant-supported prosthesis has been reported to be similar to natural dentition, and maximal biting forces are equivalent (or even higher) with such a prosthesis (Haraldson 1979, Haraldson & Carlsson 1979, Karlsson & Carlsson 1993). However, the regulation of the activity of jaw muscles in response to the gradual changes in food consistency that occur during chewing is impaired in individuals with implant-supported prostheses (Haraldson 1983, Grigoriadis et al. 2011). This is not hard to understand, because even if the osseointegrated dental implant is now as similar to a natural tooth as it can be, there are fundamental differences between a dental implant and a natural tooth.

CONTROL OF MASTICATION

Mastication, the first stage of the digestive process, involves insertion and positioning of food in the mouth for biting, crushing, and grinding by the teeth. During this chewing process, saliva is pressed into the food and, after chewing, the bolus is moved further back in the mouth for subsequent swallowing.

The masticatory muscles are involved in almost every movement of the masticatory system, for example, elevation, depression, and transverse or sagittal positioning of the mandible. Like locomotion and respiration, chewing involves highly synchronized activities by several muscle groups—those of the tongue, jaws, and facial muscles. These activities are coordinated by rhythmic signals generated by a "central pattern generator" (CPG) within the central nervous system (CNS; see Dellow & Lund 1971) and modified in response to inputs from higher brain centers (e.g., the primary motor and somatosensory cortices), as well as by signals from peripheral sensory receptors. These receptors include muscle spindles in the jaw-closing muscles, receptors in the temporomandibular (TM) joints, mucosal receptors in the

oral cavity, and skin receptors in the proximity of the mouth, as well as mechanoreceptors in the periodontal ligaments surrounding tooth roots (Lund 1991). Proper modification of the neural output from the CNS is necessary for appropriate regulation of biting and chewing through, for example, adaptation of the amplitude and rate of force production and jaw movements to the physical properties of the food being chewed (see Lund & Kolta 2006).

The innervation of human jaw muscles by several motoneurons allows effective adjustment of their activities to a specific task. In addition, when a jaw-closing muscle is stretched (such as during biting and chewing), stretch-sensitive receptors, referred to as muscle spindles, signal information about muscle length and changes in this length to the central nervous system, thereby playing an important role in both regulating contraction and allowing the brain to determine the position and movement of the mandible (i.e., providing proprioceptive information; Hulliger 1984, Hulliger et al. 1985). It has been proposed that TM joint receptors provide such information (see Klineberg 1980, Lund & Matthews 1981). However, although potentially the case, the importance of such receptors in this context is thought to be quite limited in comparison to that of muscular and cutaneous receptors, making a significant contribution only in connection with extreme positions of the joint (see Sessle 2006).

The rich mechanoreceptive innervation of the facial skin, lips, and oral mucosa responds not only to contact with objects such as food, but also to contact between the lips, changes in air pressure that occur during speech, and deformations of the facial skin and oral mucosa that accompany movements of the lips and jaws (e.g., during mastication). Thus, in addition to exteroceptive information, these afferents provide proprioceptive information concerning the position and movements of the jaw (Johansson et al. 1988, Trulsson & Johansson 2002).

Even though several different types of sensory organs in and around the mouth may signal information about loads on the teeth, the specialized periodontal mechanoreceptors (PMRs), located close to the collagen fibers in the periodontal ligament that attaches the tooth to the alveolar bone are considered to be primarily responsible for providing such information during mastication (Figure 10-1). Thus the

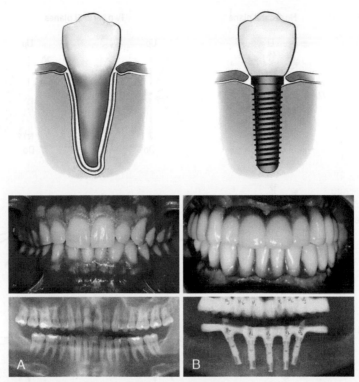

FIG 10-1 Differences between a Natural Tooth and Dental Implant Illustrations, photographs, and radiographs of a natural tooth and an individual with natural dentition (**A**) and a dental implant and an individual with bimaxillary implant-supported fixed prostheses (**B**).

periodontal ligament around each tooth is more than simply a support and contains several hundred extremely sensitive tactile receptors that are essential for fine motor control of the jaw. These receptors also provide the conscious perception of tactile forces which applied to teeth.

During biting and chewing, the teeth are subjected to complex force patterns. The slight movement of a tooth in its socket in response to a force causes nerve signals to be generated, due to tension in collagen fibers of the periodontal ligament, which probably compresses nerve terminals sandwiched between these fibers. The output from any individual PMR depends both on its sensitivity and the degree of strain on the nerve ending produced by tooth movement. As a large number of mechanical factors (including root anatomy, viscoelastic properties of the ligament, contact with adjacent teeth, etc.) influence the extent of this strain, different receptors around the same tooth are not equally sensitive to force applied in different directions to the crown of the tooth. Thus

each individual receptor is stimulated optimally by forces applied in a certain direction, dependent on its position in the periodontal ligament.

Anchoring of the surface of a dental implant directly to the alveolar bone is referred to as osseointegration. The lack of a periodontal ligament between an implant and the bone means that there are no mechanoreceptors in close proximity to the implant, a fundamental difference between a natural tooth and an implant, such as that borne by edentulous individuals with bimaxillary implant-supported prostheses. In the case of partially edentulous individuals (e.g., with an implant-supported prosthesis in only one jaw or implant-supported partial denture or single tooth or teeth) some sensory information is also missing, but forces on the remaining teeth can generate PMR signals.

Spatial Control of Masticatory Forces

Because PMRs normally respond to forces applied in several different directions to the crown of the tooth,

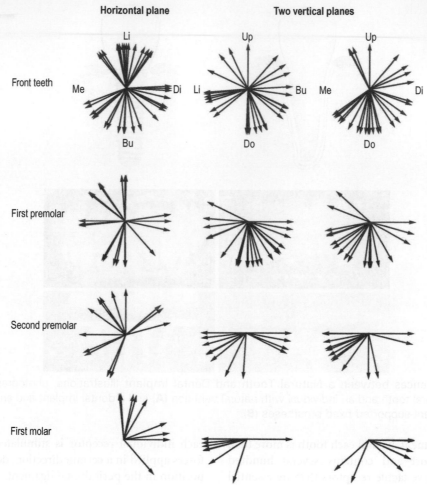

Horizontal plane

Two vertical planes

Front teeth

First premolar

Second premolar

First molar

FIG 10-2 The "preferred direction" of force to which individual periodontal mechanoreceptors around the front teeth, first and second premolars, and first molars are most sensitive. (Reproduced from Johnsen & Trulsson 2003.)

any individual mechanoreceptor provides ambiguous information about the direction of a force. However, integration of signals from small populations of periodontal mechanoreceptors provides reliable information about the precise direction of the force which is represented reliably in the activity.

The vectors in Figure 10-2 depict the directions of force to which periodontal mechanoreceptors in the human mandible are most sensitive, as determined by microneurography. Each cluster of arrows represents all such vectors for the receptors around particular teeth, and the number of vectors corresponds to the number of mechanoreceptors identified and studied.

As can be seen, the number of vectors decreases from the anterior teeth to the molars, indicating that the number of receptors in the periodontal ligaments falls distally along the dental arch, even as the average size of the teeth (and their periodontal ligaments) increases. This observation highlights the importance of well-developed mechanoreceptive innervation around the anterior teeth, which are involved in taking food into the mouth and guiding the jaw into the intercuspal position during the final phase of the chewing cycle.

In addition, the significance of appropriate sensory information from the PMRs for spatial control during

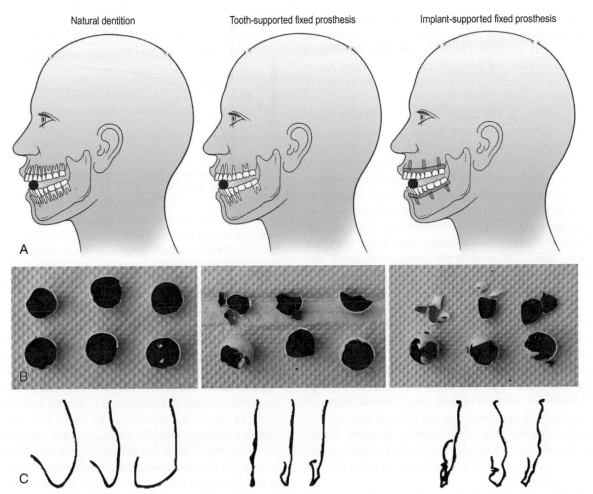

Natural dentition   Tooth-supported fixed prosthesis   Implant-supported fixed prosthesis

A

B

C

FIG 10-3 A and **B,** Examples of subjects with natural dentition or tooth- or implant-supported fixed prostheses trying to split a spherical piece of chocolate hard candy into two parts of equal size with the anterior teeth. **C,** The mandibular movements (frontal view) of these same subjects during a representative "first chewing cycle" of eating a hazelnut. (**C,** Modified from Grigoriadis et al. 2015, with permission.)

precision biting by the anterior teeth has been demonstrated experimentally (see Svensson et al. 2013). Subjects with bimaxillary implant-supported fixed prostheses, and thus lacking these receptors, exhibited clear difficulties in performing a task as demanding as splitting a spherical piece of candy into two parts of equal size between the front teeth. In contrast, the subjects with natural dentition, who received crucial information from the PMRs, could perform a precise split. Surprisingly, in that same study individuals with tooth-supported fixed prostheses in both the maxilla and mandible performed as poorly as those lacking periodontal receptors completely (Figure 10-3, *A-B*).

Apparently, when several teeth are connected, the transfer of forces applied to one of these teeth to all adjacent teeth is altered in a complex manner that perturbs the sensory information provided by the remaining PMRs.

The shift from the high sensitivity of the anterior teeth to movement in most directions to the lower distal-lingual sensitivity of the molars (Figure 10-2) reflects the corresponding functional demands. When the anterior teeth initially manipulate morsels of food and split them into pieces, they experience forces in all directions. The molars, on the other hand, only grind food by more forceful chewing during the final

135

phase of the cycle. When, while chewing, the mandibular molars on the working side approach the intercuspal position from a posterior and lateral direction, they are likely to experience distal forces directed lingually upon contact with the maxillary molars.

Nonetheless, the ability to signal different directions of tooth load appears to be important for posterior teeth as well, as shown by a recent study on subjects with natural dentitions or bimaxillary implant-supported or tooth-supported fixed prostheses eating a hazelnut (Grigoriadis et al. 2015). The first chewing cycle involves a downward movement of the mandible and proper positioning of the nut for fracturing between the upper and lower posterior teeth, which, because of the irregular shape of this food, requires a certain degree of sensorimotor skill in order to direct the closing movement optimally (as indicated by successful fracture). The subjects with implant- or tooth-supported prostheses made a larger number of slips and required additional closing movements to fracture the nut, at least in part because of the impairment or absence of sensory input from the PMRs. In addition, the wider general range of mandibular movement and larger lateral displacement during jaw closure by the subjects with natural teeth indicate that they employ a more lateral approach, which probably facilitates positioning and optimizes the area of occlusal contact with the nut (Figure 10-3, C).

Dentate individuals have been reported to use larger angles of approach to the intercuspal position during jaw closure than jaw opening. Most likely, appropriate input from the PMRs is required for optimal coordination of the mandibular muscles to allow a more lateral approach in order to attain efficient tooth-food-tooth contact during closing. The greater similarity between the closing and opening movements by individuals lacking appropriate sensory input from the PMRs thus probably reflects their use of a "safer" approach to closing the mandible.

Regulating the Magnitude of Masticatory Forces

Periodontal mechanoreceptors are exceptionally sensitive to low forces. In general, the steady-state relationship between stimulus and response for

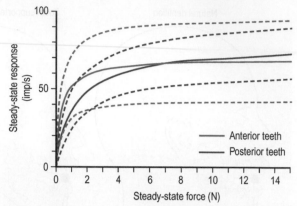

FIG 10-4 The steady-state relationship between stimulus (force) and response (impulses/sec) for periodontal receptors around anterior (*blue lines*) and posterior (*red lines*) teeth. The solid and dashed lines represent the mean ±SD, respectively. (Reproduced from Johnsen & Trulsson 2005.)

periodontal receptors around the anterior and posterior teeth is similar, with >80% of the receptors at both locations exhibiting pronounced saturation (Figure 10-4). However, receptors associated with the posterior teeth demonstrate less sensitivity at low levels of force, as illustrated by their less steep stimulus-response curve in this figure. For the anterior teeth, this slope is steepest between 0 and 1 N of force, while the corresponding value for the posterior teeth is about 3 to 4 N. Because of the rapid saturation above these limits, the receptors provide the brain with no modulated information about larger forces.

The importance of sensory information from the PMRs for regulating the magnitude of low biting forces is seen clearly in connection with the experimental "hold-and-split" task developed by Trulsson & Johansson (1996). Their subjects were instructed to hold and then bite through a peanut resting on a bar equipped with force transducers (Figure 10-5, A), employing as little force as possible during the holding phase. As shown in Figure 10-5, B, the holding force employed was below 1 N when the incisor teeth were used and about 2 to 3 N when utilizing the molar teeth. These values correspond well to the forces at which the teeth (and their PMRs) are most sensitive to change (Figure 10-4).

This same task has been applied to evaluate the significance of periodontal sensory information and

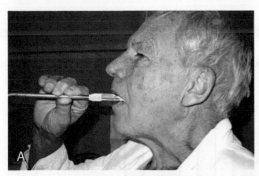 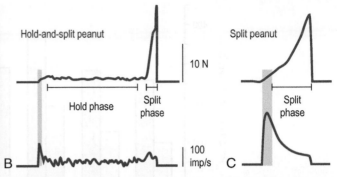

FIG 10-5 Illustration of the "hold-and-split" task developed by Trulsson & Johansson (1996). **A.** The hand-held apparatus employed to record the bite forces exerted on the morsel of food. This morsel rested on the upper horizontal plate and the apparatus was positioned between the upper and lower teeth. **B,** A representative force profile (*upper trace*) and predicted response (in impulses/sec) by the periodontal mechanoreceptors (*lower trace*) for a subject with natural teeth while holding and splitting a peanut. **C,** A representative force profile (*upper trace*) and predicted receptor response (*lower trace*) for a subject with natural teeth while splitting a peanut.

the influence of dental status, including larger prosthodontic reconstructions, on regulation of the low forces used to position and hold food between the teeth for subsequent biting (Figure 10-6). It is noteworthy that the level of force applied by subjects with complete removable dental prostheses and implant-supported fixed prostheses is similar to that for subjects with natural teeth whose sensory input from the PMRs has been blocked with local anesthesia. Subjects with tooth-supported prostheses use intermediate levels of force.

These holding forces are not only higher, but also more variable when appropriate periodontal information is not available. Together, these observations indicate that, via a sensorimotor feedback mechanism, the PMRs play an important role in regulating the force employed to hold and manipulate food between the teeth before biting. When this sensory information is not available, other, less sensitive systems for regulation dominate.

Initially, the anterior teeth are used to manipulate food, splitting it into smaller pieces and transporting it into the mouth; thereafter the jaw muscles produce high forces to allow rhythmic grinding of the food by posterior teeth. Despite their different tasks, the response characteristics of the PMRs around the anterior and posterior teeth have been shown to be similar, and a quantitative model successfully incorporating both their static and dynamic sensitivity has been

developed (Trulsson & Johansson 1994, Johnsen & Trulsson 2005). To predict the receptor discharge evoked by biting with the anterior teeth, both the "hold and split" task described previously (Figure 10-5, A and B) and a single-phase "split" task, in which subjects were instructed to bite through a morsel of food resting on a bar equipped with force transducers (Figure 10-5, A and C), have been employed.

The model predicts that the typical receptor would respond distinctly to the low force produced by initial contact with the peanut and would then provide an ongoing response while the peanut was held between the teeth (hold phase). However, in association with the higher forces exerted rapidly to split the peanut (split phase), the receptor would exhibit only a moderate and declining rate of discharge. Moreover, this simulation predicts that the rate of discharge increases rapidly upon initial contact with the food and that the receptors continue to discharge as long as there is a load on the tooth; although, because of their pronounced tendency toward saturation, poorly encoding the magnitude of and changes in large chewing forces (Johnsen & Trulsson 2005). It is noteworthy that the most rapid discharge occurs in response to the initial low force upon tooth-food contact and not to the higher amplitude or rate of force exerted during splitting of the food and that the rate of discharge falls to a saturated level even as the force continues to rise.

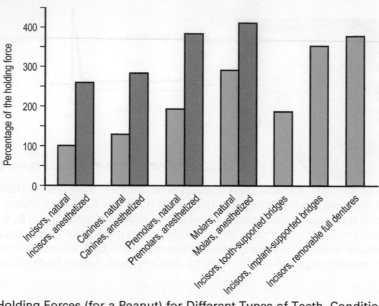

FIG 10-6 **Relative Holding Forces (for a Peanut) for Different Types of Teeth, Conditions, and Prostheses** These data are from Johnsen et al. (2007; posterior teeth); Svensson & Trulsson (2009 [incisor teeth], 2011 [tooth- or implant-supported fixed prostheses]); Trulsson & Johansson (1996; anesthetized incisor teeth) and Trulsson & Gunne (1998; implant-supported fixed prostheses and removable full dentures). In cases where more than one study has been performed under the same conditions, the mean is presented. (Modified from Svensson 2010.)

In addition to this regulation of the relatively low hold forces via sensory-motor feedback, the receptors surrounding the roots of natural teeth also provide early feedforward information concerning the properties of the food (e.g., texture, hardness, brittleness, etc.) that can be used to adjust and adapt the subsequent high biting forces. Thus, during the initial split stage of the "hold and split" task, individuals with implant- or tooth-supported fixed prostheses lack the ability to adapt the rate of bite force production to the hardness of food. In addition, investigations on chewing standardized gelatinous food of different degrees of hardness also clearly demonstrate the importance of sensory information from the PMRs for adaptation of jaw muscle activity to the hardness of the food (Grigoriadis et al. 2011, 2014; Figure 10-7).

These signaling characteristics of the PMRs (sensitivity to direction, initial tooth contact, and changes in low levels of force) indicate clearly the important role they play in the motor control of mastication. Accordingly, absence of these receptors, as in the case

of individuals with bimaxillary implant-supported fixed prostheses, will disturb this control. Although fine motor control is reduced in individuals with dental implants, there appears to be little difference in this respect between bimaxillary full-arch fixed dental prostheses supported by teeth or implants. Our present observations provide a new perspective on the use of full-arch fixed rehabilitation with implants for the management of complete edentulism. In addition, they suggest that in the case of the partly edentulous jaw, implants in between free-standing natural teeth may allow preservation of at least some of the rich sensory information provided by the PMRs.

OSSEOPERCEPTION

The term "osseoperception" is used to describe the sensation evoked by mechanical stimulation of dental implants or bone-anchored prostheses. In the absence of PMRs, this sensation must be transduced by other mechanoreceptors in the orofacial tissues (e.g., possibly those located in muscle, joint, mucosal, cutaneous, and/or periosteal tissues). As there is no evidence

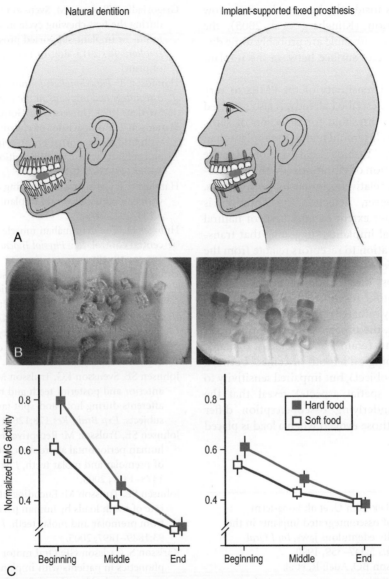

FIG 10-7 **A** and **B,** Fragmentation (after five chewing strokes) of hard (*green*) and soft (*yellow*) gelatinous candy by subjects with natural dentition or implant-supported fixed prostheses. **C,** The combined average normalized electromyographic (EMG) activity of the masseter and temporalis muscles during the three segments (beginning, middle, and end) of the masticatory sequence when chewing hard and soft test foods. The symbols depict the mean values and the error bars indicate the standard error of the mean. Overall, EMG activity was greater when chewing on hard than on soft food and declined during progression of the masticatory sequence. However, this decline was less pronounced for the subjects with implants than for those in the dentate group. Note also that the muscle activity in the implant group was less affected by the hardness of the food. (**C,** Reproduced from Grigoriadis et al. 2011, with permission.)

that nerve endings inside the bone or bone marrow make a contribution (Klineberg et al. 2005), the mechanoreceptors responsible are probably some distance from the contact surface between the implant and bone.

The pronounced sensitivity of the PMRs to very low levels of force, described already, is also reflected in reports that the threshold for detection of static force is approximately tenfold higher for implant than dentate individuals (Yoshida 1998). In contrast, the threshold for detection of vibrations (dynamic stimulation) tends to be relatively similar for both groups. Interestingly, however, detection of vibration is impaired to a greater extent by anesthesia of natural teeth than of dental implants, suggesting that transmission of the vibration to receptors remote from the tooth is more effective across the osseointegrated junction than across the periodontal ligament. Thus the mechanoreceptors responsible for osseoperception are most likely situated some distance from the implant. Moreover, the observations that individuals with dental implants retain a good sense of dynamic loads (such as tapping on a tooth or contact between a tooth and a hard object), but impaired sensitivity to static loads (e.g., spatial aspects) reveal that the sensory signals underlying osseoperception differ qualitatively from those evoked when a load is placed on a natural tooth.

REFERENCES

Adell R, Eriksson B, Lekholm U, et al: Long-term follow-up study of osseointegrated implants in the treatment of totally edentulous jaws, *Int J Oral Maxillofac Implants* 5:347–359, 1990.

Brånemark PI, Hansson BO, Adell R, et al: Osseointegrated implants in the treatment of the edentulous jaw. Experience from a 10-year period, *Scand J Plast Reconstr Surg Suppl* 16:1–132, 1977.

Dellow PG, Lund JP: Evidence for central timing of rhythmical mastication, *J Physiol* 215:1–13, 1971.

Grigoriadis A, Johansson RS, Trulsson M: Adaptability of mastication in people with implant-supported bridges, *J Clin Periodontol* 38:395–404, 2011.

Grigoriadis A, Johansson RS, Trulsson M: Temporal profile and amplitude of human masseter muscle activity is adapted to food properties during individual chewing cycles, *J Oral Rehabil* 41:367–373, 2014.

Grigoriadis J, Trulsson M, Svensson KG: Motor behavior during the first chewing cycle in subjects with fixed tooth- or implant-supported prostheses, *Clin Oral Implants Res* 2015. doi: 10.111/clr.12559. [Epub ahead of print].

Haraldson T: *Functional evaluation of bridges on osseointegrated implants in the edentulous jaw.* Thesis. Sweden, 1979, University of Gothenburg.

Haraldson T: Comparisons of chewing patterns in patients with bridges supported on osseointegrated implants and subjects with natural dentitions, *Acta Odontol Scand* 41:203–208, 1983.

Haraldson T, Carlsson GE: Chewing efficiency in patients with osseointegrated oral implant bridges, *Swed Dent J* 3:183–191, 1979.

Hulliger M: The mammalian muscle spindle and its central control, *Rev Physiol Biochem Pharmacol* 101:1–110, 1984.

Hulliger M, Nordh E, Vallbo AB: Discharge in muscle spindle afferents related to direction of slow precision movements in man, *J Physiol* 362:437–453, 1985.

Johansson RS, Trulsson M, Olsson KA, et al: Mechanoreceptive afferent activity in the infraorbital nerve in man during speech and chewing movements, *Exp Brain Res* 72:209–214, 1988.

Johnsen SE, Svensson KG, Trulsson M: Forces applied by anterior and posterior teeth and roles of periodontal afferents during hold-and-split tasks in human subjects, *Exp Brain Res* 178:126–134, 2007.

Johnsen SE, Trulsson M: Receptive field properties of human periodontal afferents responding to loading of premolar and molar teeth, *J Neurophysiol* 89:1478–1487, 2003.

Johnsen SE, Trulsson M: Encoding of amplitude and rate of tooth loads by human periodontal afferents from premolar and molar teeth, *J Neurophysiol* 93:1889–1897, 2005.

Karlsson S, Carlsson GE: Oral motor function and phonetics in patients with implant-supported prostheses. In Naert I, van Steenberghe D, Worthington P, editors: *Osseointegration in Oral Rehabilitation*, London, 1993, Quintessence, pp 123–132.

Klineberg I: Influences of temporomandibular articular mechanoreceptors in functional jaw movements, *J Oral Rehabil* 7:307–317, 1980.

Klineberg I, Calford MB, Dreher B, et al: A consensus statement on osseoperception, *Clin Exp Pharmacol Physiol* 32:145–146, 2005.

Lekholm U, Gunne J, Henry P, et al: Survival of the Brånemark implant in partially edentulous jaws: a 10-year prospective multicenter study, *Int J Oral Maxillofac Implants* 14:639–645, 1999.

Lindquist LW, Carlsson GE, Jemt T: A prospective 15-year follow-up study of mandibular fixed prostheses supported by osseointegrated implants. Clinical results and marginal bone loss, *Clin Oral Implants Res* 7:329–336, 1996. [Erratum in: *Clin Oral Implants Res* 8:342, 1997].

Lund JP: Mastication and its control by the brain stem, *Crit Rev Oral Biol Med* 2:33–64, 1991.

Lund JP, Kolta A: Generation of the central masticatory pattern and its modification by sensory feedback, *Dysphagia* 21:167–174, 2006.

Lund JP, Matthews B: Responses of temporomandibular joint afferents recorded in Gasserian ganglion of the rabbit to passive movements of the mandible. In Kawamura Y, Dubner R, editors: *Oral-Facial Sensory and Motor Functions*, Tokyo, 1981, Quintessence, pp 153–160.

Sessle BJ: Mechanisms of oral somatosensory and motor functions and their clinical correlates, *J Oral Rehabil* 33:243–261, 2006.

Svensson K: *Sensory-motor regulation of human biting behavior*. Thesis. Sweden, 2010, Karolinska Institutet.

Svensson KG, Grigoriadis J, Trulsson M: Alterations in intraoral manipulation and splitting of food by subjects with tooth- or implant-supported fixed prostheses, *Clin Oral Implants Res* 24:549–555, 2013.

Svensson KG, Trulsson M: Regulation of bite force increase during splitting of food, *Eur J Oral Sci* 117:704–710, 2009.

Svensson KG, Trulsson M: Impaired force control during food holding and biting in subjects with tooth- or implant-supported fixed prostheses, *J Clin Periodontol* 38:1137–1146, 2011.

Trulsson M, Gunne H: Food-holding and -biting behavior in human subjects lacking periodontal receptors, *J Dent Res* 77:574–582, 1998.

Trulsson M, Johansson RS: Encoding of amplitude and rate of forces applied to the teeth by human periodontal mechanoreceptive afferents, *J Neurophysiol* 72:1734–1744, 1994.

Trulsson M, Johansson RS: Forces applied by the incisors and roles of periodontal afferents during food-holding and -biting tasks, *Exp Brain Res* 107:486–496, 1996.

Trulsson M, Johansson RS: Orofacial mechanoreceptors in humans: encoding characteristics and responses during natural orofacial behaviors, *Behav Brain Res* 135:27–33, 2002.

Yoshida K: Tactile threshold for static and dynamic loads in tissue surrounding osseointegrated implants. In Jacobs R, editor: *Osseoperception*, Leuven, 1998, Catholic University of Leuven, Department of Periodontology, pp 143–156.

Zarb GA, Schmitt A: The longitudinal clinical effectiveness of osseointegrated dental implants: the Toronto study. Part I: Surgical results, *J Prosthet Dent* 63:451–457, 1990a.

Zarb GA, Schmitt A: The longitudinal clinical effectiveness of osseointegrated dental implants: the Toronto Study. Part II: The prosthetic results, *J Prosthet Dent* 64:53–61, 1990b.

CHAPTER 11

Occlusion and Principles of Oral Implant Restoration

John A. Hobkirk

SYNOPSIS

Dental implant occlusion has characteristics inherently similar to the natural and restored dentitions and should be designed to mimic nature rather than create a purely mechanical system. Its design must therefore follow similar principles. However, these principles need to be modified to allow for the different characteristics of the support mechanism and relate largely to the avoidance of mechanical overload of the patient-implant interface, the implant connecting components, and the prosthetic superstructure. Although important, occlusal features are not the principal factor in the failure of implant treatment.

Implant dentistry is a rapidly expanding and relatively novel treatment modality and

reflects sometimes entrepreneurial clinical and manufacturing skills. Not surprisingly, the evidence base for decision-making is consequently uneven, with a lack of robust data in some areas. There are, however, several established aspects:

1. The clinician has freedom to position implants in the most suitable locations, within the surgical and prosthodontic envelopes, and these should be selected to minimize nonaxial loads on the implants and reduce torqueing as a result of cantilevering of the superstructure. This can occur mesially, buccally, and distally.
2. The occlusal scheme in the partially dentate patient should normally be conformative and avoid localized stress concentration, for example by canine guidance. Where the full arch is reconstructed, then so called balanced articulation is preferred. Shallow cusp angles are associated with reduced implant loading, and a narrow occlusal platform is preferred so as to reduce loading.
3. There is no justification for using polymeric occlusal materials to solely minimize loads on implants. Ceramics or gold alloys perform better, but there

may be aesthetic or technical limitations on their use, especially in larger constructions, when a resin-based aesthetic material could be preferred.

4. Implant occlusion should be designed during treatment planning, before implant placement. It involves implant location and superstructure design, as well as occlusal configuration, and is an integral part of the process.

This book contains a wide-ranging examination of dental occlusion and is ultimately concerned with its optimization, whether using natural or artificial dentitions. The former are linked to the facial skeleton by the periodontal membranes while the latter may utilize these, or denture-bearing soft tissues, or a combination of the two. The occlusal principles associated with these loading modalities have been extensively described; however, subsequently dental implants have become a significant treatment modality. These depend for their success on the development and maintenance of an osseointegrated interface with the surrounding bone. The pioneers of modern implant dentistry largely employed conventionally accepted occlusal principles, which appeared to function well in their carefully controlled and clinically cautious studies. It has since been suggested that optimal dental implant treatment requires the adoption of different occlusal precepts. This change in thinking partly reflects the much wider use of dental implants in increasingly inventive ways, as well as a less rigid clinical framework, more inventive manufacturers, and an expanded body of research.

This chapter is an introduction to the topic of implantology and considers the potential significance of implant treatment in relation to occlusion, published evidence on the subject, and current views on how issues should be addressed. Within the context of this book,

however, it is not a treatise on implant dentistry.

CHAPTER POINTS

- Implant occlusion is inherently similar to the occlusion of any other dental prosthesis. Its design relates not only to the occlusal surface, but also to its supporting mechanisms.
- Objectives in occlusal design:
  - Maximize occlusal function
  - Minimize harm to opposing and adjacent teeth
  - Minimize wear of occlusal surfaces
  - Minimize the risk of fracture of the implant superstructure
  - Reduce the risk of fracture of the implant body and its connecting components
  - Protect the implant-host interface; currently this is synonymous with maintaining osseointegration
- Particular characteristics of implant occlusion:
  - *Location*: freedom potentially to locate implants in optimum locations
  - *Displaceability*: an osseointegrated implant is displaced very little under load and behaves elastically
  - *Immovability*: implants cannot be moved by orthodontic forces
  - *Proprioception*: proprioceptive feedback is reduced
  - *Force transmission*: high forces may be generated by a patient with an implant-stabilized fixed bridge
  - *Biomechanical overload*: this is thought to be a key factor in the loss of osseointegration
  - *Mechanical linkages*: almost all dental implants employ mechanical linkages, many of which are prone to failure due to overload
- Force management is principally through the following design features:
  - Implant location
  - Occlusal form and scheme
  - Superstructure design

IMPLANT TREATMENT

Implant treatment is currently based on the requirement to obtain and keep an osseointegrated (OI) interface between the implant body and the surrounding healthy bone. The ability to do so is multifactorial and depends on systemic and local factors, not all of which are understood. Local factors include implant design, host site, and surgical and restorative techniques. Once established, the interface is not necessarily permanent, although a small gradual loss of bone from the crestal region is considered acceptable. The OI interface is not a model of the periodontium, as it has different anatomical and functional characteristics and the maintenance of its integrity may not necessarily follow periodontal precepts. The interface is mechanically elastic, relatively stiff, and incapable of responding to orthodontic forces, in contrast to the periodontal ligament which is viscoelastic, less rigid, and anatomically adaptive, allowing tooth repositioning with orthodontic forces.

Loads applied to an implant will alter strain patterns in the bone, which may influence patterns of remodeling with overload and under-load compared with steady-state conditions, resulting in accretion or resorption of bone as proposed by Frost (2004). Much use has been made of this hypothesis in studies of strain patterns in implant-host systems, usually by computer modeling. Some clinical evidence has also been published suggesting that the insertion and loading of implants may increase bone density.

The OI interface lacks the large number of mechanoreceptors that provide crucial sensory input for masticatory control, and although there is some evidence for perception (osseoperception) related to implants, it is poorly understood and considerably less refined than that of a natural tooth. Use of implant prostheses is a learned skill reflecting the plasticity of the neuromuscular system, albeit with considerably less sophistication than in the natural dentition. Early studies on dental implant occlusion centered on measurements of masticatory forces and occlusal tactile sensibility. While some of these used force transducers placed between the teeth and were thus of little value in measuring functional loads, later studies using miniature intraoral transducers were able to demonstrate functional loads. Such investigations showed that patients could generate higher occlusal forces

with implant bridges than with conventional prostheses. It was also shown that they had a greater ability to detect thin films held between the teeth. Investigations into the phenomenon of osseoperception showed that patients with OI implants were able to detect forces applied to them, and that this changed with time. The exact mechanism is unknown, but is likely to involve nerve endings in the periosteum and mucosa, as well as those associated with the temporomandibular (TM) joints and muscles of mastication.

The spaces into which prostheses and their supporting implants may potentially be placed have been described as prosthodontic and surgical envelopes. These are three dimensional, and use of them is based partly on measurement and partly on clinical judgement. The surgical envelope is largely anatomically defined and dictates the limitations of the locations, sizes, and orientations of the dental implant bodies. The prosthodontic envelope is partly structurally based but is also influenced by clinical decisions such as optimal positions for replacement teeth. These three-dimensional spaces can influence superstructure design, implant selection, implant loading, and possibly treatment success. Anatomical and surgical constraints often severely limit implant location.

LOADING PATTERNS

OI implants, teeth, and denture-bearing tissues each have different displaceability and viscoelastic properties. Integrated implants behave elastically under load and typically displace by up to 3 to 5 µm vertically, while teeth and oral mucosa behave viscoelastically and have much higher displacements. These vary between individuals—in the case of teeth with a healthy periodontal support, typically 25 to 100 µm vertically, whereas mucosal displaceability is considerably more varied with values of 1 to 3 mm commonly observed (Figure 11-1). The different displaceabilities of these systems means that if more than one is used to stabilize a prosthesis then this can result in stress concentration in the system and subsequent mechanical failure. Superstructure design, including occlusal design, is therefore important in minimizing this risk (Kim et al. 2005).

CRITICAL FAILURES

It is sometimes assumed that implant treatment is inherently superior to so-called conventional

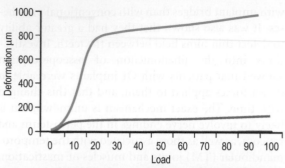

FIG 11-1 Diagrammatic Representation of OI Implants (*red*), Teeth (*blue*), and Denture-Bearing Mucosa (*green*) Under Load Units are not used on the *X* axis. *Y* axis reflects typical reported values.

techniques, yet there is considerable evidence that this is not always the case. All possible treatment alternatives must be considered before making a selection.

Occlusal errors which in the broadest sense include implant positioning and superstructure design may be implicated both in implant failure and in repeated mechanical problems within the implant-superstructure complex, both of which can be critical to long-term treatment success.

EVIDENCE BASE

Dental implant treatment has expanded exponentially in recent years, accompanied by the introduction of many hundreds of implant systems (as well as the demise of more than a few), the emergence of new designs with restricted research data, and on occasions an expansive approach to clinical applications. The sheer volume of published material on dental implantology now makes it difficult for the clinician to identify and critically analyze the material of relevance to his or her needs. Review papers, consensus conference reports, and the emergence of meta-analysis as a research tool all help to address this need. While these sources have provided invaluable information on some aspects of treatment, much current advice remains based on less-certain evidence.

There is a lack of certainty as to the significance of occlusal factors in implant success, as reflected by the successful outcomes of the pioneering studies of Brånemark, which used conventional occlusal principles. Many consider that occlusal factors, although

important, are probably not a major factor in implant treatment failure. Given the lack of extensive long-term clinical data, advice has often been based on in vitro and animal studies and small clinical investigations. It is prudent for the clinician to make use of such guidance, although the precise numerical values sometimes used are less well-grounded in valid research (Hobkirk & Wiskott 2006, Gross 2008, Carlsson 2009, Klineberg et al. 2012, Hsu et al. 2012).

FORCE MANAGEMENT

Strains occur when a material is subject to stress and are dependent on the physical properties of the material and the shape of the loaded object. In the case of bone, Frost's mechanostat theory explains a possible link between strain history and bone growth or resorption that may be relevant to the OI interface.

Strains on implant-connecting components and superstructures are typically cyclical and can lead to fatigue fracture of these components. In the case of screwed joints, loads in excess of the clamping force cause joint separation, loosening, and screw fracture.

Given that it is not easy to measure functional occlusal loads clinically or to predict their effects, the clinician must minimize unfavorable load patterns. This suggests that:

1. Occlusal forces should be directed along the long axes of the implants, which should be at 90° to the occlusal plane. It has been suggested that designs with a deviation >30° should be avoided.
2. In a dentition restored with teeth and implants, initial occlusal contacts in intercuspal contact position (ICP) ought to occur only on the natural teeth.
3. No clinical benefit has yet been shown for a particular occlusal surface material from the viewpoint of implant failure.
4. Tipping forces on implants are harmful. These can arise as a result of cusp angulation, during lateral excursions of the mandible, and most significantly due to cantilevering of the superstructure. The latter can be mesial or distal when attempting to replace posterior teeth and also buccal when there is a requirement to place maxillary teeth lateral to the residual alveolar ridge so as to provide a natural appearance and normal

relationship with the opposing teeth (Figures 11-2 and 11-3).

5. Superstructure designs with a height greater than the length of the supporting implant are considered to generate unfavorable loads on the supporting bone.

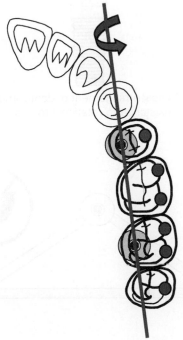

FIG 11-2 Where implants supporting a fixed prosthesis lie palatal or lingual to the occlusal platform, then vertical forces on the teeth will tend to rotate the prosthesis around its fixing points on the implants.

6. Cyclical loads are more destructive, as mechanical components are prone to fatigue failure.

7. Loads on implants in the period immediately after placement and when first loaded should be minimized. This reduces the risk of integration failing to occur because of excessive strain in the surrounding bone, or the implant being lost in the early stages before the interface between bone and implant has matured. In vitro studies have suggested that lower strain levels may stimulate favorable bone formation, although currently this cannot be quantified for clinical applications.

8. The nature of the bone at implant sites will have an impact on its load-bearing capacity. The anterior mandible is often found to be particularly favorable in this respect.

9. Some features of occlusal design, as discussed in the following, are thought to reduce unfavorable mechanical loads.

10. Implant treatment should be used with caution in patients with a bruxing habit.

IMPLANT NUMBERS

Increased numbers of implants can result in a more favorable load distribution in the bone, provided that they are adequately spaced and located so as to evenly distribute forces both to the bone and to each other. This does, however, have cost implications, and there is ample evidence of small numbers of implants being very effective over many years in some treatment procedures, for example in stabilizing removable prostheses. The decision as to the number of devices to be used is thus related partly to whether the patient is

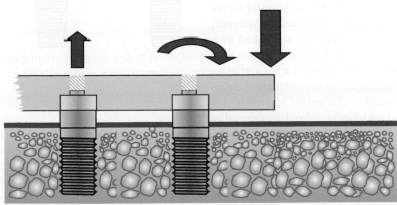

FIG 11-3 Distally cantilevered occlusal surfaces result in rotational forces when the unsupported end is loaded.

edentulous or partially dentate, the distribution of natural teeth, the desired occlusal scheme, the design of the superstructure(s), the impact of the surgical envelope on implant locations, and the quality of the bone at implant sites.

Typical general current guidelines for implant numbers include the following:

1. Interimplant spacing of 3 mm or more
2. One to four implants per quadrant
3. Two to six implants in the anterior region for fixed superstructures
4. Six to eight implants in the maxilla and five to eight in the mandible for fixed superstructures in the edentulous patient
5. Four to six implants in the maxilla and two to four in the mandible for removable superstructures in the edentulous patient

IMPLANT LOCATIONS

Implant locations are principally determined by the surgical and prosthodontic envelopes and the many factors which influence them. From the occlusal viewpoint, the most important factor is minimization of unfavorable loads on the peri-implant bone and within the implant-superstructure complex. This exercise almost always requires compromises.

SUPERSTRUCTURE DESIGN

Superstructure designs influence the loads placed on implants by cantilever effects as well as linkage between implants and possibly teeth. The prostheses themselves may also fail because of overloading as a result of design failures or lack of care in component design and construction.

Where implants are linked, then horizontal forces will be more widely distributed and torqueing reduced, especially if three or more implants are linked in a tripod fashion, as opposed to linearly (Figures 11-4 and 11-5). The problems mentioned earlier can arise as a result of cantilevering of the superstructure mesially, distally, and buccally. The extent to which this happens will depend on whether a fixed or removable superstructure is employed. In the latter situation, the linkage between the implant and the prosthesis may permit relative rotation, which will minimize torqueing. Such movement must be accommodated in the design, as it can be significant because of the disparity in the movement of different supporting tissues under

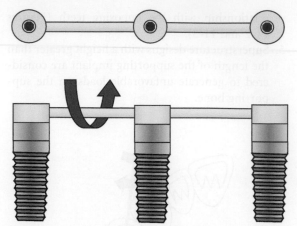

FIG 11-4 A linear arrangement of dental implants provides little resistance to rotational forces.

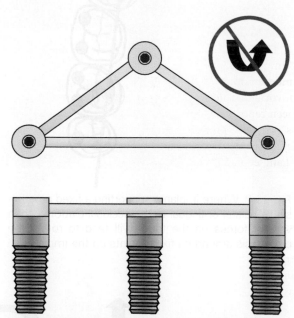

FIG 11-5 A triangular orientation of implants ("tripoidization") will effectively resist rotational forces.

load. A further effect of cantilevering is to magnify and reverse the direction of occlusal forces because of leverage effects (Duyck et al. 2000; Figure 11-6); it is for this reason that cantilever lengths are typically recommended to be 10 mm and no more than 15 mm. Indeed, Gross (2008) has recommended that fixed

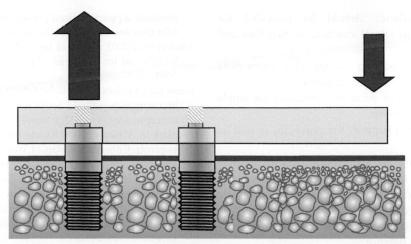

FIG 11-6 Loads on a distal cantilever are magnified by leverage effects.

superstructures in edentulous subjects be cantilevered by no more than one unit.

The linking of implants to natural teeth is a contentious issue because of differential displaceability and possible overload of the implant. Some have advocated a flexible connection; however, there have been reports of tooth intrusion and thus a rigid link is generally preferred. Currently separating support by implants from that provided by teeth is advised (Lang et al. 2004).

OCCLUSION

The design of the occlusal surfaces and the occlusal scheme is important when planning and fabricating superstructures. Occlusion should be included in treatment planning, before implant placement, and involves locations and superstructure design, as well as occlusal configuration.

There is evidence that full-arch superstructures supported either by teeth or implants can provide equivalent functional restoration, although food manipulation and biting are less effective than with free-standing teeth.

Definitive findings on occlusal precepts are somewhat restricted, but a number of general observations may be made:

1. Occlusal factors probably have less impact on implant treatment outcomes than other factors. A long-term study of mandibular implant-supported fixed prostheses indicated that factors associated with occlusal loading were of less importance for peri-implant bone loss than smoking and poor oral hygiene (Lindquist et al. 1996, 1997). Bruxism and cantilever extensions have also been reported to be more likely associated with technical complications than a number of occlusal parameters and oral parafunctions (Brägger et al. 2001).

2. There is no evidence to recommend a specific occlusal design, and traditional occlusal techniques based on physiological principles have much to commend them. Well-established procedures such as the shortened dental arch concept can be applied equally to the implant-based occlusion as to the partially dentate scenario.

3. There is little justification for using polymeric occlusal materials solely to minimize loads on implants. Ceramics or gold alloys perform better, but there may be aesthetic or technical limitations on their use, especially in larger constructions when a resin-based aesthetic material may be preferred.

4. Occlusion of implant-supported prostheses can be managed successfully by using simple methods for jaw registration and different occlusal concepts.

Within this framework there are, however, several recommendations which have been made:

1. Shallow cusp angles may be favorable.

2. Bilateral occlusal contacts in lateral excursions of the mandible should be used with large constructions.

149

3. Anterior guidance should be provided for protrusive and lateral contacts in function and parafunction.

4. Central fossa location of opposing supporting cusps will minimize lateral loads.

5. Avoid creation of excursive guidance on single implant restorations.

6. Sufficient metal support for porcelain should be established.

7. When treating an edentulous patient, employ conventional complete denture paradigms.

8. Balanced occlusion is advocated to minimize denture base displacement.

9. Lingualized occlusion may be considered to facilitate bilateral balance.

10. Balance may be difficult to achieve when using a complete denture opposing a natural dentition. Where possible, attempt to achieve a minimum of three-point balance on lateral and protrusive excursions.

11. An increased occlusal vertical dimension and altered occlusal plane relations may be required in an edentulous patient to create space for attachments and metal frameworks.

CONCLUSIONS

Planning the occlusion for an implant-supported prosthesis is an inherent part of treatment and should begin before decisions are made on superstructure design and implant locations. Many of the conventional principles used in dentistry are equally applicable; however, it is important to recognize the treatment's inherent differences in terms of force management.

REFERENCES

Brägger U, Aeschlimann S, Bürgin W, et al: Biological and technical complications and failures with fixed partial dentures (FPD) on implants and teeth after four to five years of function, *Clin Oral Implants Res* 12:26–34, 2001.

Carlsson GE: Dental occlusion: modern concepts and their application in implant prosthodontics, *Odontology* 97:8–17, 2009.

Duyck J, Van Oosterwyck H, Vander Sloten J, et al: Magnitude and distribution of occlusal forces on oral implants supporting fixed prostheses: an in vivo study, *Clin Oral Implants Res* 11(5):465–475, 2000.

Frost HM: A 2003 update of bone physiology and Wolff's Law for clinicians, *Angle Orthod* 74(1):3–15, 2004.

Gross MD: Occlusion in implant dentistry. A review of the literature of prosthetic determinants and current concepts, *Aus Dent J* 53(1 Suppl):S60–S68, 2008.

Hobkirk JA, Wiskott HWA: Biomechanical aspects of oral implants. Consensus report of Working Group 1, *Clin Oral Implants Res* 17(Suppl 2):52–54, 2006.

Hsu YT, Fu JH, Al-Hezaimi K, et al: Biomechanical implant treatment complications: a systematic review of clinical studies of implants with at least 1 year of functional loading, *Int J Oral Maxillofac Implants* 27(4):894–904, 2012.

Kim Y, Oh T-J, Misch CE, et al: Occlusal considerations in implant therapy: clinical guidelines with biomechanical rationale, *Clin Oral Implants Res* 16:26–35, 2005.

Klineberg IJ, Trulsson M, Murray GM: Occlusion on implants—is there a problem?, *J Oral Rehabil* 39: 522–537, 2012.

Lang NP, Pjetursson BE, Tan K, et al: A systematic review of the survival and complication rates of fixed partial dentures (FPDs) after an observation period of at least 5 years. II. Combined tooth–implant-supported FPDs, *Clin Oral Implants Res* 15:643–653, 2004.

Lindquist LW, Carlsson GE, Jemt T: A prospective fifteen-year follow-up study of mandibular fixed prostheses supported by osseointegrated implants. Clinical results and marginal bone loss, *Clin Oral Implants Res* 7:329–336, 1996.

Lindquist LW, Carlsson GE, Jemt T: Association between marginal bone loss around osseointegrated mandibular implants and smoking habits: a 10-year follow-up study, *J Dent Res* 76:1667–1674, 1997.

Further Reading

De Pauw GA, Dermaut L, De Bruyn H, et al: Stability of implants as anchorage for orthopedic traction, *Angle Orthod* 69(5):401–407, 1999.

Denissen HW, Kalk W, van Wass MAJ, et al: Occlusion for maxillary dentures opposing osseointegrated mandibular prostheses, *Int J Prosthodont* 6:446–450, 1993.

Duyck J, Ronold HJ, Van Oosterwyck H, et al: The influence of static and dynamic loading on marginal bone reactions around osseointegrated implants: an animal experimental study, *Clin Oral Implants Res* 12(3):207–218, 2001.

Kaukinen JA, Edge MJ, Lang BR: The influence of occlusal design on simulated masticatory forces transferred to implant-retained prostheses and supporting bone, *J Prosthet Dent* 76:50–55, 1966.

Klineberg I, Murray G: Osseoperception: sensory function and proprioception, *Adv Dent Res* 130:120–129, 1999.

Richter E-J: In vivo horizontal bending moments on implants, *Int J Oral Maxillofac Implants* 13:232–244, 1998.

Stanford CM, Brand RA: Towards an understanding of implant occlusion and strain adaptive bone modelling and remodelling, *J Prosthet Dent* 81(5): 553–561, 1999.

van Steenberghe D, Naert I, Jacobs R, et al: Influence of inflammatory reactions vs. occlusal loading on peri-implant marginal bone level, *Adv Dent Res* 13:130–135, 1999.

Weinberg LA: Therapeutic biomechanics concepts and clinical procedures to reduce implant loading. Part I, *J Oral Implantol* 27(6):293–301, 2001.

Implant Rehabilitation and Clinical Management

Steven E. Eckert

SYNOPSIS

When considering the occlusion on restorations supported and retained by dental implants, it is important to appreciate that the greatest risk to an implant-supported prosthesis is mechanical rather than biological. In this regard no specific technique has been described that is more or less favorable to the ongoing performance of the dental implant. Conversely, mechanical factors and their effect on the ongoing performance of the biomaterials is the most crucial aspect regarding implant-supported prostheses.

As dental implants are not suspended within the alveolus by a periodontal ligament, it is possible to use a smaller number of implants to support a prosthesis than would be anticipated with the natural dentition. As few as four implants may suffice to restore an entire arch of prosthetic teeth. When this occurs, however, it is incumbent upon the clinician to understand that the distance between implants will be such that flexibility of the framework will occur. Such framework flexion would have deleterious effects upon rigid and brittle veneering materials. For this reason, when the minimum number of implants are used, acrylic veneering materials are recommended. When a larger number of implants are used to support a prosthesis, the clinician has the option of using more rigid ceramic veneering materials.

The occlusal scheme that should be used is one that provides simultaneous vertical contacts of opposing teeth in the posterior quadrants when the jaw is in centric relation (Figure 12-1). In eccentric movements, the provision of a mutually protected occlusal scheme with anterior disclusion or a group function occlusal design would be appropriate (Figure 12-2). Considering the occlusion and biomaterials, a practical approach is to provide group function when the minimum number of implants and/or acrylic veneering materials are used to replace the natural teeth. When a larger number of implants are used, there is the option of group function or of mutual protection, but either approach should be provided within an occlusal scheme with flatter cuspal inclines than the natural dentition.

CHAPTER POINTS

- Dental implants have, for all intents and purposes, a direct connection to the surrounding bone
- Dental implants are for practical purposes immobile compared with natural dentition

- Adverse biological consequences associated with minor occlusal overload are generally not observed with dental implants
- Mechanical factors are more critical in the long-term survival of a dental implant-supported prosthesis than are biological factors
- The number of implants used to support a prosthesis must be considered relative to the anticipated flexion that can occur in the prosthetic framework
- When a minimum number of implants are used, the veneering materials that allow flexibility should be considered
- When a larger number of implants are used (six to eight implants), the clinician may use more rigid or brittle materials such as ceramic materials as flexibility of the framework is minimized
- Centric-relation posterior teeth should contact simultaneously in a relatively vertical position
- In eccentric movement, disclusion of the posterior teeth could be provided through the use of a mutually protected occlusal scheme or a group function with posterior and anterior teeth, providing simultaneous lateral contacts on the laterotrusive side and no contact on the mediotrusive side
- A generally low-cusp occlusal anatomy of the posterior teeth is favored

LITERATURE REVIEW

The topic of occlusion and the related topic of articulation are frequently considered relative to the biological or biomechanical factors of the static placement of teeth and the manner in which teeth or prostheses move relative to each other during masticatory function (Figure 12-1).

In understanding the complexities of functional occlusion, an initial appreciation is for the occlusal force to be within acceptable ranges. Conversely, force that is so concentrated as to lead to tissue or prosthesis breakdown is certainly possible, but is not a point of discussion in this chapter.

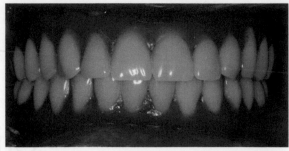

FIG 12-1 Teeth are arranged to provide maximum intercuspation when the jaw is in centric relation regardless of the number of implants or the restorative material.

When considering the contact of natural teeth, whether static or dynamic, the biological consequences deserve primary consideration. Certainly those biological factors that cause tissue breakdown must be avoided. Although occlusion is not considered to be a primary causative factor in periodontal breakdown, it is frequently described as a cofactor that could exacerbate existing periodontal disease. Tooth mobility is often described as a functional adaptation to excessive force when periodontal support is favorable; however, when support diminishes, mobility may become progressive. Biomechanical factors could lead to overload of the natural teeth that may result in abrasive wear, chronic or acute pulpitis, or natural tooth fracture.

Dental implant-supported restorations are subject to biological breakdown, but this only appears to occur when forces are grossly excessive. Severe occlusal force (generally much greater force than would be anticipated in the natural dentition) can cause the osseointegration process to fail. More likely, however, is the fracture of dental materials rather than the loss of integration. Mild to moderate force seems to have little negative effect on the bone-to-implant connection, but does appear to play a role in material failure (Figure 12-2) that may occur as a catastrophic response to a one-time impact at an unfavorable direction or to cumulative load application that results in fracture propagation. Assuming that these interpretations are correct, it appears that dental implant-supported prostheses are more likely to undergo biomechanical failure rather than biological failure.

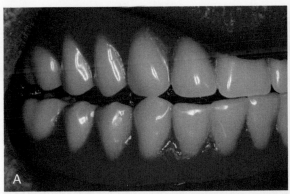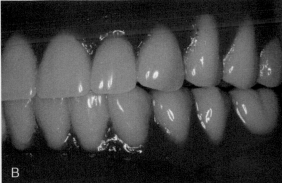

FIG 12-2 **A**, When the mandible moves laterally the clinician may select a mutually protected occlusal scheme with the incisor and canine teeth sharing the lateral guidance while the posterior teeth do not contact in lateral excursions. With ceramic materials these contacts should remain stable but with acrylic resin prosthetic teeth attrition is likely. **B**, Another alternative is to provide group function of anterior and posterior teeth during lateral jaw movement. In this situation the teeth share equally in lateral guidance. Prosthetic teeth should be adjusted in such a way as to ensure group function primarily or to ensure that a mutually protected occlusion gradually "wears" into group function.

Mechanical failure appears to be the higher risk factor in long-term functional performance of an implant-supported prosthesis. This being the case, it would seem prudent to design prostheses with careful consideration of biomechanical factors. As such, no superstructure designs should be considered unless the design features are most likely to sustain the anticipated forces.

There are a number of different factors that can affect the forces that need to be accommodated by an implant prosthesis. The variables are the number of implants, length of the edentulous span, height of the prosthesis, number of teeth being replaced, anticipated forces that may be exerted by the patient, and duration of force application. Each of these factors requires consideration.

The number of implants that are needed to retain an implant prosthesis appears to be less critical than would be the case with a traditional fixed tooth-supported prosthesis. The classic description of Ante's Law is that the peri-cemental area of teeth being replaced must be less than or equal to the peri-cemental area of the teeth used to retain the dental prosthesis. However, with implants the lack of physiological mobility creates a more favorable condition for prosthesis retention. In a similar way the rigidity of the prosthesis in the bone reduces deleterious forces that could result in conditions that previously were implicated in progressive tooth mobility.

There is an ultimate recognition that a relatively small number of dental implants can permanently retain a fixed dental prosthesis. As early as 1995, published research identified the capacity of four strategically placed implants to retain a fixed prosthesis replacing all teeth in one arch. It must be recognized, however, that with a smaller number of implants the increase in the span between implants will result in the potential for increased bending of the prosthesis.

In many instances prostheses can be strengthened, thereby reducing bending of the prosthetic framework, which is achieved by increasing the height and width of the prosthesis. Normally the framework material for dental prostheses is metal (Figure 12-3). Whether the metals are used to support a porcelain veneering material or an acrylic resin tooth replacement, the bulk of a metal and its inversely proportional bending potential must be considered when designing a prosthesis.

One way to reduce force transmission to the underlying implants is by simply reducing the number of teeth to be replaced. Another factor that may be considered is the position of the definitive prosthesis relative to the TM joint complex, as the greater the

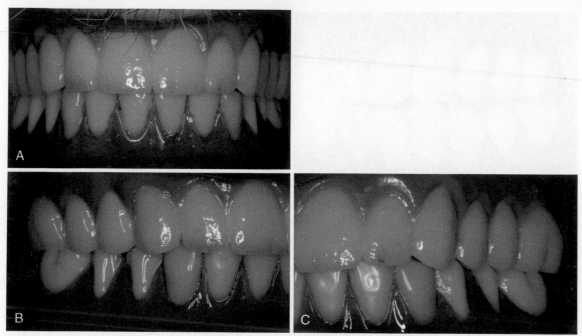

FIG 12-3 When metal-ceramic or all-ceramic prostheses are used in the maxilla and such a prosthesis is opposed by acrylic resin artificial teeth in the mandibular arch, the clinician must anticipate abrasive wear of the mandibular teeth. In this situation a group function occlusion is preferred, as maintenance of a canine disclusion or mutually protected occlusion is not realistic because wear will occur on the acrylic resin teeth.

distance from the joint the lesser the anticipated force application to the prosthesis. Greatest force is generated in the molar regions; force is reduced in the bicuspid and anterior tooth segments.

Magnitude and duration of force application will have a significant effect on the anticipated functional durability of a fixed-implant prosthesis. Low force and short duration of force application are two favorable factors related to the durability of a prosthesis. Conversely, high forces or extended time of force application increase the likelihood of material failure. Unfortunately, the identification of patients who will generate high-magnitude forces for a long application time is difficult. Clinicians may judge patients with hypertrophied masseteric musculature as high risk, a clinical impression that is often correct. The ability to identify patients who will generate force application over longer time frames, such as with bruxism, is less predictable.

Successful treatment therefore is dependent upon the selection of the appropriate dental material for specific patient needs. Application of one treatment approach for all patients will likely result in prosthesis failure for some patients.

When the minimum number of implants are used to support a fixed, full-arch prosthesis, the clinician must anticipate bending of the prosthesis. Even if the dimensions of the metal framework can be maximized, with only four implants supporting an arch of teeth framework bending is inevitable. Consequently the clinician should choose a veneering material that is matched to the supporting metal.

Currently, it is commonly believed that the most accurate fit of the prosthesis is achieved using computer-aided design and computer-aided manufacturing (CAD/CAM) technology. When the minimum number of implants are used, a titanium alloy framework may be fabricated using this technology and then this framework would support acrylic resin prosthetic teeth secured to the framework, as the deflection of the titanium alloy will be complemented by the flexibility of the acrylic resin.

When a greater number of implants are used to support a full-arch prosthesis (six to eight implants),

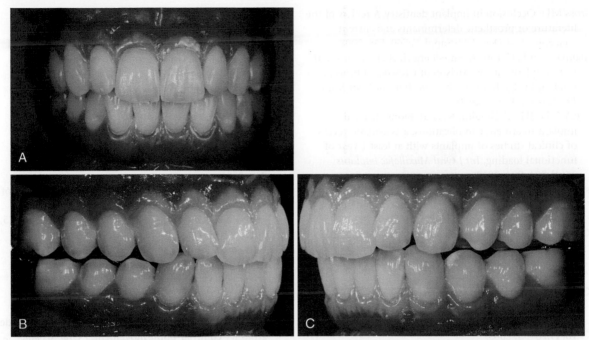

FIG 12-4 When implant-retained metal-ceramic or all-ceramic prostheses are used in the maxilla and mandible, a mutually protected occlusion is favored. **A** represents centric occlusion in which maximum intercuspation is achieved when the jaw is in centric relation. Movement of the mandible to the patient's right side (right laterotrusion) demonstrates mutual contact of the right canine and incisor teeth (**B**). When the mandible makes this movement there will be no tooth contact on the patient's left side as it moves in a mediotrusive path (**C**).

a more rigid framework will be created as the distance between any two implants is reduced. In such a situation a metal framework could be veneered with a ceramic material without a great risk of material fractures secondary to flexion within the prosthesis (Figure 12-4).

As dental implants lack the protective physiological mechanism associated with the periodontal ligament, clinicians need to recognize that lateral movement must occur without interference. In vitro biomechanical studies have consistently demonstrated stress accumulation in the coronal aspects of the implant-prosthetic system. Minimization of the lateral forces on the implants while allowing a smooth eccentric movement may be achieved by using an occlusal surface with lower cusp inclination and narrower occlusal width (see Chapter 7) than might be considered in restoring the natural dentition. Oclusal surfaces need not be flat, but their form should be designed to allow free lateral movement.

ACKNOWLEDGMENTS

The author wishes to acknowledge the reconstruction in Figure 12-3, which was delivered by Dr. Mo Taheri, DMD, and prepared by Thomas Sing, MDT.

REFERENCES

Akca K, Iplikcioglu H: Finite element stress analysis of the influence of staggered versus straight placement of dental implants, *Int J Oral Maxillofac Implants* 16(5):722–730, 2001.

Branemark PI, Svensson B, van Steenberghe D: Ten-year survival rates of fixed prostheses on four or six implants ad modum Branemark in full edentulism, *Clin Oral Implants Res* 6(4):227–231, 1995.

Duyck J, Van Oosterwyck H, Vander Sloten J, et al: Magnitude and distribution of occlusal forces on oral implants supporting fixed prostheses: an in vivo study, *Clin Oral Implants Res* 11(5):465–475, 2000.

Gross MD: Occlusion in implant dentistry. A review of the literature of prosthetic determinants and current concepts, *Aust Dent J* 53(Suppl 1):S60–S68, 2008.

Hjalmarsson L, Ortorp A, Smedberg JI, et al: Precision of fit to implants: a comparison of Cresco and Procera(R) implant bridge frameworks, *Clin Implant Dent Relat Res* 12(4):271–280, 2010.

Hsu YT, Fu JH, Al-Hezaimi K, et al: Biomechanical implant treatment complications: a systematic review of clinical studies of implants with at least 1 year of functional loading, *Int J Oral Maxillofac Implants* 27(4):894–904, 2012.

Ishigaki S, Nakano T, Yamada S, et al: Biomechanical stress in bone surrounding an implant under simulated chewing, *Clin Oral Implants Res* 14(1):97–102, 2003.

Kapos T, Ashy LM, Gallucci GO, et al: Computer-aided design and computer-assisted manufacturing in prosthetic implant dentistry, *Int J Oral Maxillofac Implants* 24(Suppl):110–117, 2009.

Kim Y, Oh TJ, Misch CE, et al: Occlusal considerations in implant therapy: clinical guidelines with biomechanical rationale, *Clin Oral Implants Res* 16(1):26–35, 2005.

Klineberg IJ, Trulsson M, Murray GM: Occlusion on implants—is there a problem?, *J Oral Rehabil* 39(7):522–537, 2012.

Lechner S, Duckmanton N, Klineberg I: Prosthodontic procedures for implant reconstruction. 2. Post-surgical procedures, *Aust Dent J* 37(6):427–432, 1992.

Lewis MB, Klineberg I: Prosthodontic considerations designed to optimize outcomes for single-tooth implants. A review of the literature, *Aust Dent J* 56(2):181–192, 2011.

Mericske-Stern RD, Taylor TD, Belser U: Management of the edentulous patient, *Clin Oral Implants Res* 11(Suppl 1):108–125, 2000.

Misch CE, Bidez MW: Implant-protected occlusion: a biomechanical rationale, *Compendium* 15(11):1330, 1332, 1334, passim; quiz 1344, 1994.

Phillips K, Mitrani R: Implant management for comprehensive occlusal reconstruction, *Compend Contin Educ Dent* 22(3):235–238, 240, 242–236; quiz 248, 2001.

Rungruananunt P, Taylor T, Eckert SE, et al: The effect of static load on dental implant survival: a systematic review, *Int J Oral Maxillofac Implants* 28(5):1218–1225, 2013.

Rungsiyakull C, Rungsiyakull P, Li Q, et al: Effects of occlusal inclination and loading on mandibular bone remodeling: a finite element study, *Int J Oral Maxillofac Implants* 26(3):527–537, 2011.

Sarinnaphakorn L, Murray GM, Johnson CW, et al: The effect of posterior tooth guidance on non-working side arbitrary condylar point movement, *J Oral Rehabil* 24(9):678–690, 1997.

Sutpideler M, Eckert SE, Zobitz M, et al: Finite element analysis of effect of prosthesis height, angle of force application, and implant offset on supporting bone, *Int J Oral Maxillofac Implants* 19(6):819–825, 2004.

Weinberg LA: Therapeutic biomechanics concepts and clinical procedures to reduce implant loading, Part I. *J Oral Implantol* 27(6):293–301, 2001.

SECTION | 4 |

Clinical Practice and Occlusion Management

CHAPTER 13

Temporomandibular Joint Disorders

Gunnar E. Carlsson

SYNOPSIS

This chapter presents a brief overview of the most common temporomandibular (TM) joint disorders, with an emphasis on their association with dental occlusion. The evidence for an occlusal etiology of TM joint disorders is weak; conversely, it is well established that several TM joint disorders can cause occlusal disturbances. The TM joint disorders presented comprise disk interference and traumatic disorders, osteoarthrosis and osteoarthritis (OA), rheumatoid arthritis, and some other less common disorders. A careful history and a clinical examination, including imaging of the TM joint, will, in most cases, be sufficient for a preliminary diagnosis. Many patients with benign TM joint disorders can be diagnosed and managed in general dental practice, whereas others will require specialist and multidisciplinary diagnosis and treatment.

CHAPTER POINTS

- Many diseases may involve the temporomandibular (TM) joints. The most common and the most studied are osteoarthrosis and osteoarthritis (OA), rheumatoid arthritis, and disk interference disorders.
- It is often claimed that occlusal disturbances can cause TM joint disorders, but the evidence for that is weak. Conversely, it is well established that several disorders affecting the TM joints may cause occlusal disturbances (e.g., occlusal instability and/or anterior open bite in patients with rheumatoid arthritis).
- Disk displacement has been considered to be the most common TM joint disorder. It involves a dysfunction of the condyle-disk relation, but the disk position is either not at all or only weakly related to clinical symptoms; the term is therefore often misleading.
- Disk derangement disorders can usually be managed with a conservative approach; more "aggressive" methods are seldom indicated or beneficial.
- Several traumatic TM joint disorders are associated with changes in occlusion,

161

which require careful consideration in diagnosis and treatment.

- Osteoarthrosis is a degeneration of the TM joint but is, in general, a benign disorder with minor or no symptoms and a good prognosis. In OA, an inflammatory component is added to the joint degeneration. Acute inflammatory phases associated with pain and dysfunction are usually reversible with simple treatment.

- A substantial proportion of patients with rheumatoid arthritis may have TM joint involvement. TM joint involvement is related to the severity and duration of the systemic disease. The proportion of patients with rheumatoid arthritis afflicted with severe occlusal disturbances and dysfunction of the masticatory system seems to decrease with improved medical treatment of the systemic disease.

- There is often a poor correlation between findings from TM joint imaging and clinical signs and symptoms of TM joint disorders.

- Investigation of a patient with a possible TM joint disorder may include a history and various clinical, laboratory, and imaging procedures; however, in most cases a careful history and a clinical examination of the masticatory system focusing on TM joint mobility, sounds, and tenderness to palpation may be sufficient for a preliminary diagnosis and initial treatment.

The role played by disorders of the temporomandibular (TM) joint in producing signs and symptoms in temporomandibular disorders (TMDs) has been much discussed. In the early development of concepts of TMD, TM joint problems were the focus. Interest then turned to the musculature as the most frequent source of pain and dysfunction of the masticatory system. During the 1980s, many clinicians thought that internal derangements of the TM joint were the major factor in TMDs. Today it is generally accepted that TMDs include a variety of different disorders involving the TM joint, the masticatory muscles, and associated structures, separately or together (Carlsson & Magnusson 1999, de Leeuw & Klasser 2013). To classify TMDs either as arthrogenous or myogenous is difficult, because patients with a primary joint disorder usually have secondary muscle dysfunction, and patients with a primary muscle disorder may exhibit joint symptoms (Stegenga 2001).

More than 100 different diseases can affect the musculoskeletal system, and many of these may also involve the TM joint. Some of these are rare and of limited interest for the general dental practitioner, but a few are relatively common, such as osteoarthrosis and osteoarthritis (OA) and rheumatoid arthritis (RA); the dentist should be familiar with them.

This chapter will focus on TM joint disorders that in various ways may be associated with changes in occlusion.

DISK INTERFERENCE DISORDERS

Of various TM joint sounds, clicking is the most common and indicative of a disk derangement. Variations from the textbook appearance of the TM joint disk have been termed disk displacements and they may occur in various directions; anterior displacements are probably the most frequently described (Figure 13-1). Among several classifications presented over the years the following is probably the most frequently cited (de Leeuw & Klasser 2013):

- Disk displacement with reduction (the displaced disk reduces on opening, usually resulting in a

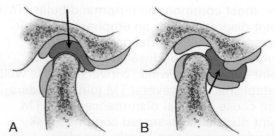

FIG 13-1 Schematic Drawings from Arthrographic Radiographs of TM Joints A, Normal position of the disk. **B,** Anteriorly displaced disk (*arrow*). (Reproduced from Carlsson & Magnusson 1999, with the permission of Quintessence Publishing Company Inc., Chicago.)

noise, clicking; this is called reciprocal clicking when the noise is heard during both the opening and closing movement)

- Disk displacement without reduction, with or without limited opening ("closed lock"); clicking ceases with locking; if the acute condition becomes chronic, pain is usually reduced and opening normalizes with time

Several recent studies have reported that there is often a lack of correlation between the structural variation of the disk-condyle complex and clinical symptoms; some patients with verified "disk displacement" may lack symptoms, and others who have symptoms and disk displacement may improve without change in the structural TM joint findings. It has been proposed that "disk displacement" is misleading, as it suggests a need for treatment, and should therefore be replaced by "disk derangement" (Stegenga & de Bont 2006).

The symptoms described in association with such disk derangements vary greatly, but usually include joint sounds, pain, tenderness to palpation of joints and/or muscles, and reduced mandibular mobility. No clear association between disk derangements and occlusion has been reported.

The etiology is not well understood but trauma, bruxism, and general joint hypermobility are frequently reported in the histories of patients with disk interference disorders. The prevalence of disk derangements presented in epidemiological studies varies much, and a recent systematic review reported a range of prevalence of clicking in population samples from 18% to 35% (Naeije et al. 2013).

Management

During the 1980s there was an enormous increase in interest in disk interference disorders. This resulted in a rapid improvement of diagnostic and therapeutic methods, but it also probably led to overdiagnosis and overtreatment; for example, overuse of magnetic resonance imaging (MRI), anterior positioning appliances followed by occlusal therapy, and various surgical methods, resulting in higher cost and sometimes increased risk for the patients. It has been repeatedly shown that many patients with TM joint disk derangements respond well to conservative treatment (Carlsson & Magnusson 1999). It is also well established that painless jaw function is possible with

deranged disks (Stegenga 2001). In the majority of patients diagnosed with disk interference disorders, the simple treatment modalities suggested for TMD patients should first be tried (i.e., counseling or reassurance, medication, and physical therapy, sometimes including an interocclusal appliance). This conservative approach has been proven effective by long-term clinical follow-up investigations (de Leeuw & Klasser 2013). In a sample of 40 patients with permanent disk displacement followed for 2.5 years without treatment, spontaneous improvement was observed in about 75% of the cases (Kurita et al. 1998).

The use of protrusive positioning splints in order to "capture the disk" is rarely indicated, as it may lead to serious changes in the occlusion, requiring extensive occlusal therapy. Some authors have even maintained that such treatment is worse than the "disease" itself. Manipulation techniques to normalize the disk position in patients with disk displacement without reduction may be successful if the "closed lock" is acute (i.e., of short duration).

A variety of surgical procedures have been applied and appear to give good results when severe pain and dysfunction continues in association with disk interference disorders. However, long-term studies are lacking, as are randomized prospective studies. Surgery is certainly not the first method of choice for treatment of disk derangement.

There is still not full consensus on the importance of and need for treatment of TM joint clicking (i.e., a disk displacement with reduction). However, a recent systematic review concluded that this is mostly a stable, pain-free, and lifelong condition of the TM joint and usually does not merit treatment. The favorable natural course of disk derangements only warrants active intervention for painful disk displacements without reduction by using conservative, nonsurgical methods to alleviate pain and improve mouth opening. "For most patients, a disc displacement is just a pain-free, lifelong lasting, 'noisy annoyance' from their TM joint" (Naeije et al. 2013).

It can be concluded that a careful history and a clinical examination, without use of sophisticated imaging techniques, and conservative management should be adequate for most patients with disk interference disorders. If severe pain and dysfunction remain after such an approach, the patient is best referred to a specialist clinic.

163

TRAUMATIC TEMPOROMANDIBULAR JOINT DISORDERS

Injury to the TM joint may result from internal forces (such as from jaw muscles) or from external forces (such as contact sport or a slamming door) applied to the joint area or along the mandible. Such trauma may produce damage to the soft tissues, the condyle, or both. The consequences may be joint dislocation, hemarthrosis, and condylar fracture; all of these have consequences for the occlusion.

Acute Dislocation

Diagnosis and treatment of an acute dislocation should be familiar to all dentists: the patient cannot close the mouth and there is an anterior open bite ("open lock"). In front of one or both auditory canals there is a depression, before which it is usually possible to palpate the condyle positioned anterior to the articular eminence (Figure 13-2). When the

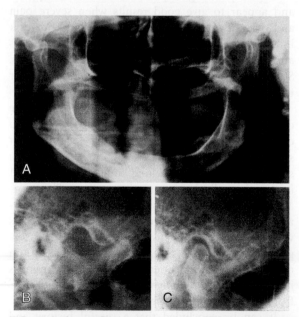

FIG 13-2 Acute Dislocation of the TM Joints in an Edentulous Patient **A,** Panoramic radiograph of a bilateral dislocation. Both condyles are anterior to the articular eminences. **B,** Transcranial radiograph of the dislocated right TM joint of the patient in **A**. **C,** The right TM joint after reduction.

dislocation is acute, reduction can often be done without anesthesia, by bimanual manipulation of the mandible from its open locked position. A classical description (similar to one found in documents from the time of Hippocrates!) suggests the following procedure: the operator stands in front of the patient and uses the thumbs to apply pressure to the molar regions in a downward direction; at the same time the chin is raised with the other fingers, after which the mandible is forced backward. If the dislocation occurred a day or days previously, there may be considerable pain and muscular tension. In such cases, local anesthetic blocks of the TM joint area(s) are performed before the manipulation, to provide patient comfort and reduce muscle guarding. In rare cases, especially after longstanding dislocation, intravenous sedation or even general anesthesia may be necessary to enable manipulation of the dislocated joint. After a successful mandibular reduction, the patient should be advised to avoid wide opening movements and heavy chewing for several days.

Hemarthrosis

A blow to the mandible or extensive stretching of the joint's soft tissues may lead to edema or hemorrhage within the joint space. When the trauma has not led to mandibular fracture, the patient will usually present with mild swelling and tenderness in the TM joint area, pain on movement, and reduced joint mobility. The patient often reports that the teeth on the injured side do not fit, which is the clinical manifestation of the lateral open bite caused by effusion and hemarthrosis within the joint space. This can be seen radiographically as an increased distance between the condyle and the fossa. This condition is sometimes referred to as *traumatic arthritis*.

If the tissue injury is not severe, the acute symptoms usually disappear within one or a few weeks. Ice may be applied intermittently to skin overlying the joint area during the first day, after which massage and careful jaw exercises may be introduced gradually to normalize joint mobility. If pain and swelling are severe, drugs with analgesic and antiphlogistic effect may be prescribed. It is important to avoid occlusal therapy during the acute phase, as the occlusion will normalize when the joint effusion resolves.

Condylar Fractures

Condylar and subcondylar fractures comprise a substantial part of all mandibular fractures. Patients will typically present with an open bite and a slight mandibular shift toward the affected side. With bilateral condyle fractures there is an anterior open bite. Patients with such fractures usually require specialist evaluation and treatment. However, the sequelae of condylar fractures on the occlusion are of general interest. In children with condyle fractures, the great capacity for TM joint remodeling results in only minor or no long-term effects on the occlusion. In adults, occlusal instability, including an increased distance between the retruded and the intercuspal jaw positions, is a frequent consequence of a previous condylar fracture (Figure 13-3). This requires special consideration in diagnosis of the occlusion for prosthodontic rehabilitation.

DEGENERATIVE TEMPOROMANDIBULAR JOINT DISORDERS

Degenerative joint disease is the most common form of rheumatoid disease affecting the human body. There are several terms used for this disease, osteoarthrosis and OA being the most frequent. It has been suggested that OA be used for disorders with clinical symptoms (indicating an ongoing inflammatory process) and osteoarthrosis where inflammation is absent or minimal and the patient is asymptomatic. There is, however, no full consensus on

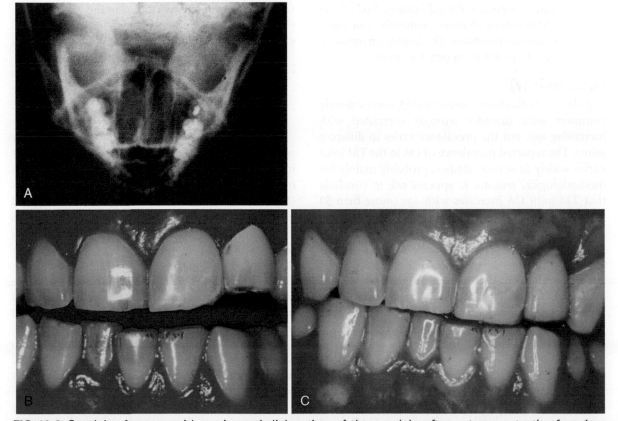

FIG 13-3 Condylar fracture with an inward dislocation of the condyle after a trauma to the face in a 29-year-old woman. **A,** Axial radiograph. **B,** Maximum intercuspal position and damages on some teeth after the trauma. **C,** One year later after some restorative treatment and occlusal adjustment.

the terminology; some maintain that this disorder involves both degeneration and inflammation and that OA is the logical term (Milam 2005, Stegenga & de Bont 2006). It can be practical to use the abridged form OA for both. The pathophysiology of degenerative TM joint diseases is described in Chapter 6.

OA is primarily noninflammatory in nature, with initial involvement of the cartilaginous and subchondral layers of the joint. It is defined as a degenerative condition of the joint, characterized by fibrillation and deterioration of the articular tissue and concomitant changes in the form of the articular components. The first changes in the articular tissues in OA are rarely visible radiographically. Radiographic evidence of changes in form will typically appear only after considerable time, which can explain the poor correlation between clinical and radiographic signs of OA. Development of OA is often a gradual non-symptomatic process, but the superimposition of secondary inflammatory changes (synovitis) can cause transitory clinical symptoms. The long-term outcome of OA in the TM joint is, in general, good.

Epidemiology

Population studies have shown that OA is an extremely common joint disorder strongly correlated with increasing age, but the prevalence varies in different joints. The reported prevalence of OA in the TM joint varies widely in several studies, probably mainly for methodological reasons. It appears safe to conclude that TM joint OA increases with age (more than 50 years), and it is more frequent in women than in men, as is also the case in other joints of the body (Zarb & Carlsson 1999). A systematic review found a mean prevalence of TM joint disorders of 30% among TMD patients and 3% in population samples (Manfredini et al. 2011). The clinician should expect a much higher prevalence among elderly individuals.

Etiology

Although overloading has been proposed to be a major etiologic factor, it is prudent to recognize that the understanding of the etiology of OA is far from complete. The literature does not contain compelling evidence for an occlusal contribution to TMDs, and this is true also for OA of the TM joint (Zarb & Carlsson 1999, Pullinger & Seligman 2000). It has been suggested that OA represents an organ failure due to an imbalance in normal tissue turnover between synthesis and breakdown. A relative increase of breakdown or degenerative activity leads to accumulation of degradation products, resulting in an inflammatory response. The previously often-proposed relationship between disk derangement and OA has been questioned, as no strong evidence is available. Present research focuses more on the molecular level of joint tissues and the failure of lubrication system leading to destruction of the articular surfaces (Stegenga 2001, Milam 2005).

Diagnosis

The signs and symptoms are very similar to those of the neuromuscular type of TMD. However, there are some features that might help with the differential diagnosis:

- They are almost always unilateral
- Symptoms often worsen during the day
- Pain is located in the joint itself
- Crepitation is a more common joint sound than clicking (but it is a late sign of the disorder)
- Radiographic changes of the TM joint are rare in the early phase of OA but increase in prevalence with time (e.g., condyle flattening, osteophytes, sclerosis, decreased joint space)

It is important to realize that there is often poor correlation between clinical and radiographic findings; many subjects with a radiographic diagnosis of OA may be asymptomatic or reveal only crepitus (Figure 13-4). Laboratory findings in synovial fluid have shown promising results in identifying markers of disease activity. The methods offer interesting research possibilities but are not yet applicable to OA diagnosis in general dental practice.

Patients with OA are characterized by a longer slide between the retruded contact position (RCP) and intercuspal position (ICP), larger overjet (horizontal overlap), and reduced overbite (vertical overlap). These occlusal characteristics have been interpreted to be the consequence of articular remodeling associated with OA, rather than its cause (Pullinger & Seligman 2000).

OA often has acute and chronic stages. It has been estimated that the average duration of the acute painful stage is 9 to 12 months. The disease process tends to "burn out," and the TM joint often shows extensive osseous changes but surprisingly good

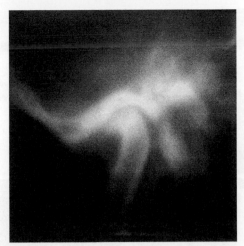

FIG 13-4 Tomogram of the Left TM Joint with Extensive Deformation Indicating OA The patient had a short period of pain some time ago and dysfunction but functioned well for many years both before and after that event.

function (Figure 13-4). The diagnosis of OA must acknowledge the usually favorable long-term prognosis of this mainly benign disorder.

Management

Because of the current knowledge of the favorable prognosis of OA, the first step in treatment is to reassure the patient about the problems associated with this benign disorder. For patients with only crepitus or mild symptoms, reassurance is the only treatment necessary. For patients with more severe symptoms, including pain and dysfunction, treatment may include one or more of the following:

- Medication—most frequently nonsteroidal antiinflammatory drugs (NSAIDs), but in cases of severe pain, intraarticular injection of glucocorticoid, hyaluronic acid, or glucosamine can be used (Kopp 2006, de Souza et al. 2012)
- Physical therapy—rest and soft diet in the most acute stage, gradually beginning jaw exercises when pain subsides, to promote normal mandibular function
- Splint therapy—interocclusal stabilization appliance (to provide reduction of a possible overloading of the joint structures)

Surgery is very seldom indicated in the treatment of TM joint OA.

RHEUMATOID ARTHRITIS

RA is a systemic inflammatory disease that involves peripheral joints in a symmetric distribution. The etiology of RA is still largely unknown, but immunological mechanisms appear to play an important role. The prevalence of RA has been reported to be about 1% to 2% of the adult population, with incidence figures of 0.03% to 0.1% per year. RA has shown a 3:1 female predilection. TM joint involvement in patients with RA depends on the duration and severity of the systemic disease, but it can be expected that about half of them will develop TM joint complaints. Severe forms of the disease with significant functional disability, including major occlusal disturbances, have been shown to occur in 10% to 15% of these patients. There is an indication that this prevalence is decreasing thanks to improved medical treatment of the systemic disease (Kallenberg 2013).

Diagnosis

Diagnosing RA of the TM joint will seldom present problems, as the systemic disease usually starts in other joints before the TM joint and the diagnosis has most probably been established when the TM joint is affected. Symptoms include pain at rest and on chewing, stiffness in the morning, and difficulty in opening the mouth. As the disease process continues, the stability of the occlusion is often destroyed, revealed as an unstable intercuspal position and an increased distance between RCP and ICP. Anterior bite opening may occur due to destruction of the condyles (Figures 13-5 and 13-6). Radiographic changes include erosion of the cortical contour of the joint components, reduced joint space, subchondral cysts, and increasingly severe destruction of the bone, eventually leading to complete loss of the condyle. Modern diagnostic methods such as analysis of TM joint fluid, laboratory tests, and thermological and arthroscopic techniques have improved our knowledge of the disease, but they are limited to specialist clinics. There is good evidence that neuropeptides take part in the modulation of TM joint arthritis and pain (Kopp 2001, Milam 2005).

Treatment

Because RA is a systemic disease, a physician must manage the primary care, while the dentist can take

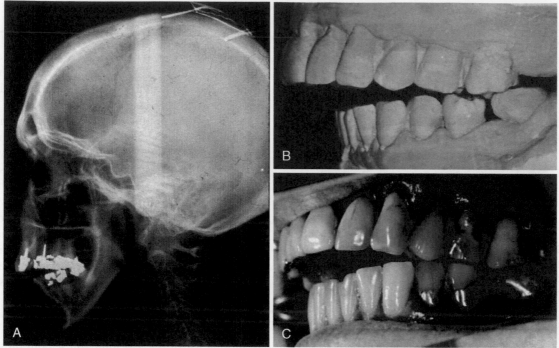

FIG 13-5 Open Bite in a Patient with Rheumatoid Arthritis Diagnosed 6 Years Ago and Starting to Affect the TM Joints 2 Years Ago **A,** Lateral cephalogram showing the open bite caused by the severe destruction of the TM joints. **B,** Casts of the patient with occlusal contacts only on the second molars. **C,** Clinical view after occlusal adjustment improving occlusal and masticatory function to the satisfaction of the patient.

part in management of local TM joint signs and symptoms. Suppression of inflammation is the general goal in treatment of RA patients. This usually involves supportive therapy to reduce pain, inflammation, and excessive joint loading.

Pain in an acute phase is most probably associated with inflammation, and therefore analgesics with antiinflammatory effects should be prescribed, for example, acetylsalicylic acid or NSAIDs such as naproxen or ibuprofen. If the pain is severe, intraarticular injection of a glucocorticosteroid often gives rapid relief.

When the acute pain has subsided or when there are only minor symptoms, physical exercises are indicated to improve joint muscle function and strength. Positive effects of physical training in TM joint-RA patients have been shown in a comparative study (Tegelberg & Kopp 1988). In a 15-year follow-up of patients with RA, subjective symptoms and function of the masticatory system were remarkably stable in

spite of the significant radiologic changes that had occurred in the TM joints during the observation period (Kallenberg 2013).

The etiological role played by occlusal factors in the development of RA of the TM joint is uncertain. From a clinical point of view it is recommended, however, to provide all patients suffering from RA with as stable an occlusion as possible, for example by eliminating gross occlusal interferences, restoring lost teeth by means of (provisional) prosthetic appliances, or temporarily with interocclusal appliances. An anterior open bite caused by RA can often be reduced by simple occlusal adjustment (Figure 13-5). If the disease has resulted in a very severe malocclusion, orthognathic surgery may be indicated.

A problem in prosthodontic rehabilitation of patients with RA is the continuing joint destruction that may disturb the occlusal stability of any reconstruction. A check of the disease activity can be obtained from the rheumatologist, and long-term

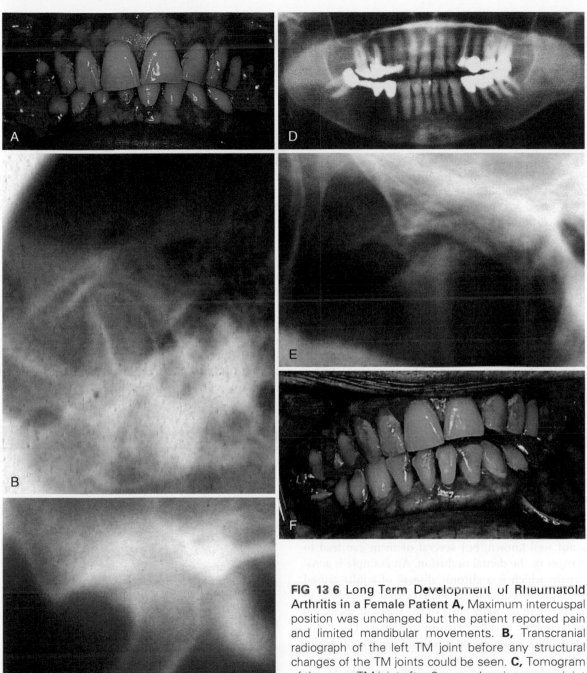

FIG 13 6 Long Term Development of Rheumatoid Arthritis in a Female Patient A, Maximum intercuspal position was unchanged but the patient reported pain and limited mandibular movements. **B,** Transcranial radiograph of the left TM joint before any structural changes of the TM joints could be seen. **C,** Tomogram of the same TM joint after 8 years showing severe joint destruction. **D,** Panoramic radiograph after 17 years when severe destruction of both TM joints has occurred. **E,** Part of the radiograph in **D** showing an almost total loss of the condyle. **F,** Maximum intercuspal position showing an anterior open bite and occlusal instability at the time of radiographs **D** and **E**.

169

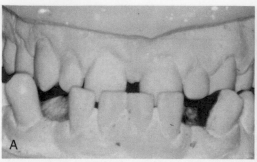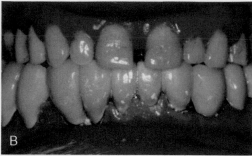

FIG 13-7 In a Patient with Acromegaly, the Extensive Growth of the Mandible has Led to Loss of Practically all Occlusal Contacts **A,** Casts with wax added on posterior mandibular teeth to see if prosthetic treatment could improve the situation. **B,** Fourteen years later the patient has multiple occlusal contacts after extensive treatment including maxillofacial surgery and prosthetic restorations.

provisional prostheses may be necessary if acute phases can still be expected. Another problem is the often substantially increased distance between the retruded and habitual occlusal positions. The retruded position cannot be used as a reference for transfer records because the disease processes have destroyed the joint structures. A more anterior position that is comfortable for the patient and acceptable to the musculature is chosen.

OTHER TEMPOROMANDIBULAR JOINT DISORDERS

The TM joint may also be afflicted in many other systemic diseases; for example, psoriatic arthritis, ankylosing spondylitis, gout, and acromegaly. The prevalence of TM joint involvement in these diseases is not well known, but several of them can lead to changes in the dental occlusion. An example is acromegaly, which is a chronic disease of adults caused by hypersecretion of growth hormone leading to enlargement of many parts of the skeleton, including the mandible and the TM joints (Figure 13-7). The importance of including questions on general health in the patient's history is obvious.

Neoplasms may be found in the TM joint. Malignant tumors are extremely rare, and when they occur they are most often metastatic. Since it has been reported that they may present with symptoms similar to TMDs, patients with a history of cancer and TM joint dysfunction must be referred for a radiographic examination of the TM joint. More common, but still

very rare, are benign neoplasms, which may change the form of the joint components and cause dysfunction and occlusal disturbances. Although not a neoplasm but a developmental disturbance, unilateral condylar hyperplasia is associated with similar consequences because of the enlarged condyle, which will also lead to facial asymmetry and malocclusion (Carlsson & Magnusson 1999).

REFERENCES

Carlsson GE, Magnusson T: *Management of Temporomandibular Disorders in the General Dental Practice*, Chicago, 1999, Quintessence.

de Leeuw R, Klasser GD, editors: *Orofacial Pain. Guidelines for Assessment, Diagnosis, and Management*, ed 5, Chicago, 2013, Quintessence.

de Souza RF, da Lovato Silva CH, Nasser M, et al: Interventions for the management of temporomandibular joint osteoarthritis, *Cochrane Database Syst Rev* (4):CD007261, 2012. doi: 10.1002/14651858.CD007261.pub2.

Kallenberg A: Long-term development of temporomandibular disorders in rheumatoid arthritis. Thesis. University of Gothenburg, Göteborg, Sweden, 2013.

Kopp S: Neuroendocrine, immune, and local responses related to temporomandibular disorders, *J Orofac Pain* 15:9–28, 2001.

Kopp S: Medical treatment of TMJ arthritis. In Laskin DM, Greene CS, Hylander WL, editors: *TMDs: An Evidence-Based Approach to Diagnosis and Treatment*, Chicago, 2006, Quintessence, pp 441–453.

Kurita K, Westesson PL, Yuasa H, et al: Natural course of untreated symptomatic temporomandibular disc displacement without reduction, *J Dent Res* 77: 361–365, 1998.

Manfredini D, Guarda-Nardini L, Winocur E, et al: Research diagnostic criteria for temporomandibular disorders: a systematic review of axis I epidemiologic findings, *Oral Surg Oral Med Oral Pathol Oral Radiol Endod* 112:453–462, 2011.

Milam SB: Pathogenesis of degenerative temporomandibular joint arthritides, *Odontology* 93:7–15, 2005.

Naeije M, Te Veldhuis AH, Te Veldhuis EC, et al: Disc displacement within the human temporomandibular joint: a systematic review of a "noisy annoyance," *J Oral Rehabil* 40:139–158, 2013.

Pullinger AG, Seligman DA: Quantification and validation of predictive values of occlusal variables in temporomandibular disorders using a multifactorial analysis, *J Prosthet Dent* 83:66–75, 2000.

Stegenga B: Osteoarthritis of the temporomandibular joint organ and its relationship to disc displacement, *J Orofac Pain* 15:193–205, 2001.

Stegenga B, de Bont LGM: TMJ disc derangements. In Laskin DM, Greene CS, Hylander WL, editors: *TMDs: An Evidence-Based Approach to Diagnosis and Treatment*, Chicago, 2006, Quintessence, pp 125–136.

Tegelberg A, Kopp S: Short-term effect of physical training on temporomandibular joint disorder in individuals with rheumatoid arthritis and ankylosing spondylitis, *Acta Odontol Scand* 46:49–56, 1988.

Zarb GA, Carlsson GE: Temporomandibular disorders: osteoarthritis, *J Orofac Pain* 13:295–306, 1999.

Further Reading

De Boever JA, Carlsson GE, Klineberg IJ: Need for occlusal therapy and prosthodontic treatment in the management of temporomandibular disorders. Part II: tooth loss and prosthodontic treatment, *J Oral Rehabil* 27:647–659, 2000.

Elfving L, Helkimo M, Magnusson T: Prevalence of different temporomandibular joint sounds, with emphasis on disc-displacement, in patients with temporomandibular disorders and controls, *Swed Dent J* 26:9–19, 2002.

Holmlund AB, Axelsson S, Gynther GW: A comparison of discectomy and arthroscopic lysis and lavage for the treatment of chronic closed lock of the temporomandibular joint: a randomized outcome study, *J Oral Maxillo Surg* 59:972–977, 2001.

Kjellberg H: Juvenile chronic arthritis, *Swed Dent J Suppl* 109:1–56, 1995.

Könönen M, Wenneberg B: Systemic conditions affecting the TMJ. In Laskin DM, Greene CS, Hylander WL, editors: *TMDs an Evidence-Based Approach to Diagnosis and Treatmen*, Chicago, 2006, Quintessence, pp 137–146.

Minakuchi H, Kuboki T, Matsuka Y, et al: Randomized controlled evaluation of non-surgical treatments for temporomandibular joint anterior disc displacement without reduction, *J Dent Res* 80:924–928, 2001.

Okesson JP: *Orofacial Pain. Guidelines for Assessment, Diagnosis and Management*, ed 4, Chicago, 1998, Quintessence.

Tanaka E, Detamore MS, Mercuri LG: Degenerative disorders of the temporomandibular joint: etiology, diagnosis, and treatment, *J Dent Res* 87:296–307, 2008.

Wenham CY, Conaghan PG: New horizons in osteoarthritis, *Age Ageing* 42:272–278, 2013.

Zarb GA, Carlsson GE, Sessle BJ, et al, editors: *Temporomandibular Joint and Masticatory Muscle Disorders*, Copenhagen, 1994, Munksgaard.

Jaw Muscle Disorders

Merete Bakke

SYNOPSIS

This chapter reviews the current knowledge
of the etiology and physiology of jaw
muscle disorders, and it presents an
approach for their clinical assessment and
treatment.

Jaw muscle disorders are characterized
by pain that is usually aggravated by
function. They are present in 45% of
patients with temporomandibular
disorders (TMDs), and women are affected
more frequently than men are. Several
contributing factors must be present for
the development of jaw muscle disorders.
No studies have yet fully explained the
relative importance of potential risk
factors.

The masseter and medial pterygoid
muscles serve primarily as sources of bite
force, whereas the temporalis and lateral
pterygoid muscles are important for jaw
movements and stability. Overuse, in terms
of sustained activity and high-level
contractions without rest periods, is
associated with raised intramuscular
pressure, and it leads to local ischemia,
increased cell membrane permeability,
edema, and eventually cellular damage.

Muscle pain is generally described as a
continuous deep dull ache, tightness, or
pressure. The onset is normally gradual,
and may vary from a feeling of tiredness to
a more severe sharp pain. The pain could
result from trauma, sustained or forceful
contractions, and stretching or ischemia but
may also be referred from other structures
(e.g., temporomandibular joints [TMJs]).
Local conditions, such as inflammation,
increase the receptivity of the pain
receptors, lowering their threshold for
activation and thus the sensation of pain.

173

A comprehensive evaluation of the jaw muscles includes a systematic history and clinical examination. The clinical examination has two main purposes: to assess jaw function and, if possible, to make controlled and standardized provoking of the patient's pain. The treatment of jaw muscle disorders is directed toward reducing pain and improving function; it should generally be reversible, evidence based, or at least based on well-established clinical practice

CHAPTER POINTS

- Jaw muscle disorders are a collection of conditions affecting the muscles, and primarily characterized by pain and limited jaw movements; they are part of temporomandibular disorders (TMDs).

- The primary masticatory muscles are the temporalis, masseter, and medial and lateral pterygoid muscles. The trigeminal nerve innervates the jaw muscles and muscle fibers associated with long contraction times, and resistance to fatigue predominates. The jaw muscles and the bite force adapt to the prevailing level of activity. Fibrosis may occur with overuse.

- The experience of muscle pain is poorly localized, but pain provoked by manual palpation more accurately identifies pain location. The intensity may be assessed by a visual analogue scale (VAS) and by rating of the response to the palpation.

- Limited mandibular opening, (less than 40 mm) is assessed by measurement between the upper and lower incisors.

- Chronic localized myalgia in terms of myofascial pain is the most frequent jaw muscle disorder. Pain from jaw muscles may also be diagnosed as headache, and it may be secondary to disk displacements, osteoarthritis, and rheumatoid arthritis of the TMJ.

- Counseling, intraoral appliances, analgesics and nonsteroidal antiinflammatory drugs (NSAIDs), and physical therapy are the main treatments for jaw muscle disorders.

EPIDEMIOLOGY AND ETIOLOGY OF JAW MUSCLE DISORDERS

Jaw muscle disorders, a collection of muscle conditions, are part of TMDs affecting the TMJs and jaw muscles. They are characterized by pain that is usually aggravated by function. There may also be limited jaw movements. TMDs affect women at least twice as frequently as men, and the condition is most prevalent in young to middle-aged adults. According to studies using the Research Diagnostic Criteria (RDC) for TMDs defined by Dworkin & LeResche (1992), muscle disorders in terms of myofascial pain with or without mouth-opening limitation are frequently found in TMDs, that is, in 45% of the patients. However, disk displacement disorders are present in 40%, and disorders of arthralgia, osteoarthritis, and osteoarthrosis are present in about 30% of the patients (Manfredini et al. 2011). The corresponding figure for myofascial pain with or without mouth-opening limitation found in epidemiological studies was 10%.

Pain in the jaw muscles, typically experienced as facial pain and headache, is the most prevalent chronic pain condition in the orofacial region. Epidemiological studies indicate that about 5% of the population suffers from jaw muscle pain (myalgia) that is sufficiently severe to require treatment (e.g., Kuttila et al. 1998). However, there is considerable fluctuation in the presence and intensity of the pain. As in other musculoskeletal conditions, jaw muscle disorders often run a recurrent or chronic course, and there may be psychological factors that can either produce or influence the pain experience. Depression, which has been shown to be present in some TMD patients, as well as multiple pain conditions, increases the risk of the development of persistent jaw muscle pain. However, symptoms can also be transient, and spontaneous pain reduction may occur.

The etiology of jaw muscle disorders is considered multifactorial, whereby several contributing factors must be present for a jaw muscle disorder to develop. No studies have yet fully explained the relative importance of potential risk factors. Thus there is presently no consensus of simple cause-effect relationships (e.g., between occlusal features and jaw muscle pain) even if occlusal parameters have been shown to influence jaw muscle activity and strength. Several occlusal features (e.g., anterior open bite) are associated with jaw muscle pain and other TMDs, but they may be a consequence of TMDs rather than their cause. Based on the present information, only loss of posterior support and unilateral cross bite appear to be true occlusal risk factors (Türp & Schindler 2012). Reduced jaw muscle strength (bite force) in patients with TMDs may also represent a risk factor, but this reduction could arise because of local pain or reduced occlusal support. Sleep bruxism has also been cited as an important factor for development of myalgia. However, in reality sporadic or a certain amount of sleep bruxism is observed in most asymptomatic adults. The prevalence is greatest in children and teenagers, and it seems to decrease with age. Interestingly, people who suffer from severe bruxism seem to have less pain than those with less frequent bruxism. In these cases, sleep bruxism is regarded as a genuine sleep disorder (Lobbezoo & Naeije 2001).

Because of the unclear etiology of jaw muscle disorders, there is no objective diagnostic method to identify the condition easily; there is no gold standard (such as tissue biopsy) against which a diagnostic test can be compared with accuracy and reliability. The best approach is a comprehensive medical and dental history and a thorough clinical examination.

FUNCTIONAL ANATOMY AND PHYSIOLOGY OF THE JAW MUSCLES

Knowledge of the functional anatomy and physiology of jaw muscles should help with diagnosis and differential diagnoses of jaw muscle disorders. Anatomical details of jaw muscles are found in anatomical texts but aspects of jaw muscle function and physiology will be briefly discussed. This section complements the comprehensive reviews of jaw muscle control and jaw movements in Chapter 5.

Jaw function during biting, chewing, swallowing, and speech is determined by a complex interaction between jaw muscles, the TMJ, and teeth through the nervous system. The primary masticatory muscles are the temporalis, masseter, and medial and lateral pterygoids. Branches from the mandibular nerve, external carotid artery, and internal jugular vein innervate and

vascularize the muscles. The jaw muscles function in concert with the suprahyoid and the infrahyoid muscles, supplemented by the tongue, lip, and cheek muscles. The cervical muscles have also an indirect role through stabilizing and changing head posture during mandibular movements (Eriksson et al. 2000).

Functional Anatomy

Jaw muscles consist of bundles of muscle fibers (muscle cells) lying side by side. They may be arranged in a relatively simple way, as in the lateral pterygoid muscle, or may be organized in architecturally complex pinnate muscles such as the temporalis and the masseter. In pinnate muscles, the bundles attach obliquely to branches of the central tendon and musculoaponeurotic layers, and this allows production of more force and has several functional compartments with capacity for selective activation. Each muscle fiber is filled with thick myosin and thin actin myofibril filaments. The numerous filaments are arranged in sarcomeres (i.e., the contractile elements constituting the basic units of muscle function). The filaments lie in parallel with an overlap between thick and thin types. When the muscle contracts, the overlap increases as the thin filaments are pulled toward the center of the sarcomere and produces force and/or movement.

The masticatory muscles are as a group among the strongest muscles in the body, and their tasks and functional activities appear to deviate from limb muscles, as they have higher capillary supply and different function of muscle receptors and reflex mechanisms. Muscle spindles are present in the jaw elevator muscles, but Golgi tendon organs are lacking and their inhibitory function on the muscle activity seem in the jaw-closing muscles to be taken over by mechanoreceptors in the periodontal ligaments (Türker 2002). In addition, the muscle fiber characteristics are different. With histochemical myofibrillar ATPase staining, the fibers can be classified according to the isoform of myosin they contain, by different staining densities. In jaw muscles, light-stained type I fibers predominate that are associated with long contraction times (slow twitch), high aerobic capability, and resistance to fatigue, whereas dark-stained anaerobic fast-twitch type II fibers predominate in limb muscles (Figure 14-1). The morphology of human jaw elevator muscle fibers is also unusual in that the type II

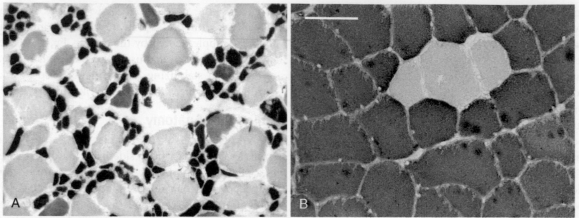

FIG 14-1 Myosin ATPase Staining of Muscle Sections from a Young Individual (Same Enlargement; Scale Bar = 62 µm) **A,** Masseter; **B,** biceps brachii. Light-stained type I fibers, dark-stained type II fibers, and intermediate-stained type IM fibers. Note the characteristic small-sized type II fibers and the type IM fibers in the masseter muscle and the equally sized type I and II fibers in the biceps brachii. (Courtesy of Associate Professor Svend Kirkeby, Faculty of Health and Medicine, University of Copenhagen.)

fibers are of smaller diameter compared with type I fibers, except in cases of increased function and hypertrophy (Sciote & Morris 2000). The masseter and temporalis muscles have a majority of type I fibers but also small-diameter fast-twitch type II fibers with low aerobic capability and low resistance to fatigue, and ATPase-intermediately stained fibers, termed IM. The type IM is characteristic for normal jaw elevator muscles but rare in trunk and limb muscles except in developing or pathological muscles. The fiber type distribution in the jaw muscles may vary with different types of occlusions and with age and sex, probably reflecting different activity patterns and functional requirements.

The muscle bulk is maintained by physical activity, as well as naturally derived steroids and growth hormones. Inactivity leads to hypotrophy and training to hypertrophy (Figure 14-2), with changes in the diameter of muscle fibers. The muscle enzymes responsible for energy release during aerobic and anaerobic muscular effort, as well as the number of capillaries, adapt to the prevailing level of activity. Overuse in terms of sustained activity and high-level contractions without rest periods is associated with raised intramuscular pressure, and it leads to impediment of muscle blood flow, local ischemia, hypoxia, increased cell membrane permeability, edema, and eventually cellular damage. Consequently, it has been proposed that low

jaw muscle strength might predispose to overuse. Even in healthy jaw muscles slight postexercise edema and hyperemia are seen after prolonged gum chewing or moderate elevator contractions more than 15% to 20% of maximum voluntary contraction. With breakdown of muscle tissue, necrosis and fibrosis may take place, as well as possible regeneration of muscle fibers from satellite cells ("resting" myoblasts), which also contribute to muscle growth. However, severe or repeated damage may induce permanent changes in the muscle tissue.

Jaw Closure and Bite Force

Elevation of the mandible is primarily due to bilateral, symmetrical activity of the masseter, temporalis and medial pterygoid muscles, whereas during chewing, the activity of the masseter muscle is asymmetric, with greater activity on the chewing side. The effect of gravity on the jaw is counteracted by the positive tone of the temporalis muscle, which is considered a significant positioner of the jaw. The mandibular elevators, especially the temporalis and the masseter, are the larger jaw muscles. The temporalis and lateral pterygoid muscles are most important for jaw stability and movements. The masseter and medial pterygoid muscles serve primarily as sources of closing power with the masseter being the strongest elevator. The two muscles work in parallel and form a common

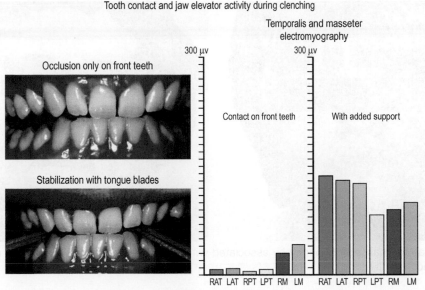

FIG 14-2 **Tooth Contact and Jaw Elevator Activity During Clenching** The facilitating effect on jaw elevator muscle activity by stimulation of low-threshold mechanoreceptors: the electromyographic activity recorded with surface electrodes during biting on the front teeth with and without posterior occlusal support obtained by tongue blades. *RAT* and *LAT*, right and left anterior temporalis muscles; *RPT* and *LPT*, right and left posterior temporalis muscles; *RM* and *LM*, right and left superficial part of the masseter muscles.

tendinous sling at the lower back part of the ramus and angle of the mandible. Low-threshold periodontal mechanoreceptors have a facilitating effect on jaw elevator muscle activity during closure to tooth contact (Figure 14-2), and high-threshold mechanoreceptors inhibit the activity. Both receptors are essential for the fine motor control of the jaw during function, as well as the conscious perception of tactile sensation when forces are applied to natural teeth.

The elevator strength is very important for the bite force, which is influenced by the thickness of the muscles and their fiber size and distribution. The bite force is generally greater in men than in women, but is also dependent on age (Figure 14-3). There is a correlation between the bite force and facial morphology, as the vertical facial relationship and jaw angle decrease with increasing strength; thus weak elevator muscles appear to be associated with long-face morphology, and strong muscles with a more square-faced appearance. Excessive use, such as with frequently ongoing sleep bruxism, leads to hypertrophy (Figure 14-4, *A*). In contrast, if the activity of the

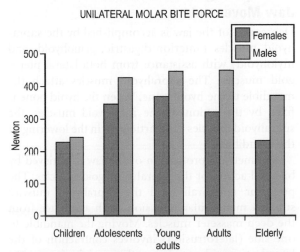

FIG 14-3 **Unilateral Bite Force Measured in the Molar Region Related to Age and Gender** Values based on data from Bakke et al. (1990) and Palinkas et al. (2010). Note the increase with age from childhood to adult life and the decrease in old age, and the lower force in females than in males.

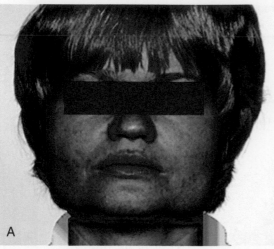 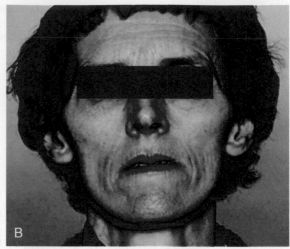

FIG 14-4 A, Bilateral masseter hypertrophy associated with heavy sleep bruxism; **B,** Bilateral masseter hypotrophy associated with ill-fitting dentures.

elevator muscles decreases due to lower chewing demands, tooth loss or ongoing pain, bite force declines and the elevator muscles may become hypotrophic, with visible hollowing of temples and cheeks (Figure 14-4, *B*).

Jaw Opening and Horizontal Jaw Movements

Depression of the jaw is accomplished by the suprahyoid muscles (anterior digastric, geniohyoid, and mylohyoid) with assistance from both lateral pterygoid muscles. The suprahyoid muscles attach the mandible to the hyoid bone. When the hyoid bone is fixed by the action of the infrahyoid muscles, the suprahyoid muscles can participate in the lowering of the mandible.

Symmetrical protrusion of the jaw is achieved by bilateral action of the lateral pterygoid muscles. The posterior temporalis and the suprahyoid muscles support mandibular retrusion, with assistance from the deep masseter muscles. Moving the mandible to one side (laterotrusion) involves contraction of the lateral pterygoid muscles on the opposite (contralateral) side from the excursion, assisted by the posterior temporalis muscle in the same side (ipsilateral). However, laterotrusion is usually performed in combination with protrusion of the contralateral side, producing anterolateral jaw movement.

JAW MUSCLE PAIN

Typical Symptoms of Jaw Muscle Disorders

Muscle pain is the most common complaint in patients with jaw muscle disorders. It is also the most prevalent cause of chronic pain of the orofacial region. The muscle pain is diffuse; it may be located at the source of pain, but may also be referred to or referred from other structures. Pain from the temporalis muscle is usually felt as facial pain or headache in the temple and forehead, from the masseter muscle in the jaw and posterior teeth, from the medial pterygoid muscle deep in the cheek and in front of the ear, and from the lateral pterygoid muscle in the zygomatic area. In addition, chronic pain in the neck and suboccipital and sternocleidomastoid muscles may spread to the facial region. The intensity of the pain felt in the jaw muscles is generally mild to moderate. The pain is described as a continuous "deep dull ache" or "tightness" or "pressure," unpleasant and often exhausting, and it is only rarely associated with a general feeling of illness or with other concomitant symptoms. The pain normally has a gradual onset, and it may vary from a feeling of tiredness to a sharper, more severe pain. It may be constant or occur both spontaneously with the jaw at rest and in response to chewing, stretching, contraction, or palpation. Besides pain, a feeling of weakness, stiffness, rigidity, or swelling and a restriction of jaw opening also often characterizes jaw muscle disorders.

Pathophysiology and Muscle Pain

Muscle pain is a form of deep somatic pain capable of causing central excitatory effects and autonomic responses. Deep pain inputs also tend to provoke referred pain, hyperalgesia, autonomic effects, and secondary muscle co-contraction, as well as emotional reactions. The information leading to the experience of jaw muscle pain is transmitted by free nerve endings, that is, nociceptors (acting as pain receptors), located in muscle, fascia, and muscle-tendon complex. Nociceptors relay to the trigeminal subnucleus caudalis and motor nucleus by small-diameter and slowly conducting primary trigeminal afferents, and local reflexes elicit motor responses. Ascending pathways to the sensorimotor cortex are the basis of nociceptive localization, discrimination, and evaluation, whereas input to the hypothalamus and limbic system provides the autonomic and emotional reactions, all of which constitute the experience of pain. When pain in the jaw muscles is long standing, it may be caused by ongoing peripheral processes inducing pain mediators. However, chronic sensation of jaw muscle pain might also be associated with a "neuropathic conversion" because of sensitization of the peripheral and central nerves. This dichotomous etiology is important for evaluation and treatment (Clark 2012).

Nociceptors respond to mechanical and chemical stimuli from mechanical forces and endogenous pain-producing substances. Under natural conditions and in patients, muscle pain may result from trauma, overuse in terms of sustained or forceful contraction, stretching, ischemia, hyperemia, or infection. However, most pain studies are performed on experimental pain in healthy subjects associated with pain-producing intramuscular injections and experimental chewing and biting tasks. Local conditions such as inflammation increase receptivity, so that stimulation becomes more evident at a lowered activation threshold, even by normally innocuous stimuli, and increased spontaneous activity in nociceptors results in soreness and pain. Such sensitization processes are most likely peripheral mechanisms for muscle tenderness and hyperalgesia (Graven-Nielsen & Mense 2001). Compression and injury to muscle result in direct activation of nociceptors. This occurs by release of prostaglandins from damaged cell membranes, which sensitize nociceptors, and by the release of inflammatory mediators and neuropeptides such as bradykinin and serotonin (from blood vessels), as well as substance P and calcitonin gene-related peptide (from nerve endings). In ischemic muscle, the induced decrease in oxygen tension and pH releases bradykinin and prostaglandin, which sensitize muscle nociceptors, so that they respond to the force of contraction. Different simultaneous stimuli may potentiate each other: for example, increased extracellular potassium concentration, which occurs in prolonged muscular work, increases sensitivity to chemical stimulation from hypoxia and to mechanical stimuli, such as increased intramuscular pressure and other effects of muscular contraction. The convergence of the neurons, processing inputs from muscles, joints, and cutaneous and visceral afferents is the basis for the poor localization and poor discrimination of muscle pain. It is also the cause of referral of pain to other tissues. The clear overlap between the symptoms from TMDs and tension-type headache indicates a common pain pathway (Caspersen et al. 2013).

In second-order neurons of the subnucleus caudalis, an altered responsiveness or sensitization may take place after long-lasting activity in afferent neurons. A range of ascending and descending modulatory mechanisms influences the transmission in the central pathways. Central sensitization and modulation are the main causes of the often-poor correlation in musculoskeletal disorders between the pain experience and the intensity and the duration of the noxious stimuli; this is also true for chronic tension-type headache. Psychological stress has also been shown to increase the pressure-pain sensitivity of the jaw muscles (Michelotti et al. 2000). The spread of muscle pain and more generalized pain conditions may also be related to central sensitization, as this phenomenon comprises not only increased excitability of neurons of the subnucleus caudalis but also an expansion of their receptive fields.

HISTORY TAKING AND EXAMINATION OF JAW MUSCLES

This is required as part of a comprehensive evaluation of jaw muscles, which includes a systematic history, as well as an examination (palpation and auscultation) of the TMJs and dental occlusion (Table 14.1). Jaw muscle disorders are often overlooked by clinicians who do not include the muscles as part of the routine dental evaluation. The use of provocation tests described in Chapter 8 might also be considered. Supplementary tests may also be helpful, for example, diagnostic injections and chewing tests. The basis of

a proper diagnosis is a thorough identification of symptoms and signs (see Chapter 13). The patient's chief complaints should be defined and listed according to their importance to the patient. It should be remembered that jaw muscle disorders often coexist with TMJ disorders, or may be a part of a general medical disorder. If a medical disorder is suspected as the primary cause of symptoms or a significant contributing factor, the patient should be referred for medical consultation.

Anamnesis or History

The history taking of jaw muscle disorders often consists of a consultative written questionnaire and an interview. The questionnaire may be mailed to the patient for completion before the initial appointment. A questionnaire would cover general medical, as well as dental problems, presence of head and face pain, location of the pain on diagrams (Figure 14-5, A), and information about restricted or painful jaw movements and chewing. Besides giving information on the history, the questionnaire provides a basis for a better clinician-patient understanding. During the interview for history taking, possible variations of facial morphology, expressions of pain, involuntary jaw movements, and the patient's attitudes should be noted. Topics for the interview are given in Box 14.1, but further details from the patient depend on the questioning and the clinician's familiarity with the signs and symptoms of jaw muscle disorders.

Table 14.1 Evaluation of Jaw Muscles

History

- Chief complaint (e.g., facial pain and headache, jaw stiffness or reduced mandibular opening, and difficulty in chewing)
- General features:
  - Medical problems including medication and social and psychosocial factors
- Local features:
  - Mandibular function—mobility, chewing, and parafunction (bruxism)
  - Muscle pain—localization, onset, course, characteristics (quality, intensity, variation, provocation, and alleviation), and concomitant symptoms, previous examination and treatment

Clinical Examination

- Orofacial examination: facial appearance; jaw muscles (jaw mobility, tenderness, and trigger points); pain referral, consistency, and volume

---

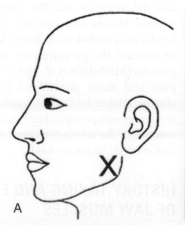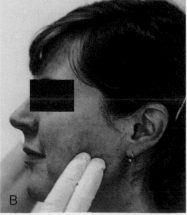

FIG 14-5 A, A patient's indication of the locations of jaw muscle pain on a diagram in a self-completed written questionnaire. **B,** Palpation of the masseter muscle with a firm pressure by two fingers, rating tenderness according to the verbal and facial expression of the patient.

As an aid in assessing the intensity of the jaw muscle pain, a 10-cm horizontal VAS (left endpoint "no pain"; right endpoint "intolerable pain") may be used, both for the initial interview and for monitoring responses to treatment (Figure 14-6). The intensity and effect of the pain may also be estimated from the following:

- Medication used
- Changes in the patient's social habits
- Pain diary listing days with pain

BOX 14.1 JAW MUSCLE DISORDERS

1. Muscle pain
   a. Myalgia
   b. Tendonitis
   c. Myositis
   d. Spasms
2. Contracture
3. Hypertrophy
4. Neoplasm
5. Movement disorders (orofacial dyskinesia and oromandibular dystonia)
6. Masticatory muscle pain attributed to systemic and central pain disorders (fibromyalgia or widespread pain)

Clinical Examination

The examination has two main purposes, as follows:
- To assess jaw function
- To reproduce the patient's pain

The assessment is achieved primarily by registration of the following:
- Jaw mobility
- Pain provocation by maximal jaw opening, by chewing, and by muscle palpation

Jaw function can be assessed routinely by measuring maximum jaw opening in the incisor region, adding the amount of overbite or subtracting the amount of open bite. The reliability of the measures of the vertical range of motion is excellent. Measurement of mandibular range of motion should include maximum comfortable opening and maximum unassisted opening regardless of pain. Generally, a maximum unassisted opening of less than 40 mm is considered moderately restricted, and less than 30 mm as severely restricted. During maximum jaw opening, muscle pain may be provoked or aggravated by stretching the elevator muscles, by the active opening itself, or during assisted opening when the clinician attempts gently to increase the interincisal

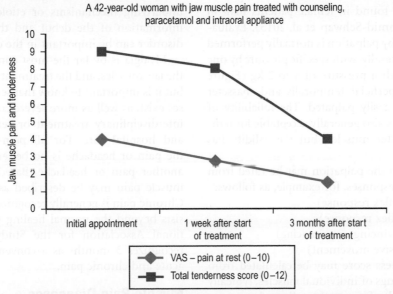

FIG 14-6 A 42-Year-Old Woman with Jaw Muscle Pain Treated with Counseling, Paracetamol, and Intraoral Appliance Overview of the effect of treatment in a patient with myofascial pain illustrated by the recordings of muscle pain by ratings from visual analogue scales (VAS) and total tenderness score from palpation of temporalis and masseter muscles on both sides.

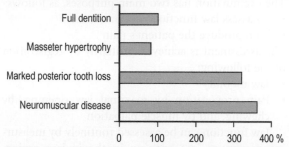

FIG 14-7 Relative chewing time of a standard apple slice in patients with different conditions compared with fully dentated and healthy subjects

distance by putting finger pressure between the upper and lower teeth. A chewing test, for example, gum or cotton rolls, may also be used to provoke or aggravate the pain for diagnostic purposes (Farella et al. 2001), but may also be used to assess masticatory function (Figure 14-7).

The patient may not easily localize the site of pain, but pain provoked by manual palpation and eventual pain referral may identify the source of pain more accurately. More jaw muscle tenderness and greater pain are generally found in female patients than in male patients (Schmid-Schwap et al. 2013). Evaluation of tenderness by palpation is normally performed unilaterally or bilaterally, with specific pressure by one or two fingers, with a pressure of 1 to 2 kg (Figure 14-5, B). The superficial temporalis and masseter muscles are most easily palpated. The reliability of manual palpation is also generally acceptable for temporalis and masseter muscles, but the validity has been questioned.

The response to the palpation may be rated from verbal and reflex responses, for example, as follows:
- 0 (none—no reflex response)
- 1 (mild—no reflex response)
- 2 (moderate—wincing or grimacing)
- 3 (severe—aversive movement)

A total tenderness score may be calculated from the sum of the ratings of individual muscles, typically including the results from temporalis and masseter muscles on both sides (Figure 14-6). Extraoral manual palpation may be supplemented by pressure algometry, to increase reliability and validity. Palpation may

also reveal changes in consistency, felt as taut bands in parallel with the fiber direction, with trigger points that are hyperirritable, may refer pain to other areas or changes in volume in terms of hypotrophy or hypertrophy. The reliability and validity of these findings are probably dubious.

Additional assessments to assist diagnosis include the following:
- Palpation of cervical muscles, as referred pain to the orofacial region is common
- Provocation tests, also described in Chapter 8
- Muscle injections with local anesthetic to confirm the location of the pain

CLASSIFICATION OF JAW MUSCLE DISORDERS

There are several classifications of jaw muscle disorders, and none is without shortcomings or criticism. The classification of jaw muscle disorders and associated pain-based signs and symptoms in this chapter is derived from the Diagnostic Criteria for Temporomandibular Disorders (DC/TMD) described by Peck et al. (2014), which is the current international classification. This classification system is based on diagnoses characterized by signs and symptoms and not underlying mechanisms or etiologies. In addition, information of the debut and the duration of the disorder can be important in the diagnostic process.

Myalgia is by far the most common diagnosis in the jaw muscles, and the treatment is relatively simple, but it is important to know that several other diagnoses exist, as well as more severe conditions that need interdisciplinary treatment or referral to physician and hospital care. For all pain-related diagnoses, the pain or headache is no better accounted for by another pain or headache. Based on the duration, muscle pain may be described as acute or chronic. Chronic pain is generally recognized as pain that persists beyond the normal healing time. The International Association for the Study of Pain (IASP) recognizes 3 months as a convenient separation of acute and chronic pain.

Muscle Pain Diagnoses

The diagnoses are defined as pain of muscle origin affected by jaw movement, function, or parafunction, and replication of this pain with provocation testing of the masticatory muscles. Limitation of mandibular movement(s) secondary to pain may be present. In addition to a diagnosis made based on examination of the masseter and temporalis muscles, a positive finding with the specified provocation tests when examining the other masticatory muscles can help to corroborate the diagnosis.

Myalgia

History: pain in the jaw, temple, in front of the ear, or in the ear AND pain modified with jaw movement, function and parafunction

Examination: confirmation of pain location(s) in the temporalis or masseter muscles AND report of familiar pain in the temporalis or masseter with at least one of the following provocation tests— palpation of the temporalis or masseter muscle(s) OR maximum unassisted or assisted opening

Local Myalgia

History: as in Myalgia

Examination: confirmation of pain location(s) in the temporalis or masseter muscle(s) AND familiar muscle pain with palpation AND pain with muscle palpation with pain localized to the immediate site of the palpating finger(s)

Myofascial Pain

History: as in Myalgia

Examination: confirmation of pain location(s) in the temporalis or masseter muscle(s) AND familiar muscle pain with palpation AND pain with muscle palpation with spreading of the pain beyond the location of the palpating finger(s) but within the boundary of the muscle

Myofascial Pain with Referral

History: as in Myalgia

Examination: confirmation of pain location(s) in the temporalis or masseter muscle(s) AND familiar muscle pain with palpation AND pain with muscle palpation beyond the boundary of the muscle

Tendonitis (Tendinitis)

The diagnosis of tendonitis is defined as pain of tendon origin affected by jaw movement, function, or parafunction, and replication of this pain with provocation testing of masticatory muscle tendons.

Limitation of mandibular movement(s) secondary to pain may be present. The temporalis tendon may be a common site of tendonitis and refer pain to the teeth and other nearby structures.

History: as in Myalgia

Examination: confirmation of pain location in any tendon in the masticatory muscles including the temporalis tendon AND report of familiar pain with at least one of the following provocation tests—palpation of the tendon OR maximum unassisted or assisted opening

Myositis

The diagnosis of myositis is defined as pain of muscle origin with clinical characteristics of inflammation or infection: edema, erythema, and/or increased temperature. It generally arises acutely following direct trauma of the muscle or from infection or chronically with autoimmune disease. Limitation of unassisted mandibular movements secondary to pain is often present.

History: as in Myalgia

Examination: confirmation as in local myalgia AND presence of edema, erythema, and/or increased temperature over the muscle. Laboratory testing: serologic tests may reveal elevated enzyme levels (e.g., creatine kinase), markers of inflammation, and the presence of autoimmune diseases

Spasm

The diagnosis of spasm is defined as a sudden, involuntary, reversible tonic contraction of a muscle. Spasm may affect any of the masticatory muscles. Acute malocclusion may be present.

History: immediate onset of myalgia as defined in local myalgia AND immediate report of limited range of jaw motion

Examination: confirmation as in local myalgia that may include any of the masticatory muscles AND limited range of jaw motion in direction that elongates affected muscle

Laboratory testing: elevated intramuscular electromyography (EMG) activity when compared with contralateral unaffected muscle

Contracture

The diagnosis of contracture is defined as the shortening of a muscle because of fibrosis of tendons, ligaments, or muscle fibers. It is usually not painful unless the muscle is overextended. A history of radiation therapy, trauma, or infection is often present. It is most commonly seen in the masseter or medial pterygoid muscle.

History: progressive loss of range of motion

Examination: unassisted and assisted jaw movements that are limited and associated with firm, unyielding resistance to assisted movements

Hypertrophy

The diagnosis of hypertrophy is defined as enlargement of one or more masticatory muscles, characterized by increased strength and volume but usually not associated with pain. It can be secondary to overuse, bruxism, and/or chronic tensing of the muscle. Diagnosis is based on the clinician's assessment of muscle size, and it needs consideration of craniofacial morphology and ethnicity.

History: enlargement of one or more masticatory muscles as evidenced from photographs or previous records

Examination: increased volume of one or more masticatory muscles (The examination may be supplemented by ultrasonography.)

Neoplasm

Neoplasms of the masticatory muscles result from tissue proliferation with histological characteristics. They are uncommon, and may be benign or malignant (e.g., metastatic). They may present with swelling, spasm, pain during function, limited mouth opening, and/or sensory/motor changes (e.g., paresthesia and weakness). Diagnostic imaging, typically using CT/CBCT and/or MRI, and biopsy are essential when a neoplasm is suspected.

Movement Disorders

Orofacial dyskinesia and oromandibular dystonia are uncommon neurological disorders with involuntary, mainly choreic (dance-like) movements, or excessive, involuntary and sustained or repetitive muscle contractions that may involve the face, lips, tongue, and/or jaw. Oromandibular dystonia is typically classified as jaw opening, jaw closing, jaw deviating, or lingual dystonia or combinations of these. There is a high prevalence of problems with mastication, swallowing, and dental attrition (Bakke et al. 2013).

BOX 14.2 TENSION-TYPE HEADACHE

At least two of the following pain characteristics:
- Pressing or tightening (nonpulsating) quality; mild or moderate intensity (may inhibit but does not prohibit activities); bilateral location; no aggravation by walking on stairs or similar routine physical activity

Both of the following:
- No vomiting
- No more than one of the following—nausea, photophobia, and phonophobia

---

Masticatory Muscle Pain Contributed to Systemic and Central Pain Disorders

Once widespread muscle pain (fibromyalgia) pain with symmetrical tenderness corresponding to at least 11 of 18 particular muscle sites with concurrent masticatory muscle pain has been diagnosed, most often the patient is familiar with the general pain condition.

Headache Attributed to Temporomandibular Disorders

Headache in the temple area may be a common tension-type headache (Box 14.2) but may also be secondary to pain-related TMD. The headache attributed to TMDs is aggravated by jaw function, or parafunction, and replication of this headache occurs with provocation testing of the masticatory system.

History: headache of any type in the temple AND headache modified with jaw movement, function or parafunction

Examination: confirmation of headache location in the area of the temporalis muscle AND report of familiar headache in the temple area with palpation of the temporalis muscle OR with maximum unassisted or assisted opening right or left lateral movements, or protrusive movements

TREATMENT OF JAW MUSCLE PAIN AND DISORDERS

The treatment of jaw muscle disorders is designed to reduce pain and improve jaw function. Ideally, the treatment of jaw muscle disorders should be evidence based and cost effective. Where evidence is lacking, treatment should be based on well-established accepted clinical practice (Kuttila et al. 1998). As there is no evidence that myalgia of jaw muscles is progressive in nature, treatment should also be based on reversible and least-invasive therapies. Such procedures are intended to facilitate the natural healing capacity of the musculoskeletal system, and to involve the patient in the management of the disorder. Regional and widespread disorders, as well as suspicion of neoplasms and general medical and neurological conditions, necessitate referral to or collaboration with primary care physicians and other medical specialists.

Depending on the type and severity of the jaw muscle disorders, a combination of several treatments may be applied, as follows:

- The first step is always counseling and education, often carried out together with medication (as required) for alleviation of pain.
- Analgesics (e.g., paracetamol and acetaminophen) and NSAIDs are normally used for treatment for musculoskeletal pain. NSAIDs (ibuprofen) have been shown to have a positive effect on muscle pain. Moreover, application of topical NSAID gel may have some effect.
- Muscle relaxants may be used, and 1 month of treatment with diazepam has been shown to reduce prolonged jaw muscle myalgia. Tricyclic antidepressants may also have a role in the treatment of chronic myofascial pain from jaw muscles. Amitriptyline has a positive effect on chronic tension-type headache, but common side effects include dry mouth, sedation, and constipation.
- Intraoral appliances such as flat occlusal stabilization splints (in hard acrylic resin) are often the main treatment for TMDs. There is controversy regarding their mode of action, and their effects are partly due to the placebo effect (Forssell et al. 1999). However, meta-analysis of randomized controlled trials have shown that hard stabilization appliances, when adjusted properly, have good evidence of modest efficacy in reducing pain in patients with TMDs affecting muscle and joint, compared with nonoccluding appliances and no treatment (Fricton et al. 2010). Other types of appliances, including soft stabilization appliances, anterior positioning appliances, and anterior bite appliances, have some evidence of efficacy in reducing TMD pain. However, the potential for adverse events with these appliances and the need for close monitoring in their use are higher. Therefore they should not be recommended generally.
- Physical therapy is often used as treatment of jaw muscle pain in association with TMDs. Symptoms of TMDs and other chronic musculoskeletal pain improve during treatment with most forms of physical therapy (Feine & Lund 1997). However, most of the therapies have not been proven more effective than a placebo. These data support the view that it may be the care and concern for the patient itself that matters. Passive exercise and stretching are likely to increase the range of jaw motion, but the effect on muscle pain is weak, and there is evidence from the treatment of other musculoskeletal disorders that active exercise of the specific painful area strengthens the muscles, improves function, and reduces pain (Feine & Lund 1997).
- Acupuncture may have a role in treatment of the jaw muscles. There is little evidence for the use of thermal agents, electrical stimulation (TENS), ultrasound, and low-intensity laser therapy for chronic muscle pain and disorders.
- Occlusal factors may contribute to TMDs, but only to a minor extent. Occlusal adjustment or prosthetic reconstructions as the treatment for jaw muscle disorders alone are not recommended.

REFERENCES

Bakke M, Holm B, Jensen BL, et al: Unilateral, isometric bite force in 8-68-year-old women and men related to occlusal factors, *Scand J Dent Res* 98:149–158, 1990.

Bakke M, Larsen BM, Dalager T, et al: Oromandibular dystonia-functional and clinical characteristics: a report on 21 cases, *Oral Surg Oral Med Oral Pathol Oral Radiol* 115:e21–e26, 2013.

Caspersen N, Hirsvang JR, Kroell L, et al: Is there a relation between tension-type headache, temporomandibular disorders and sleep? *Pain Reas Treat* 2013:845684, 2013.

Clark GT: The 30 most prevalent chronic painful diseases, disorders, and dysfunctions that occur in the orofacial region. In Clark GT, Dionne RA, editors: *Orofacial Pain. A Guide to Medications and Management*, Chichester, 2012, Wiley-Blackwell, pp 3–29.

Dworkin SF, LeResche L: Research diagnostic criteria for temporomandibular disorders, *J Craniomandib Disord* 6:301–355, 1992.

Eriksson PO, Haggman-Henrikson B, Nordh E, et al: Co-ordinated mandibular and head-neck movements during rhythmic jaw activities in man, *J Dent Res* 79:1378–1384, 2000.

Farella M, Bakke M, Michelotti A, et al: Effects of prolonged gum chewing on pain and fatigue in human jaw muscles, *Eur J Oral Sci* 109:81–85, 2001.

Feine JS, Lund JP: An assessment of the efficacy of physical therapy and physical modalities for the control of chronic musculoskeletal pain (review), *Pain* 71:5–23, 1997.

Forssell H, Kalso E, Koskela P, et al: Occlusal treatments in temporomandibular disorders: a qualitative systematic review of randomized controlled trials (review), *Pain* 83:549–560, 1999.

Fricton J, Look JO, Wright E, et al: Systematic review and meta-analysis of randomized controlled trials evaluating intraoral orthopedic appliances for temporomandibular disorders, *J Orofac Pain* 24:237–254, 2010.

Graven-Nielsen T, Mense S: The peripheral apparatus of muscle pain: evidence from animal and human studies (review), *Clin J Pain* 17:2–10, 2001.

Kuttila M, Niemi PM, Kuttila S, et al: TMD treatment need in relation to age, gender, stress, and diagnostic subgroup, *J Orofac Pain* 12:67–74, 1998.

Lobbezoo F, Naeije M: Bruxism is mainly regulated centrally, not peripherally, *J Oral Rehabil* 28:1085–1091, 2001.

Manfredini D, Guarda-Nardini L, Wincour E, et al: Research diagnostic criteria for temporomandibular disorders: a systematic review of axis I epidemiologic findings, *Oral Surg Oral Med Oral Pathol Oral Radiol* 112:453–462, 2011.

Michelotti A, Farella M, Tedesco A, et al: Changes in pressure-pain threaholds of jaw muscles during a natural stressfull condition in a group of symptom-free subjects, *J Orofac Pain* 14:279–285, 2000.

Palinkas M, Nassar MS, Cecílio FA, et al: Age and gender influence on maximal bite force and masticatory muscles thickness, *Arch Oral Biol* 55:797–802, 2010.

Peck CC, Goulet JP, Lobbezoo F, et al: Expanding the taxonomy of the diagnostic criteria for temporomandibular disorders, *J Oral Rehabil* 41:2–23, 2014.

Schmid-Schwap M, Bristela M, Kundi M, et al: Sex-specific differences in patients with temporomandibular disorders, *J Orofac Pain* 27:42–50, 2013.

Sciote JJ, Morris TJ: Skeletal muscle function and fiber types: the relation between occlusal function and the phenotype of jaw-closing muscles in human, *J Orthod* 27:15–30, 2000.

Türker KS: Reflex control of human jaw muscles, *Crit Rev Oral Biol Med* 13:85–104, 2002.

Türp JC, Schindler H: The dental occlusion as a suspected cause of TMDs: epidemiological and etiological considerations, *J Oral Rehabil* 39:502–512, 2012.

Further Reading

Bakke M: Mandibular elevator muscles: physiology, action, and effect of dental occlusion (review), *Scand J Dent Res* 101:314–331, 1993.

Bakke M, Thomsen CE, Vilmann A, et al: Ultrasonographic assessment of the swelling of the human masseter muscle after static and dynamic activity, *Arch Oral Biol* 41:133–140, 1996.

Bendtsen L, Jensen R: Amitriptyline reduces myofascial tenderness in patients with chronic tension type headache, *Cephalalgia* 20:603–610, 2000.

Dao TT, Lund JP, Lavigne GJ: Pain responses to experimental chewing in myofascial pain patients, *J Dent Res* 73:1163–1167, 1994.

Drangsholt M, LeResche L: Temporomandibular disorder pain. In Crombie IK, Croft PR, Linton SJ, et al, editors: *Epidemiology of Pain. Task Force on Epidemiology of the International Association for the Study of Pain*, Seattle, 1994, IASP Press, pp 203–233.

Dworkin SF, Huggins KH, LeResche L, et al: Epidemiology of signs and symptoms in temporomandibular disorders: clinical signs in cases and controls, *J Am Dent Assoc* 120:273–281, 1990.

Dworkin SF, LeResche L, DeRouen T, et al: Assessing clinical signs of temporomandibular disorders: reliability of clinical examiners, *J Prosthet Dent* 63:574–579, 1990.

Kreiner M, Betancor E, Clark GT: Occlusal stabilization appliances. Evidence of their efficacy (review), *J Am Dent Assoc* 132:770–777, 2001.

Layzer RB: Muscle pain, cramps and fatigue. In Engel AG, Franzini-Amstrong C, editors: *Myology*, New York, 1994, McGraw-Hill, pp 1754–1768.

Levine JD: Arthritis and myositis. In Campbell JN, editor: *Pain 1996—an Updated Review*, Seattle, 1996, IASP Press, pp 327–337.

Lund JP: Pain and movement. In Lund JP, Lavigne GJ, Dubner R, et al, editors: *Orofacial Pain. From Basic Science to Clinical Management. The Transfer of*

Knowledge in Pain Research to Education, Chicago, 2001, Quintessence, pp 151–163.

Mense S: Nociception from skeletal muscle in relation to clinical muscle pain (review), *Pain* 54:241–289, 1993.

Merskey H, Bogduk N, editors: *Classification of Chronic Pain, Description of Chronic Pain Syndromes and Definition of Pain Terms*, ed 2, Second Task Force on Taxonomy of the International Association for the Study of Pain, Seattle, 1994, IASP Press, pp xi–xiii.

Møller E: The chewing apparatus. An electromyographic study of the action of the muscles of mastication and its correlation to facial morphology, *Acta Physiol Scand* 69(Suppl 280):1–229, 1966.

National Institutes of Health: Management of temporomandibular disorders. National Institutes of Health Technology Assessment Conference statement, *J Am Dent Assoc* 127:1595–1606, 1996.

Sacchetti G, Lampugnani R, Battistini C, et al: Response to pathological ischaemic muscle pain to analgesics, *Br J Clin Pharmacol* 9:165–190, 1980.

Salmon S: Muscle. In Williams PL, Bannister LH, Berry MM, et al, editors: *Gray's Anatomy. The Anatomical Basis of Medicine and Surgery*, ed 38, Edinburgh, 1995, Churchill Livingstone, pp 737–900.

Scott J, Huskisson EC: Graphic representation of pain, *Pain* 2:175–184, 1976.

Sessle BJ: Masticatory muscle disorders: basic science perspectives. In Sessle BJ, Bryant PS, Dionne RA, editors: *Temporomandibular Disorders and Related Pain*, Seattle, 1995, IASP Press, pp 47–61.

Singer E, Dionne R: A controlled evaluation of ibuprofen and diazepam for chronic orofacial muscle pain, *J Orofac Pain* 11:139–146, 1997.

Stal P, Eriksson PO, Thornell LE: Differences in capillary supply between human oro-facial, masticatory and limb muscles, *J Muscle Res Cell Motil* 17:183–197, 1996.

Stockstill J, Gross A, McCall WD: Interrater reliability in masticatory muscle palpation, *J Craniomandib Disord* 3:143–146, 1989.

Svensson P, Houe L, Arendt-Nielsen L: Effect of systemic versus topical nonsteroidal antiinflammatory drugs on postexercise jaw-muscle soreness: a placebo-controlled study, *J Orofac Pain* 11:353–362, 1997.

Tuxen A, Bakke M, Pinholt EM: Comparative data from young men and women on masseter muscle fibres, function and facial morphology, *Arch Oral Biol* 44:509–518, 1999.

Wolfe F, Smythe HA, Yunus MB, et al: The American College of Rheumatology criteria for the classification of fibromyalgia. Report of a multicenter criteria committee, *Arthritis Rheum* 33:160–172, 1990.

CHAPTER 15

Occlusion and Periodontal Health

Jan A. De Boever and AnneMarie De Boever

SYNOPSIS

Periodontal structures depend on functional occlusal forces to activate the periodontal mechanoreceptors in the neuromuscular physiology of the masticatory system. Occlusal forces stimulate the receptors in the periodontal ligament to regulate jaw movements and the occlusal forces. Without antagonists the periodontal ligament shows some nonfunctional atrophy. Tooth mobility is the clinical expression of viscoelastic properties of the ligament and the functional response.

Tooth mobility can change because of the general metabolic influences, a traumatic occlusion, and inflammation. Premature contacts between the arches can result in trauma to periodontal structures.

A traumatic occlusion on a healthy periodontium leads to an increased mobility but not to attachment loss. In inflamed periodontal structures traumatic occlusion contributes to a further and faster spread of the inflammation apically and to more associated bone loss. Occlusal adjustment before periodontal therapy may result in more attachment gain.

A traumatic occlusion, as in a deep bite, may cause stripping of the gingival margins. Gingival recession and noncarious cervical lesions have a multifactorial etiology, including prematurities and steep occlusal guidance.

CHAPTER POINTS

- Healthy periodontal structures and occlusal forces
- Physiology and clinical aspects of tooth mobility
- Tooth mobility
- Types of occlusal forces
- Trauma from occlusion:
  - Primary trauma in healthy noninflamed periodontium
  - Primary trauma in healthy but reduced periodontal structures
  - Secondary trauma in the progression of periodontitis
- Tooth migration
- Noncarious cervical lesions and occlusal trauma
- Clinical consequence and procedures

HEALTHY PERIODONTAL STRUCTURES AND OCCLUSAL FORCES

Healthy periodontal structures, including root cementum, periodontal ligament, and alveolar bone, constitute a functional unit or organ. The periodontal ligament is a highly specialized interface between teeth and the alveolar bone. It serves as a structural, sensory, and nutritive unit supporting the normal oral functions of chewing, swallowing, speaking, etc. It has a very dense network of interconnecting fibers attached to the bone. The supracrestal fibers are especially important because they maintain the relative position of the teeth in the arch. The collagen fibers in the periodontal ligament are very dense and represent up to 75% of the volume. These so-called Sharpey's fibers are apically oriented and embedded both in the alveolar bone and the root cement. The natural dentition has been compared, because of these interconnecting supracrestal fibers, to beads on a string. Teeth function together but have their individual mobility in the alveolus. The entire periodontal ligament has viscoelastic characteristics. The ligament provides tooth fixation and force absorption. The thickness of the periodontal ligament is directly related to the forces exerted on it.

The periodontal ligament has a rich and dense vascular and nervous network. The ligament contains proprioceptors for movement and positioning and mechanoreceptors for touch, pain, and pressure. They regulate muscle function and occlusal forces to avoid overload and damage of the teeth and alveolar bone. The periodontal ligament distributes and absorbs forces. Under physiological conditions the occlusal forces are transferred to alveolar bone and further to the mandible, maxilla, and entire skull. The alveolar process has a pronounced capacity for modeling and remodeling under functional loading. The alveolar process remodels at a rate of 20% per year. The basal bone does not have this capacity. The periodontal ligament and alveolar bone need the functional stimulus of the occlusion to maintain their physiological, healthy condition.

TOOTH MOBILITY

Physiological tooth mobility is the result of the histological characteristics of the periodontal ligament.

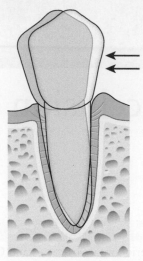

FIG 15-1 Physiological tooth mobility in healthy periodontium is determined by the bone height, form of the root, and magnitude of the applied force, and the extent is limited.

Physiological tooth mobility, horizontally as well as vertically, is different between single-rooted and multirooted teeth and is determined by the width, height, and quality of the periodontal ligament (Figure 15-1).

In the vertical direction the displacement is 0.02 mm by small forces up to 1 N. Under larger vertical forces the tooth is moved in an apical direction because venous fluid and blood of the periodontal structures is pushed toward the venous lacunae and cancellous bone. It takes 1 to 2 minutes before the tooth returns to its normal position after releasing an applied occlusal force. This explains why tooth mobility is decreased after chewing, and the tooth is then in a more apical position.

In healthy conditions the teeth move in a horizontal plane under a force of 500 g, as follows (Mühlemann 1960):

- Incisors: 0.1 to 0.12 mm
- Canines: 0.05 to 0.09 mm
- Premolars: 0.08 to 0.1 mm
- Molars: 0.04 to 0.08 mm

Tooth mobility can also be estimated using the Periotest (Siemens AG, Benscheim, Germany), an electronic device that measures the reaction of the periodontium to a small dynamic force of short duration in the range of milliseconds. This dynamic force is similar to the masticatory force in velocity and duration.

Under higher occlusal loads, forces are transmitted to the bone, with slight deformation of the alveolar process as a result. The force is also transmitted to neighboring teeth through the interproximal contacts.

Evaluation of Tooth Mobility

The exact measurement of individual tooth mobility (periodontometry) is necessary for research purposes. Clinically an estimation of tooth mobility is performed by loading the tooth in an anterolateral direction with two instruments.

Four possible grades of tooth mobility are considered:

- Grade 0: physiological mobility
- Grade 1: increased mobility but less than 1 mm in total
- Grade 2: pronounced increase; more than 1 mm in total
- Grade 3: more than 1 mm displacement combined with a vertical displacement (tooth can be intruded)

Increased mobility can also be observed on radiographs: there is a widening of the periodontal space without vertical or angular bone resorption and without increased probing depth of the periodontal pocket (Figures 15-2 and 15-3).

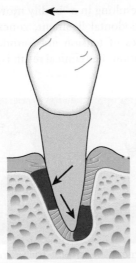

FIG 15-2 Forces applied in one direction on the tooth give a widening of the periodontal ligament at the bone margin at the opposite side and in the apical area on the same side of the force.

Etiological Factors of Hypermobility and Hypomobility

Excessive occlusal forces or premature contacts on teeth are primary etiological factors for hypermobility. There is an increased mobility during pregnancy because of the increase in the fluid content of the periodontal structures due to a higher level of progesteron, increased vascularity, and proliferation of capillaries into the periodontal tissues. This physiological phenomenon can also be observed during puberty and with the use of oral contraceptives. Systemic diseases, such as non-Hodgkin's lymphoma, scleroderma, and Cushing's syndrome, may lead to increased mobility. Normal physiological mobility is decreased in the elderly and in the absence of antagonist teeth. In cases of severe bruxism and clenching, mobility remains unchanged or it may decrease ("ankylosing effect"). Even in cases with pronounced occlusal attrition, hypermobility is seldom found. Without antagonists and therefore without functional stimulation, teeth will either overerupt or become ankylosed. The periodontal ligament becomes thinner and nonfunctional.

Hypermobility may be observed in cases of severe periodontal inflammation (periodontitis), teeth with a healthy but reduced periodontal support (i.e., in patients after successful periodontal treatment), or in the first weeks after periodontal surgery. Chewing movements deviating from normal chewing movements also increase tooth mobility.

Evaluation of the changes in occlusal mobility can be helpful in the diagnosis of occlusal dysfunction

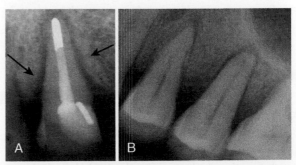

FIG 15-3 A, B, Widening of the periodontal space as observed on radiographs of the maxillary canine and second premolar.

191

and parafunction and in the evaluation of occlusal treatment procedures.

TYPES OF OCCLUSAL FORCES

The reaction of the bone and ligament depends on the magnitude, duration, and direction of the forces. Clinically different types of occlusal forces can be recognized:

- *Physiologically normal occlusal forces in chewing and swallowing:* small and rarely exceeding 5 N. They provide the positive stimulus to maintaining the periodontium and the alveolar bone in a healthy and functional condition.
- *Impact forces:* mainly high but of short duration. The periodontium can sustain high forces during a short period; however, forces exceeding the viscoelastic buffer capacities of the periodontal ligament will result in fracture of tooth and bone.
- *Continuous forces:* very low forces (e.g., orthodontic forces) but continuously applied in one direction are effective in displacing a tooth by remodeling the alveolus.
- *Jiggling forces:* intermittent forces in two different directions (premature contacts on, for example, crowns, fillings) result in widening of the alveolus and increased mobility.

Frost (1992) developed a physiological model to explain the different bone reactions to loading:

- Trivial loading: inadequate stimulus to the bone resulting in bone loss
- Physiological loading: a balance between bone formation and resorption
- Mild overload: preservation of existing bone and new bone formation resulting in more bone mass
- Severe overload: microdamage results in repair bone

These types of bone reaction to loading play a role in the preservation of periodontal structures clinically expressed by the height of the alveolar bone and tooth mobility.

TRAUMA FROM OCCLUSION

Trauma from occlusion has been defined as structural and functional changes in the periodontal tissues caused by excessive occlusal forces. Some of these changes are adaptive, whereas others should be considered pathological. Occlusal trauma can be acute if caused by external impact forces or chronic if caused by internal occlusal factors (premature contacts, grinding). *Occlusal trauma* is the overall process by which *traumatic occlusion* (i.e., an occlusion that produces forces that cause injury) produces injury to the attachment apparatus.

Premature contacts exist in centric and excentric positions; they prohibit a stable occlusal position. Epidemiological studies showed that 80% to 90% of individuals in the Western population have such prematurities or/and supracontacts. However, in only a small number of people these prematurities may lead to functional and/or morphological complications. Chronic occlusal trauma can be understood as primary and secondary trauma.

Primary Occlusal Trauma

Primary occlusal trauma (Figure 15-4) is caused by excessive and nonphysiological forces exerted on teeth with a normal, healthy, and noninflamed periodontium. The forces may be exerted on the periodontal structures in one direction (orthodontic forces) or as "jiggling" forces.

Forces in One Direction: Orthodontic Forces

Forces in one direction cause tipping of the tooth in the opposite direction or tooth displacement parallel to the force, resulting in a "bodily movement."

In the periodontal ligament, zones of compression and zones of tension are found, inducing increased resorption. The clinical result is a (temporary)

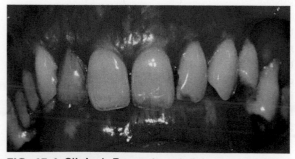

FIG 15-4 Clinical Example of Primary Occlusal Trauma Frontal view of deep bite. In closing, mandibular anterior teeth and canines traumatize and strip palatal gingiva of maxillary anterior teeth, which show increased tooth mobility.

increased mobility. However, there are no changes in the supracrestal fibers, no loss of periodontal attachment, or an increased probing pocket depth. The increased tooth mobility is a functional adaptation to the forces exerted on that tooth. If the forces are too high and above the adaptation level, an aseptic necrosis in the tension zone of the periodontal ligament occurs, characterized by hyalinization. In the compression zone, pressure stimulates osteoclasts in the adjacent bone, and the alveolar wall is resorbed until a new connection is formed with the hyalinized bone ("undermining resorption"). In the tension zone, bone apposition and rupture of the collagen fibers occur. After removal of the force the periodontal ligament is reorganized and after some time develops a normal histological appearance. If the applied forces are too high, root resorption occurs in the middle of the hyalinized tissues. This resorption continues for a variable time, resulting in shorter roots, frequently seen after orthodontic treatment.

Jiggling Forces

Jiggling forces, coming from different and opposite directions, cause more complex histological changes in the ligament. Theoretically the same events (hyalinization, resorption) occur; however, they are not clearly separated.

There are no distinct zones of pressure and tension. Histologically there is apposition and resorption on either side of the periodontal ligament, resulting in a widening of the periodontal space (Figures 15-3 and 15-5). This may be observed on radiographs. This phenomenon explains the increased mobility without pocket formation, migration, and tipping.

The clinical phenomena are not only dependent on the magnitude of the forces, but also on the crown-root relationship, position in the arch, direction of the long axis, and pressure of tongue and cheek musculature. The interarch relationship (e.g., deep bite) influences the extent of the trauma caused by jiggling forces. The hypermobility is found as long as the forces are exerted on the tooth: there is no adaptation. Hypermobility is therefore not a sign of an ongoing process, but may be the result of a previous jiggling force.

The long-term prognosis of teeth with increased mobility is poor and is a complicating factor if they are used as abutment in prosthodontic reconstruction.

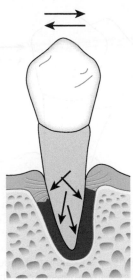

FIG 15-5 Under jiggling forces in a healthy periodontium, the periodontal ligament space is widened, resulting in more tooth mobility but not in marginal bone resorption or attachment loss.

Successful periodontal treatment leads to healthy but reduced periodontal structures. Jiggling forces exerted on the teeth in this condition result in a pronounced increase in tooth mobility because the point of rotation (fulcrum) is closer to the apex than normal. This is uncomfortable for the patient and might be an indication for splinting of teeth (Figure 15-6).

Secondary Occlusal Trauma

Secondary trauma from occlusion is defined as the trauma caused by excessive and premature occlusal forces on teeth with an inflamed periodontium. A number of animal experiments and clinical epidemiological studies investigated the role of occlusion in the pathogenesis of periodontitis. In his original studies in the 1960s Glickman & Smulow (1967) formulated the hypothesis that premature contacts and excessive occlusal forces could be a cofactor in the progression of periodontal disease by changing the pathway and spread of inflammation into the deeper periodontal tissues. Glickman hypothesized that the gingival zone was a "zone for irritation" by

193

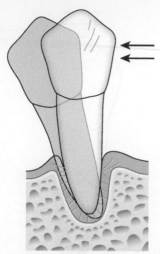

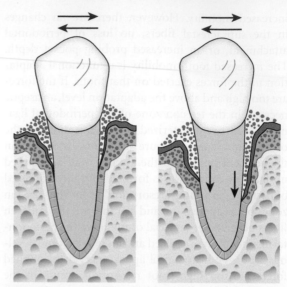

FIG 15-6 In cases of a healthy but reduced periodontium the tooth mobility (measured at the crown level) is increased for the same force, as compared with a tooth with a complete periodontium, because of the more apical position of the fulcrum.

FIG 15-8 In applying jiggling forces on an inflamed, untreated periodontium with existing infrabony pockets (**A**), the bone destruction is accelerated and the bacteria move more apically (**B**).

Animal Experiments

Animal experiments investigating the influence of a faulty occlusion on the progression of periodontal disease were published by Swedish investigators between 1970 and 1980 using the beagle dog model and by American investigators using the squirrel monkey model. In spite of the many remaining questions and controversies, few animal studies have been published since then.

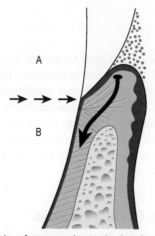

FIG 15-7 Role of traumatic occlusion in the progression of periodontitis according to Glickman & Smulow (1967). In the presence of microbial plaque and inflammation, **A** is the "zone of irritation" and **B** the "zone of codestruction" where the prematurities are codestructive by changing the inflammatory pathway.

From these studies the following conclusions may be drawn:

- In the absence of marginal inflammation, jiggling forces do not induce more bone resorption or a shift of the epithelial attachment in an apical direction.
- In the case of marginal inflammation (gingivitis), occlusal overload has no influence.
- Jiggling forces on teeth with periodontal disease result in more bone loss and more loss of connective tissue attachment (Ericsson & Lindhe 1982).
- Jiggling forces induce a faster shift of microbial plaque in the apical direction in the pocket (Figure 15-8).

the microbial plaque; the supracrestal fibers were then considered to be a "zone of codestruction" under the influence of a faulty occlusion (Figure 15-7).

Clinically, vertical bone resorption and the formation of infrabony defects should be an indication for occlusal trauma.

- One single trauma does not influence pathogenesis; the forces have to be chronic.
- Treatment of periodontal inflammation without elimination of the premature contacts results in decreased tooth mobility, an increase in bone density, but no change of bone level.
- After periodontal treatment with scaling and root-planing, the presence or absence of prematurities have no influence on the microbial repopulation of the periodontal sulcus. However, over a longer period of maintenance, mobile teeth showed greater attachment loss than nonmobile teeth (Wang et al. 1994).

It must be mentioned that some animal studies did not reach the same definitive conclusions due to differences in experimental set-up and different animal models. The results of experimental animal studies (usually short-term studies) cannot therefore be directly extrapolated to the human situation. Ligature-induced periodontitis in animals develops fairly rapidly, whereas periodontal disease in humans tends to be slow progressing.

Clinical Epidemiological Studies

Given the complexity of the occlusal and periodontal interaction and the multifactorial aspect of the pathology, few human studies have been published. Also, ethical concerns prohibit human experimental studies in this field. Furthermore, a well-defined and generally accepted standard for a so-called ideal or physiological occlusion is not existing. Most studies have a limited number of subjects, and the results are analyzed on a subject basis rather than on a tooth basis. By reporting on a patient basis rather than on a tooth basis, results tend to average over the whole mouth the influence of occlusal prematurities on the periodontal structures. It has been demonstrated (in animal experiments) that premature contacts do not result in a histological attachment loss but rather in deeper probing depth. Clinically increased probing depth is therefore not only the result of inflammation but also of increased tooth mobility.

Human studies have been summarized by Hallmon & Harrel (2004). A number of cross-sectional epidemiological studies found no relationship between the presence of premature contacts and increased probing depth or bone loss, whereas others reported that mobility and radiographic evidence of a widened periodontal ligament were associated with increased pocket depth, attachment loss, and bone loss (Jin & Cao 1992). By comparing periodontally healthy subjects with patients having different severities of periodontitis, a relationship has been found between trauma from occlusion and the severity of the disease. The number of occlusal discrepancies increased with the level of attachment loss (Branschofsky et al. 2011). In longitudinal studies (Harrel & Nunn 2001) teeth with premature contacts at initial examination had a deeper probing pocket depth, increased mobility, and worse prognosis. At the 1 year examination, teeth originally without premature contacts or teeth where premature contacts had been removed showed a 66% reduced chance of a worsening periodontal situation. After a few months, teeth with prematurities showed an increased probing depth compared with the teeth receiving occlusal adjustment. It was concluded that premature contacts are a "catalyst" in the progression of periodontal disease. In a later study the same authors (Harrel & Nunn 2009), using a tooth-based analysis, defined the types of occlusal discrepancies associated with deeper pockets: prematurities in centric occlusion and centric relation, nonworking contacts, and contacts on the molars in protrusive movements. In using a four-scale system to describe the prognosis of a tooth (from good to hopeless), teeth with premature contacts never had a "good" prognosis. This worse prognosis can probably be explained by the larger probing depth found in hypermobile teeth and the fact that less gain in connective tissue attachment has been found. In a German cross-sectional epidemiological study a weak correlation was found between nonworking contacts and the status of periodontal disease (Bernhardt et al. 2006). Therefore occlusal adjustment has been advocated before plaque-related periodontal therapy in order to gain more attachment (Sanz 2005).

It has also been shown that in the same patient more periodontopathogens (*Campylobacter rectus, Porphyromonas gingivalis, Peptostreptococcus micros*) are found in pockets around hypermobile teeth than in teeth with normal mobility, even if they have a similar probing pocket depth. This leads to the hypothesis that the increased mobility changes the ecosystem in the pocket, favoring growth of these bacteria (Grant et al. 1995).

TOOTH MIGRATION

Migration of teeth in the posterior zone followed by spread of anterior teeth (collapsed bite syndrome) is often part of severe periodontal pathology (Figure 15-9). Tooth migration is a common symptom for the loss of occlusal stability after extraction of teeth and/ or loss of periodontal structures in peridodontal disease. In at least 30% of patients with severe periodontitis, tooth migration (flaring) of teeth in the frontal region is the main reason for patients to seek periodontal treatment. Tooth migration is multifactorial: bone loss due to periodontitis, premature contact in centric and eccentric positions, class II jaw relationship with deep bite, shortened dental arches, and posterior collapsed bite (Brunsvold 2005). Oral habits, such as tongue thrusting and lip biting, can contribute to pathological tooth migration. After resolving the plaque-related inflammation and the resolution of deep (intrabony) pockets, an interdisciplinary approach combining orthodontic and prosthodontic therapy to correct the migration is often necessary. Orthodontic treatment can realign the anterior teeth and create occlusal stability. Intrusion of teeth in a reduced but healthy periodontium results in the formation of new connective tissue attachment (Greenstein et al. 2008). However, the treatment is often extensive and cumbersome. Therefore early diagnosis of tooth migration is recommended, and the occlusion (as important etiological factor) should be adjusted during the periodontal maintenance phase. Because of the high percentage of relapse, splinting (semidefinitive or definitive) should always be considered (Figure 15-10, *A* and *B*).

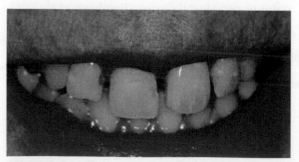

FIG 15-9 Flaring of maxillary anterior teeth after loss of posterior zone in a patient with progressive adult periodontitis.

Migration of teeth also includes tipping after extraction of neighboring teeth and overeruption if antagonists are lost (Figure 15-11). These changes lead to occlusal interferences and difficulties in planning restorative therapy in the antagonistic arch. Overeruption of maxillary molars and premolars occurs in up to 83% of an adult population, but the extent varies considerably (Sarita et al. 2003; Craddock & Youngson 2004). Tipping of molars occurs mainly in the lower jaw, whereas rotations are more frequent in the upper jaw. Control sessions should not only include caries detection and bleeding of the gingiva on probing as an indicator of inflammation, but also the occlusion and occlusal changes.

GINGIVAL AND NONCARIOUS CERVICAL LESIONS

Gingival recession may be provoked by direct contact of the teeth and gingiva. In severe deep bites the upper incisors damage the buccal gingiva of the lower incisors. Likewise a severe overbite might strip the palatal gingiva of the upper incisors. This, as a common symptom of loss of occlusal stability, is not easy to solve and may require orthodontic treatment, orthognathic surgery, or extensive prosthetic rehabilitation to obtain a normal vertical dimension.

Noncarious cervical lesions are defined as the loss of tooth substance at the cementoenamel junction very often combined with gingival recession, erosion, and loss of periodontal structures. Three distinct types have been identified: erosion, abrasion, and abfraction. Erosion is caused by drinking acidic drinks and abrasion mainly by an incorrect, frequent tooth brushing with excessive force. Abfraction is the breaking away of layers of enamel and dentine in the cervical area. In this area the flexure of these layers are under pressure and mainly excentric occlusal forces (e.g., grinding). Epidemiological studies show that up to 39% of the population between 20 and 59 years of age have these lesions. The frequency increases with age. The largest concentration is found in the canines and maxillary premolars (Bernhardt et al. 2006).

In most patients a combination of these three mechanisms has been found. It has been impossible to find a specific causal agent for these lesions (Senna et al. 2012). However, clinical and in vitro experiments have shown that in many patients, occlusal

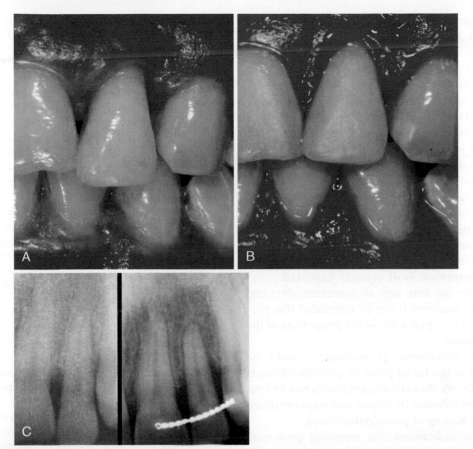

FIG 15-10 Flaring of Lateral Incisor with Loss of Bone and Supraocclusion in Centric and Eccentric Position **A**, Before orthodontic intrusion. **B**, After intrusion. **C**, Radiographs before and after periodontal-orthodontic treatment.

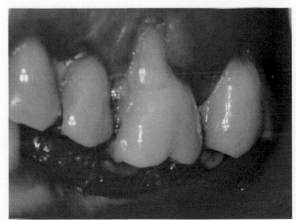

FIG 15-11 Overeruption of maxilllary molars 6 years after extraction of molars in the mandible.

factors, such as a steep lateral canine guidance, wear facets, clenching, and high chewing loads, are responsible or at least a cofactor. Consequently, in some patients at least, a limited change of the occlusion and lateral guidance to avoid further damage should be part of a multifactorial therapy. Therapy should include counseling on not only dietary habits and tooth-brushing techniques but also control of the occlusion-related habits.

PRACTICAL CLINICAL CONCLUSIONS AND GUIDELINES

- In a healthy noninflamed dentition, traumatic occlusion leads to hypermobility of some teeth; if hypermobility, radiological widening of periodontal ligament space or pronounced cervical abfraction is found, the occlusion should be analyzed and corrected. Simple, uncomplicated, procedures are in most cases adequate to restore a physiological situation and to reduce hypermobility.

- In cases of a healthy but reduced periodontium, increased mobility may also be reduced by occlusal adjustment; it should be recognized that tooth mobility in such cases, based on the mechanical situation, is nevertheless increased. It may be necessary to splint the teeth to increase functional comfort and to avoid direct fracture. This may include very mobile teeth with a healthy but reduced periodontium but complicates the clinical procedures.
- In cases of secondary occlusal trauma, treating the inflammation is of primary importance and should be the first step in treatment planning. From the literature it can be concluded that prematurities may play a role in the progression of the periodontitis.
- Occlusal adjustment, if necessary, should be included in the initial phase of periodontal treatment. This results in more gain in attachment level during periodontal treatment and may contribute to better healing of periodontal tissues.
- There are indications that removing premature tooth contacts improves the prognosis of periodontally involved tissues.
- If some teeth do not react to conventional periodontal treatment as expected, further investigation should not only include periodontal reexamination and microbiological testing but also more extensive occlusal analysis.
- The relationship between occlusal trauma and periodontal disease (progression, outcome of therapy, prognosis) should be included in undergraduate and postgraduate teaching.

REFERENCES

Bernhardt O, Gesh D, Look JO, et al: The influence of dynamic occlusal interferences on probing depth and attachment level: results of the Study of Health in Pomeriana, *J Periodontol* 77:506–516, 2006.

Bernhardt O, Gesh D, Schwahn C, et al: Epidemiological evaluation of the multifactorial aetiology of abfractions, *J Oral Rehabil* 33:17–25, 2006.

Branschofsky M, Beikle T, Schäfer R, et al: Secondary trauma from occlusion and periodontitis, *Quintessence Int* 42:515–522, 2011.

Brunsvold MA: Pathologic tooth migration, *J Periodontol* 76:859–866, 2005.

Craddock HL, Youngson CC: A study of the incidence of overeruption and occlusal interferences in unopposed posterior teeth, *Brit Dent J* 196:314–318, 2004.

Ericsson I, Lindhe J: The effect of long standing jiggling on the experimental marginal periodontitis in the beagle dog, *J Clin Periodontol* 9:495, 1982.

Frost HM: Perspectives: bone's mechanical usage windows, *Bone Miner* 19:257–271, 1992.

Glickman I, Smulow IB: Further observation on the effects of trauma from occlusion, *J Periodontol* 38:280, 1967.

Grant D, Flynn M, Slots J: Periodontal microbiota of mobile and non-mobile teeth, *J Periodontol* 66:386–390, 1995.

Greenstein G, Cavalarro J, Scharf D, et al: Differential diagnosis and management of flared maxillary anterior teeth, *J Am Dent Assoc* 139:715–723, 2008.

Hallmon WW, Harrel SK: Occlusal analysis, diagnosis and management in the practice of periodontics, *Periodontol 2000* 34:151–164, 2004.

Harrel SK, Nunn ME: The association of occlusal contacts with the presence of increased periodontal probing, *J Clin Periodontol* 36:1035–1042, 2009.

Harrel SK, Nunn ME: The effect of occlusal discrepancies on periodontitis (II): Relationships of occlusal treatment to the progression of periodontal disease, *J Periodontol* 72:495–505, 2001.

Jin L, Cao C: Clinical diagnosis of trauma from occlusion and its relation with severity of periodontitis, *J Clin Periodontol* 19:92–97, 1992.

Mühlemann HR: Ten years of tooth mobility measurements, *J Periodontol* 31:110–122, 1960.

Sanz M: Occlusion in the periodontal context, *Int J Prosthodont* 18:7–8, 2005.

Sarita PT, Kreulen CM, Witter DJ, et al: A study on occlusal stability in dental arches, *Int J Prosthodont* 16:375–380, 2003.

Senna P, Del BelCury A, Rösing C: Non-carious cervical lesions and occlusion: a systematic review of clinical studies, *J Oral Rehabil* 39:450–462, 2012.

Further Reading

Beertsen W, McCulloch CAG, Sodek J: The periodontal ligament: a unique, multifunctional connective tissue, *Periodontol 2000* 13:20–40, 1997.

Burgett FG, Ramfjord SP, Nissle RR, et al: A randomized trial of occlusal adjustment in the treatment of periodontitis, *J Clin Periodontol* 19:381–387, 1992.

Foz AM, Artese P, Horliana AR, et al: Occlusal adjustment associated with periodontal therapy—a systematic review, *J Dent* 40:1025–1035, 2012.

Gher ME: Changing concepts. The effects of on periodontitis, *Dent Clin North Am* 42:285–299, 1998.

Giargia M, Lindhe J: Tooth mobility and periodontal disease, *J Clin Periodontol* 24:785–791, 1997.

Grant DA, Flynn MJ, Slots J: Periodontal microbiota of mobile and non-mobile teeth, *J Periodontol* 66:386–390, 1995.

Kaufman H, Carranza FA, Enders B, et al: Influence of trauma from occlusion on the bacterial re-population of periodontal pockets in dogs, *J Periodontol* 55:86–92, 1984.

McCulloch CAG, Lekic P, McKee MD: Role of physical forces in regulating the form and function of the periodontal ligament, *Periodontol 2000* 24:56–72, 2000.

Polson AM II: Co-destructive factors of periodontitis and mechanically produced injury, *J Periodontal Res* 9:108–113, 1974.

Schulte W, Hoedt B, Lukas D, et al: Periotest for measuring periodontal characteristics. Correlation with periodontal bone loss, *J Periodontal Res* 27:181–190, 1992.

Svanberg GK, King GJ, Gibbs CH: Occlusal considerations in periodontology, *Periodontol 2000* 9:106–117, 1995.

Wang H, Burgett FG, Shyt Y, et al: The influence of molar furcation involvement and mobility on future clinical periodontal attachment loss, *J Periodontol* 65:25–29, 1994.

CHAPTER 16

Occlusion and Orthodontics

Om P. Kharbanda and M. Ali Darendeliler

PART 1: CHILDREN AND YOUNG ADULTS

CHAPTER OUTLINE

SYNOPSIS

An overview of concepts of normal occlusion and malocclusion is presented from an orthodontic viewpoint. Orthodontists perceive occlusion as tooth alignment and interarch alignment in relation to the underlying skeletal bases and facial soft tissues. Functional and dynamic aspects of occlusion are now also being incorporated into objectives of orthodontic treatment. A classification of malocclusion and its characteristics is presented. Features of postorthodontic optimal occlusion following treatment with fixed appliances are presented.

CHAPTER POINTS

- Orthodontics is aimed at providing a well-functioning and anatomically optimal occlusion that is in harmony with the underlying skeletal base, is aesthetically pleasing, and functionally stable with age.
- Malocclusion is not an organic disease but a deviation from normal that can have infinite variations.
- Malocclusion has aesthetic, functional, and superimposed psychological implications.
- Development of normal occlusion and malocclusion is the outcome of complex interactions of jaw growth, growth of the cranium and face, development of the dentition, eruption timing and sequence of eruption, and soft-tissue function and maturation. These features are governed by genetic architecture and yet are greatly influenced by environmental factors, including nutrition, mode of respiration, habits, and integrity and maintenance of the deciduous dentition.
- Early recognition of malocclusion and its timely interception can minimize or eliminate certain forms of malocclusion.
- Growth modification of growing class II malocclusion is now a recognized and accepted modality of treatment.
- Growth modification in growing class III malocclusion is relatively less predictable yet recommended in certain types of maxillary hypoplasia.
- Full-banded, fixed appliance therapy is the most effective mode of treatment of

malocclusions of dental origin and some variations of skeletal malocclusions.

OPTIMAL OCCLUSION: PHILOSOPHY OF EVIDENCE FOR ORTHODONTICS

The concept and philosophy of "normal" occlusion in orthodontics developed in relation to the teeth having a "specific arrangement" in the dental arches (intraarch) and in relation to opposing arches (interarch). The well-aligned dental arches that have "normal" labial and buccal overjet, some overbite, and a "normal" anteroposterior relationship between maxillary and mandibular arches constitute normal occlusion.

Historically, cusp-to-fossa relationships of upper and lower teeth were regarded as being of special significance. In the late nineteenth and early twentieth centuries, Angle (1899) emphasized the relationship of the mesiobuccal cusp of the maxillary first molar to the buccal groove of the mandibular first molar as the "key factor" in the establishment of a class I molar "normal" relationship. He considered the maxillary first molar to be a stable tooth, which occupied a distinct relationship in the maxillary bone. The position of each dental unit in the arch was also described in terms of its unique "axial inclination".

Clinical observations on occlusion were considered both within an arch and in relation to the opposing arches. Within the arch the following were considered: tight proximal contacts, labiolingual and buccolingual placement, rotation, and labiolingual and mesiodistal inclination. Angle also believed that a full complement of teeth was essential for teeth to be in balance with facial harmony.

Following Angle, clinical research evidence was considered. Studies from the University of Illinois reported that the maxillary first molar did not always have a distinct relationship with the key ridge in the maxilla. The research by Begg (1954) on the occlusion of Australian Aborigines suggested that reduction in tooth substance by proximal and occlusal wear was physiological. Tweed (1954) considered the face and the occlusion from the perspective of axial inclination of the lower incisors and their relationship with the mandibular plane as a guide for determining normal or abnormal relationships of other dental units to their basal bones. His cephalometric studies provided

evidence that in order to achieve a balance of lower incisors with basal bone it may be necessary to extract some teeth.

The advent of cephalometrics and studies on "facial variations" reconfirmed many of the earlier empirical clinical observations that normal occlusion may exist in harmony with skeletal bases only if the skeletal bases and facial bones follow normal growth and development. Cephalometric studies provided an understanding of how the dentition and the occlusion and underlying skeletal structures grow over time and differentiated normal and abnormal growing faces and occlusion.

In 1972 Andrews' analysis of dental casts of normal (nonorthodontic normal occlusion/no history of orthodontic treatment) subjects generated a database of occlusal characteristics that have been grouped into "six keys of occlusion":

1. *Molar relationships*: In addition to the previously described features of the mesiobuccal and mesiolingual cusps of the maxillary first molar with the mandibular first molar, Andrews added that the distal surface of the distobuccal cusp of the maxillary first molar occluded with the mesial surface of the mesiobuccal cusp of the mandibular second molar.

2. *Crown angulations (mesiodistal tip)*: Andrews reconfirmed the axial inclination of the teeth and termed it "tip". The crown tip is expressed in degrees and is variable for each tooth.

3. *Crown inclination (labiolingual or buccolingual)*: Each tooth crown in the arch has a distinct buccolingual and labiolingual inclination, designated as "torque", which is distinct for each tooth crown.

4. *Rotations*: In optimal occlusion, there should be no tooth rotation. A rotated molar occupies more space in the arch and does not allow optimal occlusion.

5. All teeth in the arch should have tight proximal contact.

6. Flat or mild curve of Spee is a prerequisite of normal occlusion. A deep curve of Spee is suggestive of malocclusion.

The "six keys" are meaningful for normal occlusion (Figure 16-1) not because they are consistently seen in all cases but because the "lack of even one" may suggest incomplete orthodontic treatment. Orthodontic treatment goals should aim to attain Andrews'

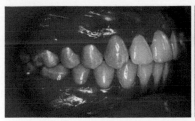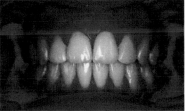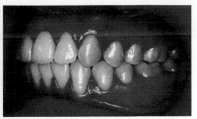

FIG 16-1 Normal Occlusion: Occlusion Following Nonextraction Orthodontic Treatment (Source: *Orthodontics* 2E by O.P. Kharbanda, with permission from Reed Elsevier India Pvt. Ltd.)

six keys. Andrews' proposals on tip and torque values have been incorporated into orthodontic brackets and tubes of fixed appliances. Such appliances are generically called "preadjusted" because they facilitate tooth movement in optimal inclinations and angulations without requiring many adjustments.

Tip and torque values suggested by Andrews are supposedly more suitable for Caucasians. There are variations in Asians, African-Americans, and other races, but they follow similar features.

Roth (1981) suggested that orthodontic treatment goals should also include intercuspal contact position (ICP) or centric occlusion coincident with retruded contact position (RCP) or centric relation. In protrusive excursions, eight lower anterior teeth should ideally contact six upper anterior teeth and provide smooth lateral and anterior guidance.

MALOCCLUSION

Any significant deviation from normal occlusion may be termed "malocclusion." Current orthodontic understanding of occlusion necessitates that teeth should have normal intraarch and interarch relationships, be in harmony with the underlying skeletal bases, and exhibit a well-balanced face. In addition, deviations in normal functional relationships suggest malocclusion.

Malocclusion may be of dental or skeletal origin or both. Deviations could occur in all the dimensions (i.e., anteroposterior, vertical, or transverse), in isolation, or in combinations of varying severity.

Deviations range from minor, such as slight alterations in arch position, tooth tip, or tooth rotation, to more severe forms of crowding, spacing, or abnormal overjet and overbite and their combinations of varying severity. Minor malocclusions may have insignificant

functional consequences, yet may generate psychosocial concerns for child or adult. Although more severe malocclusion in other individuals may or may not be of any concern, it may be associated with functional problems.

Classification of Malocclusion

In order to standardize description and treatment planning, malocclusion based on molar relationships was grouped into three classes (Angle 1899), using Roman numerals (I, II, III) to denote the classes and Arabic numerals (1, 2) to denote divisions. A malocclusion that exists unilaterally is termed a subdivision. Using the maxillary first molar as a reference, the classification is: normal mesiodistal (anteroposterior) relationship of the upper and lower first molars (class I); and variations, that is, a distal lower arch (class II), or mesial lower arch (class III) relationship. Figure 16-2, *A*, illustrates dental classes I, II, and III.

- Class I malocclusion exists when maxillary and mandibular first molar teeth have a normal cusp-to-fossa relationship, but there may be deviations in the arrangement of teeth, intraarch, interarch, or both. The common features of class I malocclusions include:
  - Maxillary protrusion
  - Crowding and spacing
  - Anterior and posterior crossbites
  - Deep and open bite
  - Midline shift
  - Combinations of the above
- Class II malocclusion (also called distal occlusion) exists when the lower first molar is distal to its normal relationship with the maxillary first molar; the mesiobuccal cusp of the maxillary first molar falls mesial to the buccal groove of the mandibular

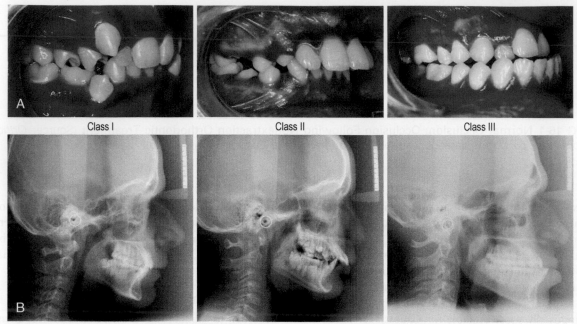

FIG 16-2 A, Three types of dental malocclusion: left to right, classes I, II, and III. **B,** Corresponding cephalograms exhibiting skeletal pattern: left to right, classes I, II, and III. (Class III, Source: *Orthodontics* 2E by O.P. Kharbanda, with permission from Reed Elsevier India Pvt. Ltd.)

first molar. The usual features of such malocclusions are:

- Distal positioning of lower canines (class II canine)
- Maxillary protrusion
- Deep bite
- Interarch and/or intraarch deviations in teeth
- Class II malocclusions associated with proclined maxillary incisors are called division 1 or with retroclined maxillary incisors division 2.
- Class III malocclusion exists when the lower arch (mandibular first molar) is mesial to its normal relationship with the maxillary first molar, that is, the mesiobuccal cusp of the maxillary first molar falls distal to the buccal groove of the lower first molar.

The advent of cephalometrics allowed study of the morphology of the cranium, face, and jaws, which provided a better understanding of the skeletal and dental components of malocclusion. This allowed classification of skeletal jaw relationships. Figure 16-2, *B*, describes three types of skeletal malocclusion.

- *Skeletal class I:* Orthognathic or normal—maxillary and mandibular skeletal bases are in a normal anteroposterior relationship. Skeletal class I jaw relationship does not necessitate a dental class I relationship. A dental class II or class III malocclusion may occur on a skeletal class I base.
- *Skeletal class II:* Distal jaw relationship exhibits an anteroposterior discrepancy between the maxillary and mandibular bases. A skeletal class II relationship could arise from a smaller (or posteriorly positioned) mandible or an anteriorly placed (or larger) maxilla, or a combination of both. A class I or class II dental malocclusion may be observed on skeletal class II bases, but a dental class III relationship on a skeletal class II base is extremely unusual.
- *Skeletal class III:* Mesial jaw relationship exists when the mandibular skeletal base is mesial to the maxillary base in an anteroposterior relationship. Such a relationship could arise when there is a normal maxilla and a large mandible or as a pseudo-class III with a small maxilla and a

normal-sized mandible. A varying combination of maxillary deficiency and mandibular prognathism also occurs. Depending on the severity and location of the skeletal class III dysplasia, a class I or class III dental relationship might exist.

OCCLUSION FOLLOWING ORTHODONTIC TREATMENT

Nonextraction Era

The development of a more scientific approach from the beginning of the twentieth century was mainly devoted to refinement of "appliance(s)", which could effectively move teeth into the preconceived concept of "normal dental relationship." The treatment by expansion and alignment could provide normal alignment and cusp-to-fossa relationships but was not always in harmony with the underlying skeletal bases and facial soft tissues.

Extraction Era: Search for the Evidence

Tweed (1945) reviewed his treated cases that (1) did not result in good facial aesthetics, (2) had relapsed, and (3) showed facial balance and a stable occlusion. Clinical observations were supported by cephalometric studies; in subjects with a balanced face and good occlusion (orthodontically treated), mandibular incisors were approximately 90° to the mandibular plane (IMPA) and their Frankfort mandibular plane angle (FMA) was approximately 25°. Accordingly the maxillary arch required alignment to normal overjet with the mandibular incisors. To upright mandibular incisors (bringing close to 90°), space was required in the arch, which could be obtained with extracting first premolars. Tweed's extraction approach was further supported by Begg, who reported that proximal reduction of tooth surfaces was an essential part of physiological occlusion (Begg 1954). Similarly, maxillary expansion may be insufficient in the correction of large overjet or crowding, and alignment and extraction of some teeth may be unavoidable.

This resulted in extractions being performed without the necessary consideration of the remaining growth in children and their effect on the adult facial profile. The long-term growth studies that are now available need to be considered in orthodontic treatment planning, together with specific racial and ethnic characteristics, which show variations in cephalometric parameters. It has since been realized that extractions should only be used with caution following a comprehensive assessment that includes space requirements, growth trend or anticipated growth, soft-tissue profile, and treatment mechanics.

Occlusion without Extraction

The occlusal relationships following nonextraction orthodontic treatment are similar to that of an occlusion with a full complement of teeth (Figure 16-3).

Occlusion with Extraction
Four First Premolars
Class I Malocclusion

The extraction space achieved following premolar extraction in both arches is used for arch alignment and establishment of optimal overjet and overbite. With the use of preadjusted appliances, normal mesiodistal angulation (tip) and labiolingual inclinations (torque) of the teeth may be achieved. However, in some cases proximal contact of the distal surface of the canine with that of the mesial surface of the second premolars will be less than ideal, due to the smaller convexity of the mesial surface of the second premolar. The maxillary second premolars are usually smaller than the first premolars.

Class II Malocclusion

The extraction space in the maxillary arch is used to correct overjet and crowding. The extraction space in the lower arch is used to reduce the curve of Spee, crowding, and mesial movement of lower molars to achieve class I molar relationship (Figure 16-4).

Maxillary First Premolars and Mandibular Second Premolars

Lower second premolar extractions provide greater mesial movement of the lower first molars for the correction of class II to class I molar relationships where space requirements in the lower anterior segment are small. This approach is common in treatment of class II division 1 dental malocclusion.

Maxillary First Premolars Only: Therapeutic Class II Occlusion

In certain forms of class II malocclusion, where the lower arch is well aligned, protrusion may be corrected by extraction of first premolars in the upper

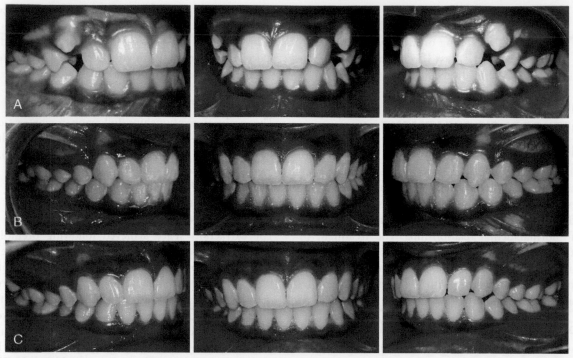

FIG 16-3 A, Pretreatment: bilateral mild class II, buccally placed canines, midline change. **B**, Occlusion at post-debond: bilateral class I molar and canine relation, normal over jet, and overbite. **C**, Occlusion at 3 years postretention.

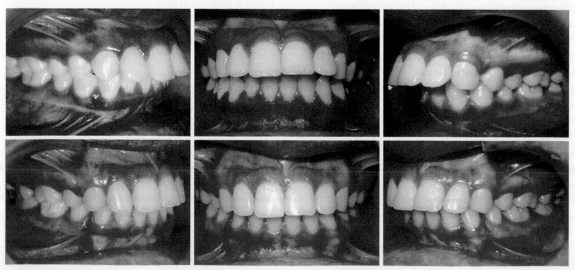

FIG 16-4 Occlusion following extraction of four premolars: before (top row) and after (bottom row) treatment. (Source: *Orthodontics* 2E by O.P. Kharbanda, with permission from Reed Elsevier India Pvt. Ltd.)

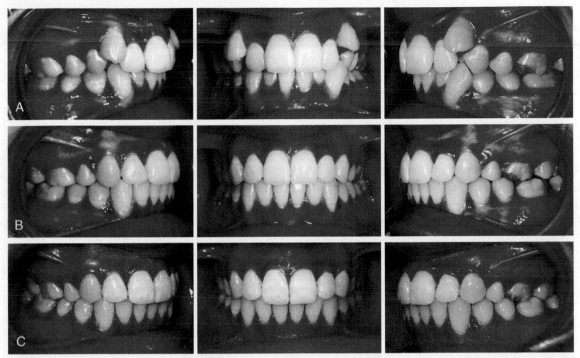

FIG 16-5 A, Pretreatment. **B**, Post-debond. **C**, Two year-follow up. (Source: *Orthodontics* 2E by O.P. Kharbanda, with permission from Reed Elsevier India Pvt. Ltd.)

arch only. The postorthodontic occlusion would have a normal overjet and overbite, with maxillary second premolars and molars in a full cusp class II relationship with the mandibular arch. Under these conditions the mesiobuccal cusp of the maxillary first molar articulates in the embrasure between the mandibular first molar and second premolar. The distobuccal cusp of the maxillary molar articulates with the mandibular first molar mesiobuccal groove (Figure 16-5). Earlier it was suspected that finishing in class II molar relationship can lead to temporomandibular joint disorder and compromised occlusal stability. However, studies have found that occlusal stability of class II malocclusion finished in class II molar relationship was at par with those finished in class I molar relationship (Jason et al. 2010).

Mandibular First Premolars: Therapeutic Class III Occlusion

In certain forms of class III malocclusion, treatment might involve alignment of the maxillary arch, proclination of the upper anteriors, and retraction of the mandibular incisors, whereas the molars are maintained in a class III malocclusion. The space for retraction and retroclination of the lower incisors may need to be obtained by extraction of lower first or second premolars. Postorthodontic occlusion will have a class III molar and premolar relation and class I canine relation with normal overjet and overbite. Farret et al. (2009) observed good occlusal stability and tissue health in patients with therapeutic class III after 13 to 14 years of treatment.

Extraction of First Molars

The permanent first molars are highly important in schemes of normal occlusion. However, in certain types of malocclusion cases, extraction of permanent first molars can be preferred over other teeth. In addition to extracting the first permanent molars in a systematic orthodontic treatment approach, there are certain objective indications for first molar extractions. These include extensive caries lesions, large fillings, endodontic or periodontal problems, or grossly hypoplastic teeth.

Extraction of first molars, especially those with questionable long-term prognosis, could help retain more healthy teeth, gain satisfactory orthodontic results, and improve posttreatment occlusion (Stalpers et al. 2007, Tian et al. 2009). Extraction of a carious first molar is considered only in situations in which healthy second and third molars are present and the second molar can be orthodontically aligned to occupy the position of the first molar.

Occlusion with Missing Maxillary Laterals

Orthodontic treatment with missing maxillary laterals may include regaining space and restoration of laterals. In other situations in which extraction space may be required for the correction of the malocclusion, the lateral incisor space can be closed by moving the maxillary canines mesially. Postorthodontic (normal) occlusion in such a case would substitute the first premolars for the maxillary canines and the canines for the laterals. Canines need to be modified for aesthetics and would require reshaping of the labial surface, cusp tip, and proximal surfaces to more closely resemble the laterals. The mesial and distal slopes may be modified with composite resin. The functional anterior guidance would necessitate some adjustment of the lingual surface. The maxillary first premolar may substitute for the maxillary canine, and the intraarch "canine" relationship has the mesial slope of the maxillary first premolar with the distal of the lower canine. The maxillary first premolar may need reshaping of the mesiobuccal slope and some reduction of the lingual cusp (Figure 16-6).

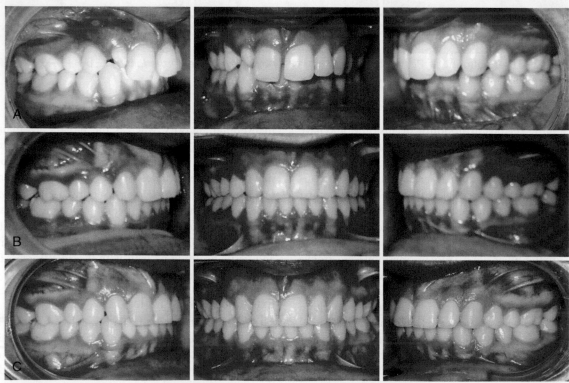

FIG 16-6 Case of Microdontic Maxillary Right Lateral Incisor and Palatally Impacted Canine Microdontic lateral incisor is extracted and space is managed with substitution of right maxillary canine. Slight space seen distal to substituted canine can be effectively managed with tooth colored restoration. The final occlusion necessitated finishing of molar relation to full cusp class II on right side and class I relationship on left side. **A**, Pre; **B**, post; and **C**, 22 month-follow up. Note stable outcome with class II buccal relations on right and class I on left side.

PART 2: ADULTS

SYNOPSIS

This section provides an overview of the combined orthodontic and orthognathic treatment options in cases of severe malocclusion with underlying skeletal problems. Treatment considerations and objectives of adult orthodontic occlusion are summarized. The concepts related to postorthodontic retention—philosophy, methods, and prevention of relapse—are introduced.

CHAPTER POINTS

- The occlusion is in a constant state of biological adaptation, with age changes in the dentition, periodontal tissues, and supporting structures.
- Orthodontic treatment goals in adult occlusion are aimed at achieving a functionally and aesthetically acceptable occlusion within the limitations of each case. These are imposed by periodontal health, missing teeth, health of the existing teeth, and general health of the individual.
- More severe forms of malocclusion, such as severe mandibular retrognathia, maxillary hypoplasia, mandibular prognathism, extreme vertical dysplasia (long face syndrome), large transverse discrepancies, and jaw deviations, can

only be managed with a combined orthodontic and surgical approach (orthognathic surgery). The outcome(s) are rewarding in suitable patients and require careful treatment planning.
- Orthodontic treatment (including surgical orthodontic treatment) shows some relapse with time.
- The severity of the relapse is governed by many factors, including the nature of the initial malocclusion, type of treatment, quality of treatment, retention protocol, residual growth of the face, type of face, presence of third molars, soft-tissue behavior, and periodontal health.
- Choice of a retention appliance and specific retention protocol are governed by the type and severity of the initial malocclusion, the age of the patient, and any individual predisposing factors for relapse.
- Relapse is associated with and may be amplified by the natural aging process.

ADULT OCCLUSION

Adult occlusion changes continuously throughout life and adapts to intrinsic and extrinsic factors.

Physiological Changes

Physiological tooth migration is the lifelong ability for teeth and their supporting tissues to adapt to functional demands and as a result move through the alveolar process. In humans teeth in the posterior segments tend to migrate mesially to compensate for wear of interproximal contact surfaces. Further tooth movement may occur following changes in occlusal equilibrium with loss of a neighboring or antagonistic tooth. In addition to mesial migration, teeth exhibit continued eruption. Studies have demonstrated continuous eruption of upper incisors by 6.0 mm/yr between the ages of 19 and 25 (Iseri & Solow 1996). Growth and development of the craniofacial skeleton is a continuing, long-term process with periods of exuberance and relative quiescence, but the biological mechanisms that regulate growth changes remain intact and active throughout life.

ORTHODONTIC TREATMENT IN ADULTS

In recent years, altered lifestyles and improved dental and orthodontic awareness have led to an increased demand for orthodontic treatment by adults. The ideal treatment objectives of aesthetics, function, and stability may need to be modified for adult patients, and many cases require an interdisciplinary approach. To facilitate placement of fixed or removable prostheses and a healthy periodontal status, parallelism of abutment teeth, intraarch and interarch space distribution, adequate embrasure space and root position, and occlusal vertical dimension change need to be achieved in comprehensive treatment in conjunction with other specialities.

Aesthetics of hard and soft tissues are often the main concern for adults. The harmony of smile line, gingival level, and dental alignment need to be considered as part of interdisciplinary treatment. Adults tend to be anxious about lip competency and support; many adults have a thin upper lip that may be increased in length; changes to the upper lip, with inadequate tooth, bone, and soft-tissue support, create an aged appearance. The maintenance of upper lip support precludes significant retraction of maxillary incisors, and, in class II division 1, advancement of the mandibular dental arch may be the preferred treatment objective to develop incisal guidance.

Periodontal health is accomplished by improving the crown:root ratio in patients who have bone loss and by correcting mucogingival and osseous defects by repositioning prominent teeth to improve gingival topography. The reduction of clinical crown length together with orthodontic extrusion will improve the crown:root ratio. Location of gingival margins is determined by the axial inclination and alignment of teeth. Clinically there is improved self-maintenance of periodontal health when teeth are correctly positioned. The aim is to level crestal bone between adjacent cementoenamel junctions because this creates a more physiological osseous architecture and the potential to correct osseous defects.

There is a delayed response to mechanical forces in adults as a result of age-related changes of the skeleton and alveolar bone. However, there is no evidence to suggest that teeth move at a slower rate. In a healthy periodontium, bone will remodel around a tooth without damage to the supporting tissues. This principle is used to create favorable alveolar bone changes in patients with periodontal defects, for example, the uprighting of molars to reduce pocket depth and improve bone morphology.

Extrusion, together with occlusal reduction of clinical crown height, is reported to reduce infrabony defects and reduce pocket depth. This procedure is advocated for the treatment of isolated periodontal osseous defects, which may be eliminated when marginal bone heights are leveled. Intrusion of teeth to improve periodontal support has been proposed, but the evidence in the literature is conflicting.

OCCLUSION AFTER TREATMENT WITH COMBINED FIXED APPLIANCE AND ORTHOGNATHIC SURGERY

Severe dysplasia of skeletal malocclusion—skeletal class II, class III, or extreme open and deep bite, long face, and jaw deviations—can only be corrected in a combined approach of orthodontic treatment and orthognathic surgery for surgical correction of the deformity. Where a severe skeletal class III malocclusion presents, orthodontic treatment alone is insufficient and treatment requires reduction in jaw length. A number of surgical lengthening or shortening procedures of the mandible and relocation of the maxilla are used in clinical practice. Bilateral sagittal split osteotomy (BSSO) is the most common for the mandible and Le Fort I and II (fracture of the maxilla and subsequent fixation in the required position) for the maxilla. A number of variations or combinations of occlusal relationships are governed by the type and extent of the skeletal and dental malocclusion and the orthodontic treatment and surgical options. In general the objectives are to provide a well-balanced harmonious face (skeletal and soft tissue) and an acceptable functioning occlusion in a class I, class II, or class III molar relationship. Ideally the occlusion at the end of treatment should match specifications of a normal occlusion; however, depending on the severity of the discrepancy, dental compensations are accepted. Dental compensations may camouflage the extreme nature of the discrepancy in the sagittal, transverse, and vertical planes.

In the sagittal plane, upper and/or lower incisors are proclined or retroclined in class II and class III orthognathic surgery cases to decrease the amount of surgical movement of the maxilla and/or mandible.

In the transverse plane, upper and/or lower posterior teeth are buccally and/or lingually tipped in posterior crossbite and buccal bite cases to decrease the amount of surgical movement of the maxilla and/or mandible.

In the vertical plane, upper and/or lower posterior teeth may be extruded or intruded; upper and/or lower incisors may be extruded or intruded in open-bite and deep-bite cases to decrease the amount of surgical movement of the maxilla and/or mandible.

Skeletal class III: These cases require shortening of the mandibular base and occasionally maxillary advancement.

Skeletal class II: These cases require lengthening of the mandibular base and occasionally maxillary impaction.

ORTHODONTIC OCCLUSION IN THE LONG TERM: RELAPSE AND RETENTION

Relapse is the tendency for teeth to move from the positions in which they were placed by orthodontics, whereas retention is "the holding of teeth following orthodontic treatment in the treated position for the period of time necessary for the stability of the result".

Long-term studies of treated cases at the 10- to 20-year postretention period have shown that orthodontic results are potentially unstable due to:

- Physiological mesial migration of teeth (age-related changes)
- Periodontal and gingival health
- Residual growth
- Neuromuscular influences
- Specific orthodontic tooth movements
- Developing third molars

A retention phase following orthodontic treatment is required to:

- Allow time for periodontal and gingival reorganization
- Minimize changes in the orthodontic result from subsequent growth
- Permit neuromuscular adaptation to the corrected tooth position
- Maintain unstable tooth positions

Normal developmental changes occur in the dentition in both untreated individuals and those who have undergone orthodontic treatment. The changes in the craniofacial structures, including the dental arches, are not simply due to, or the result of, orthodontic and orthopedic treatment but are also due to aging. There is an increase in intercanine width until eruption of the permanent canines, after which this width decreases. The intermolar width, however, appears to be stable from 13 to 20 years. Mandibular arch length decreases with time and the lower incisors become increasingly irregular, particularly in females. These arch changes are observed before 30 years of age; lower incisor crowding continues beyond 50 years of age.

Periodontal and Gingival Tissues

The stability of tooth position is determined by the principal fibers of the periodontal ligament and the supraalveolar gingival fiber network. These fibers contribute to a state of equilibrium between the tooth and the soft-tissue envelope. Orthodontic tooth movement causes disruption of the periodontal ligament and the gingival fiber network, and a period of time is required for reorganization of these fibers after removal of the appliances:

- Reorganization of the collagen fiber bundles in the periodontal ligament occurs over a 3- to 4-month period; at this stage tooth mobility disappears.
- The gingival fiber network is made up of both collagenous and elastic-like oxytalan fibers. Reorganization of this network occurs more slowly than in the periodontal ligament; the collagenous fibers remodel in 4 to 6 months, whereas the oxytalan fibers may take up to 6 years to remodel.
- It is believed that the slow remodeling of the supraalveolar fibers of the gingival complex contribute to the relapse of teeth after orthodontic treatment, especially in those teeth that were initially rotated.

The direction of relapse will tend to be toward the original position of the tooth; thus full-time retention for 3 to 4 months following removal of orthodontic appliances is required to allow time for reorganization of the periodontal tissue structures. Retention should be continued part-time for at least 12 months to allow time for reorganization of the gingival fibers.

To minimize rotational relapse, the following has been suggested:

- Early correction of the rotation to allow more time for reorganization
- Overcorrection of the rotation if the occlusion allows. In the premolar region overcorrection is possible, especially during early stages of the treatment. However, overcorrection at the anterior region, especially toward the achievement of the normal occlusion, when an ideal incisor relationship is obtained, is practically impossible.
- Circumferential supracrestal fiberotomy or pericision at or just before removal of appliances. This procedure involves transection of the supraalveolar fibers, allowing reattachment in the corrected position.

Neuromuscular Influences

The soft tissues of the lips, cheeks, and tongue at rest contribute to the equilibrium and therefore stability of tooth position following orthodontic treatment. The initial mandibular intercanine and intermolar arch widths are believed to be accurate indicators of the individual's muscle balance between lips, cheeks, and tongue. The initial position of the lower incisor has also been shown to be the most stable position for the individual. Permanent retention for the first 3 to 4 months is required to allow time for soft tissues of cheeks, lips, and tongue to adapt to the new tooth positions. Wherever possible the initial intercanine width and lower incisor positions should be maintained. Permanent retention is essential if advancement of the lower incisors is an objective of treatment.

Effect of Residual Growth on Orthodontic Occlusion

Skeletal problems will tend to relapse if growth continues beyond completion of orthodontic treatment. In late adolescence, and even adulthood, continued growth in the pattern that caused a class II, class III, deep-bite or open-bite problem is a major cause of relapse and requires careful management during retention. As a result of the residual mandibular growth, the lower incisors, contained by the upper incisors, cannot accommodate forward movement of the mandible and tend to tip lingually, causing lower incisor crowding. Clinical observation suggests finishing either with a small overjet at the end of treatment or fixed retainers for the lower canine-to-canine area. Some clinicians rotate the mesial side of the lower canine lingually to prevent mesial movement of the canines after the retention period.

Late mandibular growth has been considered a major cause of relapse of crowding in the mandibular arch in late adulthood. Figure 16-7 illustrates both removable and fixed retention appliances.

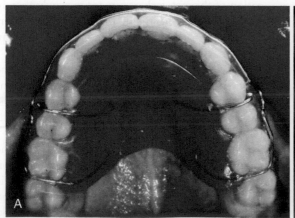 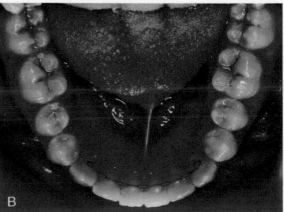

FIG 16-7 Retention Appliances **A**, Removable maxillary Begg retainer. **B**, Fixed lower lingual retainer. (Source: *Orthodontics* 2E by O.P. Kharbanda, with permission from Reed Elsevier India Pvt. Ltd.)

REFERENCES

Andrews LF: The six keys to normal occlusion, *Am J Orthod* 62:296–309, 1972.

Angle EH: Classification of malocclusion, *Dental Cosmos* 41:248–264, 1899.

Begg PR: Stone age man's dentition, *Am J Orthod* 40:298–312, 373–383, 462–475, 517–531, 1954.

Farret MM, Farret MM, Farret AM: Strategies to finish orthodontic treatment with a Class III molar relationship: three patient reports, *World J Orthod* 10:323–333, 2009.

Iseri H, Solow B: Continued eruption of maxillary incisors and first molars in girls from 9–25 years, studied by implant method, *Eur J Orthod* 18:245–256, 1996.

Janson G, Camardella LT, Araki JD, et al: Treatment stability in patients with Class II malocclusion treated with 2 maxillary premolar extractions or without extractions, *Am J Orthod Dentofacial Orthop* 138:16–22, 2010.

Kharbanda OP: *Orthodontics: Diagnosis and Management of Malocclusion and Dentofacial Deformities*, ed 2, New Delhi, India, 2013, Elsevier.

Roth RH: Functional occlusion for the orthodontist, *J Clin Orthodon* 15:32–51, 1981.

Stalpers MJ, Booij JW, Bronkhorst EM, et al: Extraction of maxillary first permanent molars in patients with class II division 1 malocclusion, *A J Orthodon Dentofacial Orthop* 132:316–323, 2007.

Tian YL, Qin K, Zhao Y, et al: First molar extraction in malocclusion: an analysis of 20 consecutive cases, *Shanghai Kou Qiang Yi Xue* 18:375–379, 2009.

Tweed CH: The Frankfort-Mandibular Incisor Angle (FMIA) In Orthodontic Diagnosis, Treatment Planning and Prognosis, *Angle Orthod* 24:121–169, 1954.

Tweed CH: A philosophy of orthodontic treatment, *Am J Orthodont Oral Surg* 31:74–103, 1945.

Further Reading

Behrents RG: *An Atlas of Growth in the Aging Craniofacial Skeleton*, vol 18, Ann Arbor, 1985, Center for Human Growth and Development, University of Michigan.

Blake M, Bibby K: Retention and stability: a review of the literature, *Am J Orthodon Dentofacial Orthop* 114:299–306, 1998.

Clark JR, Evans RD: Functional occlusion: a review, *J Orthodon* 28:76–81, 2001.

Farret MM, Farret MM, Farret AM: Strategies to finish orthodontic treatment with a Class III molar relationship: three patient reports, *World J Orthodon* 10:323–333, 2009.

Graber TM, Vanarsdall RL Jr, editors: *Orthodontics: Current Principles and Techniques*, ed 3, St Louis, 2000, Mosby, pp 29–30.

Horowitz SL, Hixon EH: Physiologic recovery following orthodontic treatment, *Am J Orthodon* 55:1–4, 1969.

Kasrovi PM, Meyer M, Nelson GD: Occlusion: an orthodontic perspective, *J Calif Dent Assoc* 28:780–790, 2000.

Kharbanda OP: *Orthodontics: Diagnosis and Management of Malocclusion and Dentofacial Deformities*, ed 2, New Delhi, 2013, Elsevier India.

Little RM, Riedel RA, Artun J: An evaluation of changes in mandibular anterior alignment from 10 to 20 years post-retention, *Am J Orthodon* 93:423–428, 1988.

Moyers RE: *Handbook of orthodontics*, ed 4, Chicago, 1988, Yearbook.

Nangia A, Darendeliler MA: Finishing occlusion in class II or class III molar relation: therapeutic class II and III, *Aust Orthodon J* 17:89–94, 2001.

Proffit WR, White RR Jr, editors: *Surgical Orthodontics*, St Louis, 1991, Mosby, pp 248–263, 264–282.

Reitan K: Tissue behavior during orthodontic tooth movement, *Am J Orthodon* 46:881–900, 1960.

Richardson ME: The role of the third molar in the cause of late lower arch crowding: a review, *Am J Orthodon Dentofacial Orthop* 95:79–83, 1989.

Richardson ME: Prophylactic extraction of lower third molars: setting the record straight, *Am J Orthodon Dentofacial Orthop* 115(1):17A–18A, 1999.

Richardson ME: A review of changes in lower arc alignment from seven to fifty years, *Sem Orthodon* 5:151–159, 1999.

Richardson ME, Gormley JS: Lower arch crowding in the third decade, *Eur J Orthodon* 20:597–607, 1998.

Roth RH: The straight wire appliance 17 years later, *J Clin Orthodon* 21:632–642, 1987.

Staley RN, Bishara SE, editor: *Text Book of Orthodontics*, Philadelphia, 2001, Saunders, pp 98–104.

Strang RHW: *A Textbook of Orthodontia*, ed 2, Philadelphia, 1950, Lea & Febiger, pp 24–51, 78–106.

Thilander B: Orthodontic relapse versus natural development, *Am J Orthodon Dentofacial Orthop* 117:562–563, 2000.

Vaden JL, Dale JG, Klontz HA: The Tweed–Merrifield appliance: philosophy, diagnosis and treatment. In Graber TM, Vanarsdall RL Jr, editors: *Orthodontics: Current Principles and Techniques*, ed 3, St Louis, 2000, Mosby, pp 647–707.

213

CHAPTER 17

Occlusion and Fixed Prosthodontics

Terry Walton

SYNOPSIS

This chapter presents the rationale for establishing tooth contact patterns during fixed prosthodontic procedures, that is, for establishing a therapeutic occlusal form.

In the absence of scientific data, various "philosophies of occlusion" have evolved in an effort to describe the relationship that should be developed between the teeth during restorative procedures or adjustment of the natural dentition. With little evidence these philosophies or concepts often involve complicated and expensive instrumentation and are promoted with almost religious zeal rather than scientific rigor. These philosophies have also been applied to implant-supported prostheses—with little scientific data to verify their effectiveness.

Form that supports function is the rationale for the occlusal form outlined in this chapter. Evidence for its effectiveness is provided by the outcomes—biological, physiological, and mechanical—of up to 15 years of longitudinal assessment of fixed metal-ceramic dental prostheses and up to 25 years of longitudinal assessment of metal-ceramic single unit crowns.

There is a need for further long-term studies evaluating the outcome of fixed prosthodontics. It is accepted that prospective, randomized clinical trials with adequate controls and well-defined criteria are very difficult to carry out. In addition, clinical studies of less than 5 years have little relevance (Creugers et al. 1994) and can lead to incorrect conclusions (Walton 2002). It is therefore imperative that clinicians document and publish information from their clinical practice. The resultant collective data would facilitate a more evidence-based approach to procedures used in fixed prosthodontics.

CHAPTER POINTS

• Intraarch stability effected by firm interproximal contacts

- Interarch stability effected by at least one contact on each opposing tooth in the intercuspal contact position (ICP)
- Bilateral synchronized contacts in ICP
- Absence of posterior contacts during protrusive movements
- A flat occlusal plane
- Maintenance of inherent physiological tooth mobility where possible
- Slight clearance (10 μm foil thickness) between the incisors in maximum intercuspation (MI)
- Minimal cusp height and fossa depth
- Lateral gliding contacts restricted to the canines or effected as far forward in the arch as possible

RATIONALE FOR ESTABLISHING TOOTH CONTACTS DURING FIXED PROSTHODONTICS

Occlusion is the dynamic interplay of various components, including the teeth, their supporting tissues, the jaw muscles, the temporomandibular joints (TMJs), the central pattern generator, and other associated cortical interactions. This interplay involves the application of forces of varying magnitude and duration. Resistance against resultant strain or pathology of these components will be reduced by any compromise to their integrity (Figure 17-1). As in any physiological system, a "normal" state includes a degree of adaptability with a range of form and the absence of pathology. The magnitude of any changes and the duration over which they occur will influence whether adaptation or pathology ensues (Figure 17-2). Slow changes will facilitate adaptation even when the changes eventually lead to a significant deviation from ideal form. Fixed prosthodontics, however, may involve relatively instantaneous changes in form, thus challenging the adaptive capacity of the occlusal system. A resultant therapeutic occlusal form that requires minimal adaptation will less likely initiate pathology, and the health of the occlusal components will be determined to a great extent by the subsequent stability of the teeth.

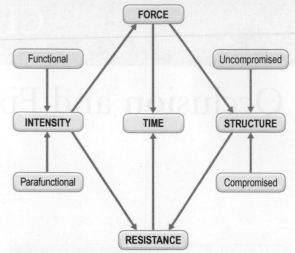

FIG 17-1 The interrelationship between force and resistance associated with the components of occlusion. The intensity of the force and integrity of the structures (teeth, periodontal tissues, alveolar bone, muscles of mastication, and temporomandibular joints) will determine the physiological or pathological response. Time provides an accumulated effect.

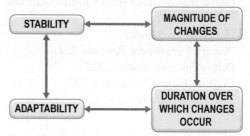

FIG 17-2 The interrelationship of changes in form and adaptation of structures. Adaptation occurs with time, but there are limits to this adaptive capacity, and it is patient dependent. In contrast to small changes over a long duration in the natural dentition, a therapeutic occlusal form involves large changes over a short duration.

Tooth Contacts

There has been debate regarding the number and position of contacts required to maintain individual tooth stability. Contacts on natural teeth occur on flat surfaces, marginal ridges, cusp tips, cusp inclines, and in fossae. They may be point or plane contacts.

Philosophies of occlusion that prescribe specific and multiple points per tooth contact pattern, assume a required precision that does not occur naturally. It has not been demonstrated that such precision results in any greater long-term stability of tooth position than that which occurs in the natural unrestored dentition.

Contacts between teeth result in vertical and lateral forces. The resilience of the periodontal ligament dissipates some of this stress through physiological tooth movement. Peak impact loads are dampened and forces are spread over many more teeth as a consequence of this jiggling. These physiological movements are exacerbated in periodontally compromised teeth but absent in implant-supported prostheses, both occurrences necessitating some modification in therapeutic occlusal form. Significant tipping and rotations may occur if tooth position is unstable. Maintaining interproximal contacts facilitates intraarch stability, whereas interarch tooth stability is facilitated by bilateral contacts between opposing teeth in the intercuspal position (ICP). However, the relatively short time that opposing teeth contact in function also indicates that other forces arising from the tongue and facial musculature, the periodontal ligament, and alveolar bone transceptal fibers may also influence long-term tooth stability.

Form That Supports Function

The functions performed by components of the occlusion include suckling, mastication, swallowing, speech, and parafunction. They also contribute to self-image (aesthetics) and emotional expression.

Suckling

Suckling is an innate reflex, which does not involve the teeth. However, in its mature form sucking might be considered a parafunction if habits, such as finger or tongue sucking, become prolonged. The forces involved during such parafunction and other habits, such as tongue thrusting, can affect the position and stability of the teeth, especially those with reduced periodontal support, and may be linked to specific skeletal jaw morphology. Therefore, although these forces have little bearing on considerations of tooth form in fixed prosthodontics, it is important to

recognize their existence when assessing and effecting long-term follow-up. For example, the overcontoured palatal form of a crowned maxillary central incisor in conjunction with a tongue thrust habit may result in mobility or migration of the tooth even in the absence of any opposing tooth contact.

Swallowing

Swallowing is also an innate reflex response, which does not necessarily involve the teeth. An important aspect of swallowing involves bracing of the jaw to support the suprahyoid muscles. This is achieved during the infantile swallow pattern by bracing the tongue against the palate. Although the tongue is sometimes used for jaw bracing by children and adults, for example when drinking, the more common means of jaw bracing during swallowing involves contact between the teeth in the ICP. The forces involved are relatively light. Thus contact between only a few teeth would be unlikely to involve excessive loading leading to symptoms within the teeth or periodontal tissues. Tooth contacts during swallowing will also vary with head posture. The occlusal form of the teeth and their interarch contacts would seem to have little bearing on swallowing. However, bilateral synchronized tooth contacts in centric occlusion (CO) may facilitate optimum physiological neuromuscular activity during swallowing.

Phonetics

The arrangement of the anterior teeth will affect phonetics as well as aesthetics. The proximity of the upper and lower anterior teeth during protrusive movements, for example, will determine the "c," "s," and "t" sounds. The relationship of the upper anterior teeth and the lower lip will affect "f" and "v" sounds. As well as facilitating interpersonal communication, there is a social expectation that phonetic patterns will be effected in a specific way. Thus the absence of anterior teeth or any impediment, such as posterior contacts that prevent anterior tooth approximation when protruding the jaw for speech, can affect self-image as well as speech.

Excessive lateral deviation or torquing around posterior teeth to develop socially acceptable speech patterns will require adaptation of the jaw neuromuscular system. Exceeding the physiological "adaptability" of one or more of these components may result in pain or dysfunction. The length of the incisors, degree of overbite and overjet, angle of condylar inclination, and curve of the occlusal plane will influence anterior tooth approximation during protrusion. These factors, except condylar inclination, may be modified by restorative procedures. Tooth form and arrangement should therefore ensure an absence of posterior contacts during protrusive jaw movements, and this will be facilitated by developing a flat occlusal plane. Thus restorative procedures that affect phonetics may also influence the patient's psychological and physiological wellbeing.

Mastication

Mastication usually involves an approximation, but not necessarily contact between posterior teeth. It is possible to prepare a food bolus for swallowing without tooth contact. The efficiency of comminution of the food bolus will be influenced by the contour of the occlusal surfaces. Steep cuspal inclines may or may not promote chewing efficiency but will increase lateral loading on the teeth. The need for chewing efficiency (and posterior teeth) has decreased significantly with modern food handling techniques. Thus the actual occlusal form provided during restorative procedures would seem to have minimal efficiency of mastication. The effect on lateral loading on teeth may be more significant, especially if the restored teeth have reduced periodontal and bony support. In these circumstances, low cusp height and shallow fossa depth appear to be beneficial to reduce lateral loads. In implant-supported prostheses the incapacity to dissipate these lateral forces through dampening movements will result in high loads to the restorative materials and may result in strain evidenced by veneer chipping or significant veneer or supporting core and frame fracture.

Parafunction

Tooth clenching and grinding (bruxing) are common forms of parafunction involving tooth contacts. However, it may be difficult to distinguish between what is normal physiological activity and what is parafunctional activity. Clenching during power activities, such as weight lifting, is more likely a normal physiological action than parafunction. Clenching and bruxing during tooth eruption or during stress may

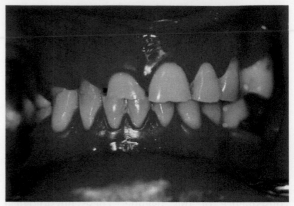

FIG 17-3 Severe tooth wear resulting from parafunctional forces. This patient had no symptoms of pain or discomfort and functioned adequately. A changed social status prompted presentation to improve the aesthetic appearance of the teeth.

also be part of normal physiological activity. It is generally agreed that forces generated during these activities are greater than during other forms of tooth contact. It is likely that these forms of parafunction are universal. Their amplitude and frequency, however, vary significantly between individuals and result in various forms of adaptability and morphological changes including muscular hypertrophy, tooth movement, tooth intrusion and wear, periodontal ligament thickening, increased periodontal bone density, and TMJ remodeling (Figure 17-3). They may possibly also result in pathological changes, including neuromuscular and TMJ dysfunction, tooth and periodontal ligament sensitivity, pulpal inflammation, and tooth fracture. In implant-supported prostheses they may result in mechanical failures of materials and components (veneer fracture, screw loosening and fracture, frame fracture) and also biological failure (loss of integration).

It should be assumed that all patients at some time engage in tooth clenching and grinding, either physiological or parafunctional, and that dental restorations will be subjected to the relatively high magnitude of forces involved. The intensity and duration of these parafunctional forces will vary dramatically between individuals (Figure 17-4). It therefore seems prudent to apply an occlusal scheme that promotes

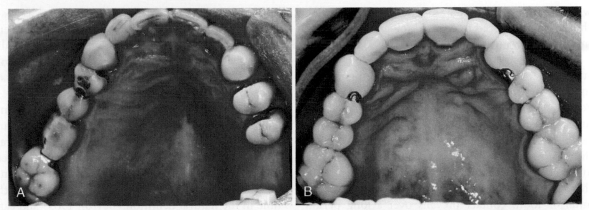

FIG 17-4 Different reactions to force in patients with maxillary tooth-supported rehabilitations. Both maxillary tooth-supported reconstructions have been in situ for 21 years. **A,** Patient A is a heavy bruxer. The intensity and duration of the applied forces have resulted in both mechanical failures of the veneering porcelain and biological failures (loss of vitality and root fractures of the supporting teeth. **B,** Patient B is not a bruxer, and functional forces have resulted in little change in material and biological structures.

the integrity of the occlusal components assuming the presence of such forces.

Tooth Wear

Tooth wear by itself cannot be considered a pathological consequence of parafunctional activity. Only when the rate of wear exceeds the response of the pulp and results in pain can it be considered pathological. However, tooth wear and increased tooth mobility may become psychologically debilitating and socially unacceptable. There are cultural differences between what is considered acceptable tooth wear because there are cultural differences in what is considered acceptable tooth color. Just as commercial marketing has promoted the concept that all teeth should be "white," there is a perception that teeth should maintain their adolescent form throughout life.

Maintaining Tooth Integrity

The periodontal ligament is structured to convert compressive forces to tensile strain between the tooth and supporting bone and does this most efficiently when the forces are applied along the long axes of the teeth. Bone resorbs under compression, but its structural integrity is stimulated under moderate tensile forces. The inherent resilience imparted by the periodontal ligament acts as a shock absorber during the application of force, thus lowering the impact loads

(dampening) that have to be sustained by bone, teeth, and restorative materials. In addition, movement of the teeth away from an applied force can allow other teeth to accept the load. Initial contact in or around CO is often limited to one or two teeth, but as the biting force increases, more teeth accept the load (Riise & Ericsson 1983). Thus physiological tooth mobility is a "protective" mechanism and helps to ensure tooth and bone integrity. It will also help preserve the mechanical integrity of restorations. Splinting of teeth may be necessary, especially if they are periodontally compromised, but maintaining individual tooth mobility where possible rather than joining teeth together for restorative purposes would seem to be a worthwhile goal. The use of a nonrigid connection in fixed dental prostheses may assist in achieving this goal and help maintain the mechanical integrity of any prosthesis (Walton 2003).

Excessive lateral loading can result in structural failure of teeth (fracture) or breakdown of supporting structures. Teeth that are structurally weakened through dental caries and resultant restorative procedures or have lost support through periodontal disease are particularly affected by increased lateral loading. Forces applied to the teeth during clenching and grinding will be higher than those applied during any other function. Thus the loading on tooth form and contacts developed during restorative treatment will be greatest during parafunction. Lateral loading should be minimized to ensure biological health and mechanical integrity.

The maxillary anterior teeth are most likely to be subjected to increased lateral loading during clenching and chewing because of their inclination (Wiskott & Belser 1995). This will be further exacerbated following posterior tooth wear (and possibly restoration) and any associated loss in occlusal vertical dimension (OVD). Excessive contact between the anterior teeth results in fremitus when closing into the ICP. Anterior flaring may also occur if excessive anterior tooth contact prevails over a long period especially if there is associated loss in periodontal support. Splinting of teeth may reduce fremitus, but because of its limiting effect on inherent tooth mobility, it may also increase tooth fracture. Tooth fracture has been shown to be the most common form of failure associated with fixed dental prostheses (Walton 2003). Given that it is not possible to measure the intensity of contacts clinically, it would seem prudent to establish and maintain slight clearance (10 μm foil thickness) between the anterior teeth in ICP.

All teeth are potentially subjected to increased lateral loading during eccentric bruxism. It is assumed that the shallower the cuspal inclines and fossae the less lateral loading will be developed during gliding tooth contacts.

Lateral Tooth Guidance during Function

Canine teeth are well adapted to accept lateral loading (see Chapter 1). They have a favorable crown-to-root ratio, are broad buccolingually, are encased in dense and well-buttressed bone, and the cuspal inclination is relatively shallow. In other animals the canine is most laterally loaded during tearing of food. This evolutionary adaptation is redundant in humans for food gathering, but has established the canine as capable of withstanding lateral forces involved in parafunction. This fact can be used in restorative procedures. Unless the canine is structurally weakened or canine contact is not possible during eccentric movements (Angle class 11 division 1 anterior tooth arrangement), it appears to be reasonable to concentrate lateral gliding contacts on the canines during restorative procedures. When this is not possible it is clinically prudent to distribute lateral forces over several teeth but furthest away from the point of application of maximum biting force, that is, as far forward in the arch as possible. When canine guidance is not possible then eccentric gliding contacts may be distributed simultaneously over several teeth, that is, "group function" involving incisors and premolars to distribute lateral forces on less biomechanically robust teeth.

It is inevitable that changes in restored tooth form will subsequently occur due to differential wear, muscle forces, and skeletal changes. As with a natural dentition, adaptation to these relatively small changes over a long duration will likely occur. Development of group function has been shown to develop with time in the natural dentition (Beyron 1969) and can occur in the restored dentition. Although the therapeutic occlusal form may incorporate canine guidance for convenience and to facilitate physiological adaptation, a "slow" development to group function following these changes need not be modified and indeed may be desirable if it involves a wider distribution of forces. The prerequisite, however, is that the restored teeth involved must have adequate structural integrity, resistance form, and periodontal support to withstand any destructive lateral forces.

Posterior teeth may act as pivoting fulcrum points during gliding movements. This may result in distraction and negative pressure within the ipsilateral TMJ in association with tensile stress on capsular attachments, as suggested by Hylander (1979). Repeated stress may lead to strain involving stretching or tearing of the attachments and result in "looseness" in the joint. This may result in internal joint derangement and affect condylar and associated meniscus movements. Developing a flat occlusal plane will help to avoid posterior eccentric contacts.

Supporting Evidence from Clinical Outcome Studies

As a result of these considerations, recommendations are proposed only for establishing tooth form and contacts during restorative procedures. There are no prospective studies confirming that a particular design promotes physiological and mechanical stability in fixed prosthodontic treatment. There are few longitudinal outcome studies that detail the occlusal contact pattern used as part of the study protocol. However, a retrospective 10-year review of single crowns and fixed dental prostheses incorporating these recommendations into the treatment protocol resulted in only 2% of 344 patients developing temporomandibular dysfunction (TMD) subsequent to treatment (Walton 1997). Of these patients 78% had experienced TMD before treatment, and the development of posttreatment symptoms may have been part of the cyclical nature of TMD. In addition, only 0.6% of 2340 metal-ceramic single unit crowns up to 25 years (Walton 2013) and 1.0% of 1208 abutments in 515 metal-ceramic fixed dental prostheses up to 15 years (Walton 2002, 2003) mechanically failed (lost retention, fracture of the materials). These data suggest that the guidelines for occlusal form as described above contributed to physiological and mechanical stability.

Harm Versus Benefit

Dental treatment involves a degree of iatrogenic injury. The benefits of dental restoration must therefore be weighed against the injury caused. In the absence of signs or symptoms of dysfunction associated with the occlusion, compromised tooth structure integrity, or poor aesthetics (teeth or supporting structures), it is difficult to justify any restorative procedures (or occlusal adjustment). Cultural demands to restore tooth wear, discoloration, or other perceived tooth imperfections and even tooth replacement may result in overtreatment, in which the benefits are outweighed by the iatrogenic consequences or financial costs of the procedures and necessary long-term maintenance. The concept of "the shortened dental arch" as a viable treatment option had its genesis in the reality that tooth replacement in the posterior segments often results in iatrogenic injury to remaining hard and soft tissues without significant improvement in function. A review (Kanno & Carlsson 2006) of the outcomes of the shortened dental arch attested to its effectiveness in restoring adequate patient comfort and functional satisfaction.

"Centric" Treatment Position

There has been much confusion and debate regarding the correct maxillomandibular relationship (MMR) to be used during restorative procedures. Initial consideration of MMR was applied to the construction of complete dentures where there were no naturally occurring interdental relationships. Jaw closure around the TMJs at a specific vertical dimension was

the reference point, and instrumentation was developed to simulate this arc of closure. The actual position of the condyle in the glenoid fossa became a controversial topic (see Chapter 1).

Recording retruded jaw position (RP) or centric relation (CR) has also been a contentious issue. Jaw guidance by the dentist to ensure correct condyle-fossa relationships has been strongly advocated by some clinicians. However, it is difficult to assess what guidance force should be applied to the resilient TMJs to prevent a strained joint position. In addition, different operators will inevitably apply different guiding force. It is difficult to accept that a physiological MMR would be obtained. Furthermore, to assess when the condyles are in a "desired" position in the fossae is not clinically possible. Other clinicians advocate a nonguided closure, provided that deflective tooth contacts are either absent or eliminated. However, in this case, it is difficult to assess if habitual neuromuscular patterns mask the optimum physiological closure path and possibly perpetuate recording of a strained TMJ relationship. Interarch recording materials that eliminate tooth contacts can be used to relate casts in RP at a given OVD. Further opening or closure of articulated casts along this arc will only represent the clinical situation if the hinge axis has been determined and the orientation of the casts in relation to the hinge axis is identical to that which occurs clinically.

Intercuspal contact position (ICP) will be determined in part by biting force and head posture. Following initial contact the tooth surfaces may cause a deviation in the arc of closure and individual tooth movement may result in more teeth contacting as bite force increases. Indeed it is well established (see Chapter 1) that only approximately 10% of the population have an ICP that is coincident with RP (CO) at the clinical level.

Maximum interdigitation of teeth on casts is repeatable for a given set of casts but will be determined by the position of the teeth recorded in the impressions. In most instances it will very closely simulate the clinical ICP, resulting with moderate biting force. It is a convenient and acceptable reference for indirect restorative procedures provided that individual teeth have minimal mobility and there are sufficient tooth contacts to stabilize the casts. Deflective tooth contacts may result in this reference position being anterior or lateral to the MMR in RP (CR). In severely periodontally compromised teeth with increased mobility, casts may not accurately record true in vitro tooth position and therefore their interdigitation may not simulate the clinical ICP.

The recorded maximum interdigitation of teeth on casts should be used for single tooth restorations, fixed dental prostheses involving one or unilateral posterior teeth, or fixed dental prostheses involving anterior tooth restoration or replacement. This assumes an absence of either signs or symptoms of dysfunction or a significant deviation (>2.0 mm) from the RCP position. It also assumes that tooth position will not be altered during impression taking.

Tooth contact relationships may be altered by occlusal adjustment or by changes to the contour of provisional restorations and may result in an area of possible tooth contacts rather than point contacts. The resultant contact area may even include the ICP position at the same vertical dimension. There is no scientific evidence to specify that such an adjustment is necessary before carrying out restorative procedures. It may be indicated to enhance individual tooth integrity where contacts occur on inclines of teeth that have become structurally weakened by previous restorative procedures or have significantly reduced periodontal support. Occlusal adjustment (see Chapter 1) may then result in a reduction in the lateral component of the applied force.

Role of Instrumentation

Instruments used in fixed prosthodontics should allow development of a physiological occlusion and should not require a specific tooth contact pattern. Irrespective of the degree of sophistication of the instrumentation, harmony of the various occlusal components must be established. It is prudent to simplify the role and type of any instrumentation employed given the possibilities for inaccuracies developing in the many procedures involved (see Chapter 6).

Changes to the occlusal form during restorative procedures may preclude the use of ICP as a treatment position. Prior elimination of deflective tooth contacts by occlusal adjustment or with the use of provisional restorations would likely unmask any habitual neuromuscular patterns. Subsequently, a patient-directed recording would likely result in a physiological RCP (CR) and avoid the variables associated with active jaw guidance by the clinician. Recording the MMR at the anticipated restored OVD then eliminates the need to accurately record the hinge axis. It has been claimed, however, that when an arbitrary hinge axis is used, rotational changes of the articulated casts up to 2 mm (measured at the teeth) will not induce errors above clinically tolerable levels (Morneburg & Pröschel 2002). Providing the recording medium itself does not cause jaw deflection, the subsequently restored tooth contact pattern (ICP) will approach CO.

The need to accurately record and reproduce lateral jaw movements can be eliminated by restricting lateral gliding contact patterns between as few teeth as possible, minimizing cusp height and fossa depth and developing a flat occlusal plane. Average value settings on an articulator may be appropriate to ensure adequate clearance of posterior teeth during lateral movements. A facebow oriented along an arbitrary hinge axis is a convenient method for locating casts relative to the intercondylar axis through the condyle spheres of an articulator. Furthermore, this can closely simulate the actual position of the jaws in the frontal, sagittal, and vertical planes relative to the TMJs. A flat occlusal plane indicator may be just as effective for some clinical procedures (Shodadai et al. 2001). It has been mathematically derived that when average value articulator settings are used there is a relatively low risk of inducing occlusal errors at premolar and molar regions during lateral movements (Pröschel & Morneburg 2000). Thus even if group function involving posterior teeth is indicated (e.g., Angle class 11 division 1 tooth relationships) only minor intraoral adjustment would be necessary to ensure appropriate tooth contacts.

There are no published data validating improved outcomes in fixed prosthodontics when complex jaw movement-recording devices and fully adjustable articulators are used. In contrast, use of instrumentation as described in this chapter for fixed prosthodontic treatment has been found to be appropriate to ensure optimum outcome of prostheses up to 15 years (Walton 2002). There has also been minimal physiological disharmony of the occlusal components in monitoring patient treatments for up to 10 years (Walton 1997).

Occlusal Plane Orientation

There has been much emphasis in the past on orientation of the occlusal plane. Initial consideration related to facilitating stability of full dentures by minimizing posterior space between the prostheses in eccentric movements. The compensating curves (curve of Spee and curve of Wilson) facilitated obtaining balanced occlusion for a given anterior overjet and overbite. Other concepts, such as the Monson curves, have been used to orient the occlusal plane in fixed prostheses to achieve multiple contacts in eccentric movements, such as group function.

There is no evidence that there is any relationship between occlusal plane orientation and either function or outcome of fixed prostheses.

In the natural dentition the most significant feature of the occlusal plane relates to aesthetics rather than function. The anteroposterior cant, measured by reference to the incisal edges and buccal cusp tips of the maxillary teeth, mostly follows the curve of the lower lip when in the smile pose, and this has an association with an aesthetic appearance. Thus a "steep" cant will often be associated with an Angle class 11 skeletal pattern and an obtuse gonial angle. A flat cant is often associated with a more acute gonial angle. Where it is possible to change the orientation of the occlusal plane in fixed prosthodontics, than it should be related to aesthetic rather than any perceived functional considerations.

Long-Term Maintenance

The recommendations outlined in this chapter are designed to result in relative stability of the dentition to minimize adaptation and/or the development of pathology in the occlusal components. It must be accepted that changes will inevitably occur with time. Minor changes in tooth position, even in intact arches, have been demonstrated. Differential wear between anterior and posterior teeth will occur due to varying forces applied. Many dentitions will have several materials (natural and artificial) forming occlusal contacts and different toughness, abrasion resistance, and erosion resistance will result in differential wear of these materials. Long-term monitoring of the teeth and supporting structures should include adjustments to reestablish the described contact patterns, thus maximizing biological, physiological, and mechanical stability.

REFERENCES

Beyron H: Optimal occlusion, *Dent Clin North Am* 13:537–554, 1969.

Creugers NH, Kayser AF, van't Hof MA: A meta-analysis of durability data on conventional fixed bridges, *Community Dent Oral Epidemiol* 22:448–452, 1994.

Hylander WL: An experimental analysis of temporomandibular joint reaction force in macaques, *Am J Phys Anthropol* 51:433–456, 1979.

Kanno T, Carlsson GE: A review of the shortened dental arch concept focusing on the work by the Käyser/Nijmegan group, *J Oral Rehabil* 33:850–862, 2006.

Morneburg TR, Pröschel PA: Predicted incidence of occlusal errors in centric closing around arbitrary axes, *Int J Prosthodont* 15:358–364, 2002.

Pröschel PA, Morneburg TR: Predicted incidence of excursive occlusal errors in common modes of articulator adjustment, *Int J Prosthodont* 13:303–310, 2000.

Riise C, Ericsson SG: A clinical study of the distribution of occlusal tooth contacts in the intercuspal position in light and hard pressure in adults, *J Oral Rehabil* 10:473–480, 1983.

Shodadai SP, Türp JC, Gerds T, et al: Is there a benefit of using an arbitrary facebow for the fabrication of a stabilization appliance?, *Int J Prosthodont* 14:517–522, 2001.

Walton TR: A ten-year longitudinal study of fixed prosthodontics: 1. Protocol and patient profile, *Int J Prosthodont* 10:325–331, 1997.

Walton TR: An up to 15-year study of 515 metal-ceramic fixed partial dentures: Part 1. Outcome, *Int J Prosthodont* 15:439–445, 2002.

Walton TR: An up to 15-year study of 515 metal-ceramic fixed partial dentures Part 11. Modes of failure and influence of various clinical characteristics, *Int J Prosthodont* 16:177–182, 2003.

Walton TR: The up to 25-year survival and clinical performance of 2340 high gold-based metal-ceramic single crowns, *Int J Prosthodont* 26:151–160, 2013.

Wiskott HW, Belser UC: A rationale for a simplified occlusal design in restorative dentistry: Historical review and clinical guidelines, *J Prosthet Dent* 73:169–183, 1995.

Further Reading

Helsing G, Helsing E, Eliasson S: The hinge axis concept: A radiographic study of its relevance, *J Prosthet Dent* 73:60–64, 1995.

Picton DC: Tilting movements of teeth during biting, *Arch Oral Biol* 7:151–159, 1962.

Sarver DM: The importance of incisor positioning in the esthetic smile: The smile arc, *Am J Orthod Dentofacial Orthop* 120:98–111, 2001.

Tradowsky M, Kubicek WF: Method for determining the physiologic equilibrium point of the mandible, *J Prosthet Dent* 45:558–563, 1981.

Wood GN: Centric relation and the treatment position in rehabilitating occlusions: A physiologic approach. Part 11: The treatment position, *J Prosthet Dent* 60:15–18, 1998.

Occlusion and Removable Prosthodontics

Rob Jagger

SYNOPSIS

Occlusal considerations for removable prostheses are essentially the same as for fixed restorations.

The approach to establishing occlusion for partial dental prostheses (PDPs) is usually conformative. Partial dentures should not transmit excessive forces to supporting tissues nor interfere with any contacts in intercuspal contact position (ICP) or in functional movements. Occasionally, a reconstructive approach using onlays is used.

Occlusion for complete dental prostheses has three significant differences from partial dental prostheses:
- The absence of natural teeth in edentulous patients may present significant difficulties in determining an acceptable occlusal vertical dimension.
- Complete denture occlusion is always a reorganized occlusion.
- Absence of teeth produces problems of denture stability (resistance to displacement by lateral forces), particularly of the mandibular complete denture. The stability of complete dentures is optimized by a balanced occlusion/articulation.

This chapter provides an overview of occlusion for partial and complete removable prostheses, including discussion of both clinical and laboratory procedures.

CHAPTER POINTS

- PDPs should not transmit excessive forces to supporting tissues nor interfere in intercuspal position or in functional movements. The occlusal form is usually conformative with the natural teeth. Occasionally, for example in relation to extensive tooth wear, a reorganized approach is used.

- The occlusion of complete dental prostheses is always a reorganised occlusion.
- The absence of natural teeth in edentulous patients can present significant difficulties in determining an acceptable occlusal vertical dimension (OVD). Several methods may be used. Experienced clinicians usually rely on a combination of methods.
- There is little evidence to support assertions of the superiority of various occlusal schemes. It has been said that stability of complete dentures may be optimised by a balanced occlusion and articulation. Balance may achieved by developing a balance occlusion and articulation on an average value articulator and by making occlusal correction when the dentures are fitted.

PARTIAL DENTAL PROSTHESES

Occlusion: Conformative and Reorganized Approaches

The usual goal of treatment with partial RDPs (Removable Dental Prosthesis) (in respect of the occlusion) is to position the artificial teeth so that there is simultaneous bilateral posterior tooth contact in intercuspation (ICP). For more extensive partial dentures, such as bilateral distal extension prostheses, the aim might also be to achieve a balanced occlusion and articulation. Occasionally—for example, when there has been extensive tooth wear—instead of this conformative approach, a reorganized approach is used when dentures are provided in conjunction with crowns or bridges or when an onlay prosthesis covers some or all of the occlusal and incisal surfaces of the dental arch.

Treatment Planning for Partial Dental Prostheses

When replacing missing teeth, it is important that treatment is based on a comprehensive treatment plan. The treatment plan must be derived from a careful history and examination and the use of appropriate special investigations. For the partially dentate patient, special investigations often include radiographs, tooth sensibility tests, and articulated, surveyed study casts. The treatment plan for the partially dentate patient must include a detailed design of any prosthesis that is to be made.

Occlusal Analysis

It is important to analyze the occlusion during the treatment planning phase to detect any tooth alignment problems, such as overeruption, that might prevent the construction of a prosthesis with a satisfactory occlusion.

A decision must be made as to whether any preprosthetic occlusal adjustments or alterations are necessary. Occlusal analysis involves a critical analysis of the existing dentition through clinical observation and by the use of articulated study casts. A detailed account of clinical occlusal analysis is given in Chapter 8.

Study casts may be articulated without an occlusal record if there are sufficient teeth to provide stable intercuspation of the casts. If there are insufficient teeth, wax occlusal rims should be used to provide a stable intercuspal record for articulation.

Clinical Stages
Recording Centric Jaw Relation

Wax occlusal rims are used if there are insufficient teeth to provide a stable relationship. If the denture being constructed has a metal base, wax rims may be formed on the metal framework. It is important to ensure that the framework fits accurately and does not interfere with the occlusion in ICP, retruded contact position (RCP), or in lateral excursions before the occlusal record is made.

Insertion—Occlusal Correction

Minor occlusal interferences are often present at insertion due to clinical or laboratory errors during construction. The dentures must be adjusted so that the natural teeth meet in precisely the same way both with and without the dentures in place. Often chairside adjustment by selective grinding is sufficient. Marks produced by articulating paper must be interpreted with caution, by visual confirmation and by asking the patient for his or her perception of how the teeth contact. The patient should be asked whether the teeth contact evenly or meet on one side first. If the patient is aware of a premature contact, can the patient detect which tooth or teeth meet first? Again, this information must be used with caution.

When both maxillary and mandibular removable dental prostheses are being inserted, each denture must be checked and corrected separately. A final occlusal correction is done with both dentures in place.

Very occasionally at insertion the occlusal errors are so large that chairside correction is not possible. In these cases, the artificial teeth causing the interferences should be ground off. Wax can be placed on the denture base in the regions that the teeth were removed, and the jaw relation can be re-recorded. If the denture has been returned to the clinic with the casts, a new occlusal record can be taken, the casts remounted, and the occlusion corrected in the laboratory. Otherwise an overall impression should be taken with the denture(s) in place. The impressions should be cast and the dentures rearticulated, reset, and retried before being finished. This is particularly important when a significant error has been detected at insertion.

Onlay Dentures

An onlay is a restoration that restores one or more cusps and adjoining occlusal surfaces. When a component of a partial denture extends to cover the occlusal or incisal surface of a tooth, it may be called an onlay prosthesis. The denture may be made of acrylic resin or of a cast-metal denture base material. An alternative method is to add acrylic resin onto retention tags in metal that are cast to the fitting surface of the teeth. This has the advantage that the acrylic resin occlusal surface may be easily adjusted. A diagnostic or temporary onlay denture may be constructed in acrylic resin.

Onlay dentures, sometimes in conjunction with extracoronal restorations, may be used to correct an overclosed occlusion (reduced OVD) or to improve an occlusion, for example when there is a gross discrepancy between RCP and the intercuspal position. The use of an onlay denture to correct extensive toothwear is shown in Figure 18-1.

Extensive coverage of teeth by occlusal onlays can predispose to dental caries. Fixed restorations are the preferred treatment option if clinical conditions allow.

COMPLETE DENTAL PROSTHESES
Occlusion

A detailed overview of the literature of occlusal considerations in complete dentures concluded that patients' satisfaction with complete dentures is a complex phenomenon and that the occlusion plays only a minor role (Palla 1997). Further, there is little evidence to support commonly held views on the advantages or disadvantages of tooth form, tooth arrangement, or occlusal schemes. Patient satisfaction with dentures does not correlate closely with technical quality (Fenlon & Sherriff 2004). For example, patients with greatly decreased vertical dimension and severely worn occlusal surfaces may have no complaint about their prostheses. Indeed they may be unable to adapt to new and "better," more technically correct prostheses. Nevertheless, it is important to understand the principles of occlusion related to complete dentures to try to provide optimum treatment best suited to each individual. The clinician should have a clear picture of the occlusion that he or she is trying to achieve for each patient.

Recommended Occlusion for Complete Dental Prostheses

- Recommended practice is to develop maximum intercuspation of complete dentures in the retruded arc of closure at an acceptable OVD (Occlusal Vertical Dimension). Failure to achieve that can lead to denture intolerance, usually because of instability of the dentures or because of pain of the alveolar mucosa as a result of uneven load distribution and high stress concentrations.
- It is also recommended that a *balanced articulation* (cross-arch harmonious contacts between maxillary and mandibular teeth in all excursive movements) is provided to help provide occlusal stability.

Occlusal Vertical Dimension

There is much evidence to show that it is possible to increase OVD without adverse consequences in both

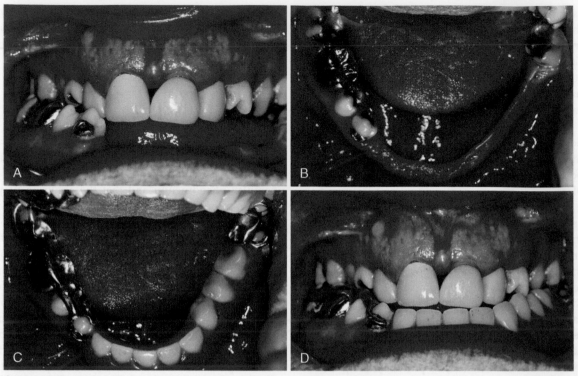

FIG 18-1 A-D, A mandibular partial onlay denture. The prosthesis replaces one of similar design that had been worn for approximately 20 years.

the natural dentition and in complete denture wearers (Palla 1997). There are limits to an individual's ability to adapt to opening or closing an OVD. The OVD has a great influence on facial appearance. Complete dentures with insufficient freeway space also cause difficulties with speech and may result in pain in alveolar mucosa beneath the denture.

It can be very difficult to determine an acceptable OVD once natural tooth contacts are lost, and many methods have been developed to help establish OVD (Box 18.1). These are described in detail in standard prosthetic dentistry texts. Perhaps the most commonly used method has been to determine postural jaw position at the so-called resting vertical dimension (RVD). OVD is then established at 2-4 mm less than RVD. RVD is not constant, however, and methods used to measure it generally have poor reproducibility. RVD varies with, among other things, head posture, the instructions given to the patient to achieve "rest," level of patient fatigue, and time. It is

> **BOX 18.1 SOME METHODS USED TO DETERMINE OCCLUSAL VERTICAL DIMENSION**
>
> - RVD, postural jaw position (PJP); OVD is approximately 2 to 4 mm less
> - Measure OVD of satisfactory previous dentures
> - Aesthetics
> - Ridge parallelism—paralleling the crests of maxillary and mandibular edentulous ridges plus a 5° posterior opening gives an indication of correct vertical dimension
> - Preextraction records
> - Lateral skull radiographs
> - Facial measurement
> - Phonetics
> - Patient reported position of comfort
> - Intraoral central bearing pin

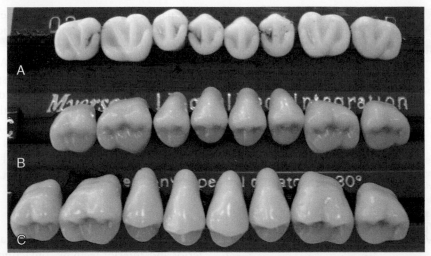

FIG 18-2 Artificial Posterior Teeth **A,** Zero degree teeth. **B,** 10° cusps. **C,** Anatomical teeth.

also known that altering an OVD may lead to the establishment of a new RVD.

The clinician must select and register an OVD and pass that information to the technician. Experienced clinicians usually rely on a combination of methods at the registration stage; for example, measuring RVD, observing patient appearance at selected OVD, receiving feedback from the patient regarding tactile appreciation of the appropriate OVD, and measuring the OVD of previously satisfactory dentures. Clinicians must then try to verify the dimension at try-in stage, again by the use of a similar combination of methods.

It is usually possible, if required for aesthetics, to provide a patient with new dentures with a greater OVD than that of the previous old dentures. It has been suggested that a patient's ability to tolerate an increased OVD can be tested by the progressive addition of autopolymerizing acrylic to the occlusal surfaces of the artificial teeth of the old dentures. This is however time-consuming, and it may be difficult to restore the dentures to their original occlusal contour.

Artificial Teeth

Artificial teeth are made from either acrylic resin or porcelain. The quality of acrylic teeth has improved greatly in recent years, and porcelain teeth are no longer commonly used. Two types of posterior cusp form are produced by manufacturers of artificial teeth (Figure 18-2):

- Anatomical teeth—may have different cuspal angulations, for example, 20°, 30°, or 40° cuspal angle; 20° cuspal angle teeth are commonly used for complete dentures
- Zero-degree teeth (flat-cusped, cuspless)—are said to be indicated for cases with flat alveolar ridges, with retrognathic or prognathic maxillomandibular relations, or where there is great difficulty recording centric relation (CR)

Research has not provided much evidence to support commonly held views on advantages and disadvantages of artificial tooth forms. A systematic review found weak evidence that it may be advantageous for dentists to prescribe dentures for posterior teeth with cusps, as patient satisfaction is greater compared with cuspless teeth. However it was noted that this conclusion may only be made tentatively until further well conducted trials comparing different occlusal schemes for complete dentures are undertaken (Sutton et al. 2005).

Balanced Occlusion and Articulation

Balanced occlusion and articulation refers to occlusion with simultaneous bilateral contacts of the occlusal surface of the teeth in all mandibular

BOX 18.2 HANAU'S QUINT—INTERRELATED OCCLUSAL VARIABLES USED TO BALANCE ARTICULATION

1. *Orientation of occlusal plane*: Average value articulators have preset distances between the condylar components and the incisal tips. The orientation of the occlusal plane is determined by the clinician when trimming the upper occlusal rim using anatomical landmarks to achieve parallelism with the interpupillary line anteriorly and parallelism with Campers Plane (ala-tragus line) posteriorly.
2. *Condylar guidance*: Condylar angles of average value articulators are also preset, usually at 30° although it is possible to record the condylar inclination through protrusive records. Lateral and protrusive wax records can be used to set condylar angles.
3. *Incisal guidance*: Incisal guidance is commonly set arbitrarily at 10° or 15° and could also be achieved by positioning the anterior teeth for aesthetics and phonetics.
4. *Cuspal angle or cusp height (Hanau)*: The cuspal angles of the artificial teeth are produced by the manufacturer.
5. *Compensating curve*: The dental technician sets the artificial teeth with a compensating curve that develops the balanced occlusion.

positions. Balance is developed by the dental technician on the articulator.

The five determinants or interrelated variables affecting occlusal contacts are known as Hanau's quint (Box 18.2).

The extent to which the balanced occlusion and articulation developed on an articulator will be present in the mouth will obviously depend on the accuracy of the centric jaw relation record. Balanced articulation is dependent upon lateral and protrusive records used to program the articulator and correlate with the third reference point used in the facebow transfer. It will also depend on the degree to which the settings of the articulator replicate the corresponding parameters of the patient's jaws. The accuracy of centric jaw relationship records will define the clinician's ability to accurately establish maximum intercuspation in centric occlusion. If this is not correct, it will be impossible to balance the articulation in lateral positions; even if it is correct, if the

articulator cannot mimic the movements made by the patient, all lateral movements will be inaccurate. In most cases, when inserting a denture it will therefore be necessary to adjust the occlusion. Articulating tape may be used in the mouth and specific occlusal adjustment completed at the chairside to produce a balanced occlusion. It must be noted that the evidence for the benefits of balanced occlusion is limited. It has been suggested that further studies are needed to determine if there are specific clinical conditions that may benefit from balanced occlusion (Farias-Neto & Carreiro 2013).

Canine Guidance

Canine guidance refers to the disengagement of posterior and anterior teeth by contacting canines on the working side during lateral excursive mandibular movement. Canine guidance is commonly present in the natural dentition of young patients; however, throughout life attrition of the natural dentition generally leads to the establishment of a unilateral group function. Canine guidance is also used commonly in occlusal reconstruction of fixed prosthodontics (see Chapter 17). While canine guidance has not been recommended by prosthodontists as an occlusal scheme for complete dentures, studies have shown little difference in patient satisfaction between groups of patients having complete dentures with either canine guidance or balanced occlusion (Heydecke et al. 2008, Paleari et al. 2012, Farias-Neto & Carreiro 2013).

Lingualized Occlusion

In conventional artificial tooth arrangement, the mandibular artificial buccal cusps occlude with the fossae of the opposing maxillary teeth. The maxillary palatal cusps occlude with the fossae of the mandibular teeth. In a so-called lingualized occlusion, the mandibular buccal cusps are reduced so that there is only contact on the maxillary palatal cusps.

This scheme allows for ease in obtaining a balanced occlusion comparable with the use of zero cusped teeth, together with the advantage of retaining posterior tooth cusp form and therefore a pleasing appearance. The benefits of lingualized occlusion have been advocated by many; however these benefits have not been confirmed by clinical studies (Heydecke et al. 2007).

Clinical Considerations Relating to Occlusion

Determining Occlusal Vertical Dimension

As described above, determining an acceptable OVD can be difficult. As discussed, the clinician has, however, to register an OVD and pass that information to the technician. Experienced clinicians usually rely on a combination of methods at the registration.

Recording Centric Jaw Relation

Centric jaw relationship is a reproducible position that is used to articulate edentulous casts. The artificial teeth are arranged in centric occlusion; it is the same as ICP for complete dental prostheses. Many different methods have been described for recording CR (Table 18.1). They may be classified as static or functional.

Most methods are capable of giving accurate results, but functional techniques such as "chew-in" techniques are not commonly used as it is difficult to maintain a consistent OVD while performing the "chew-in." The most common method is the use of interocclusal wax occlusal rims.

Selecting an Articulator for Complete Denture Prosthodontics

As discussed previously, an average value articulator can be used with good results.

Table 18.1 Methods Used to Record Centric Relation for Complete Denture Construction

STATIC	FUNCTIONAL
Wax occlusal rims	Chew-in techniques
Extraoral tracing	Swallowing techniques (gothic arch) technique
Intraoral tracing devices	
Wax occlusal rims	Chew-in (functionally generated path)
Intraoral or extraoral tracing (gothic arch) technique	Swallowing techniques

Tooth Arrangement for Complete Dental Prostheses

Tooth arrangement procedures for artificial teeth have been described in detail elsewhere (Zarb et al. 2012). Arrangement of teeth requires considerable skill. Occlusal requirements and the determinants of a balanced occlusion have been described above.

Split-Cast Technique

During the processing of complete dental prostheses, the artificial teeth can move slightly in the molds, producing occlusal errors. A split-cast technique is recommended to relocate the complete dental prosthesis on the articulator following processing. This allows any minor occlusal errors that have occurred during processing to be corrected.

Occlusal Correction at Insertion

There are often occlusal interferences at the insertion stage as a result of inaccuracy of recording CR and limitations imposed by the articulator. Three methods are used to correct the occlusion: selective grinding, precentric (check) record, and re-recording CR.

1. *Selective grinding*: Minor errors are commonly detected with the use of articulating foil and corrected at the chairside. Because of the inherent instability of the prosthesis bases, caution must be used when interpreting the marks made by the paper. There are two stages to chairside occlusal adjustment:

    The *first* objective is to ensure maximum intercuspation (MI) occurs in CR. Two possible errors may be present. One error occurs when the cusp-fossa relationships are correct but one or more teeth meet prematurely. To correct this type of error, the opposing fossae should be deepened until there is even bilateral contact. The other error is when there is misalignment of cusp-fossa relationships. This is corrected by first grinding mesial and distal slopes of opposing teeth, until cusp-fossa realignment is regained. The opposing fossae can then be deepened until even contact is established.

    The *second* objective of occlusal adjustment is to obtain a balanced occlusion. To readily achieve this, the BULL (buccal upper, lingual lower) rule is recommended. It is the contacting surfaces of these

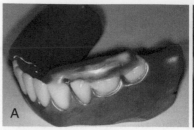 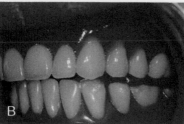 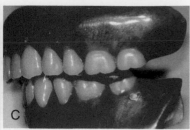

FIG 18-3 Precentric Check Record A, Softened wax on the posterior mandibular teeth. **B,** Patient has closed into the wax in the retruded arc of closure. Closing has stopped before the artificial teeth contact. **C,** Precentric record removed from the mouth.

cusps (the palatal surface of the upper buccal cusps and the buccal surfaces of the lower lingual cusps) that are ground, rather than the cusp tips. When prosthesis contact occurs on the nonworking side, adjustments will need to occur on the buccal incline of the maxillary lingual cusp and on the lingual incline of the mandibular buccal cusp. If there is misalignment of cusp-fossa relationships, the cusps and their opposing embrasures should be adjusted by grinding the mesial and distal cusp slopes of opposing teeth. The adjustment process should be continued until balance is achieved.

Some clinicians consider that any adjustments should only be made with the use of a precentric (check) record as described in the following.

2. *Precentric (check) record*: More extensive errors can be eliminated using a precentric record. To do this, two layers of warm softened baseplate wax are placed on the lower premolars and molars. The patient is instructed or guided to close into the wax (but not to close into tooth contact) in the retruded position. The prostheses are then articulated using this record and any errors are removed (Figure 18-3). When the prostheses are inserted, minor errors can be readily corrected as described.

3. *Re-recording CR*: Occasionally the occlusal errors may be so large that chairside adjustment or even a check record cannot correct the problem. In these cases, if the appearance of the anterior teeth is satisfactory, the posterior teeth should be removed, wax placed on the base in those regions, and CR re-recorded. The prostheses can then be rearticulated, teeth re-arranged, and a try-in repeated, with the teeth processed onto the base when the trial is satisfactory.

Occlusal Maintenance. It is important that the integrity of prostheses is included in regular dental check-up appointments. They should be examined for any deterioration of fit or function, and the mouth examined to ensure that there are no adverse effects caused by the prostheses.

The occlusal surfaces may wear with time. Articulation that was not balanced may become balanced. The bases that are mucosa-borne or tooth- and mucosa-borne will move toward the tissues where alveolar resorption has taken place. Tooth contacts will change or be lost.

Prostheses can be "refurbished" by relining, and the artificial teeth that have become worn can be replaced.

REFERENCES

Farias-Neto A, Carreiro A: Complete denture occlusion: an evidence-based approach, *J Prosthodontics* 22:94–97, 2013.

Fenlon MR, Sherriff M: Investigation of new complete denture quality and patients' satisfaction with the use of dentures after two years, *J Dent* 32:327–333, 2004.

Heydecke G, Akkad AS, Wolkewitz M, et al: Patient ratings of chewing ability from a randomised crossover trial: lingualised vs. first premolar/canine-guided occlusion for complete dentures, *Gerodontology* 24:77–86, 2007.

Heydecke G, Vogeler M, Wolkewitz M, et al: Simplified versus comprehensive fabrication of complete dentures: patient ratings of denture satisfaction from a randomized crossover trial, *Quintessence Internat* 39:107–116, 2008.

Paleari AG, Marra J, Rodriguez LS, et al: A cross-over randomised clinical trial of eccentric occlusion in complete dentures, *J Oral Rehab* 39:615–622, 2012.

Palla S: Occlusal considerations in complete dentures. In McNeil C, editor: *Science and Practice of Occlusion*, Chicago, 1997, Quintessence, pp 457–467.

Sutton AF, Glenny AM, McCord JF: Interventions for replacing missing teeth: denture chewing surface designs in edentulous people, *Cochrane Database Syst Rev* (1):CD004941, 2005.

Zarb G, Hobkirk JA, Eckert SE, et al: *Prosthodontic Treatment for Edentulous Patients*, ed 13, St Louis, 2012, Mosby.

CHAPTER 19

Occlusion in Maxillofacial Prosthetics

Rhonda F. Jacob and Thomas J. Vergo Jr

SYNOPSIS

Maxillofacial prosthetics are prosthetic treatments for patients with craniofacial abnormalities resulting from cancer surgery, trauma, or congenital anomalies. These abnormalities are often skeletal and may or may not affect the muscles of mastication. The altered envelope of mandibular motion in the maxillofacial patient can be attributed to the abnormal facial form and muscular impairment. Predictions of the synergy of the ipsilateral and contralateral muscles, and therefore occlusal contact, can be based on the etiology and site of the abnormality or deformity.

Abnormalities of the maxilla usually affect the position of maxillary teeth and possibly vertical dimension. In these situations, the envelope of motion is rarely affected. The exception would be ablation of maxillary posterior tumors that involve the pterygoid plates and therefore the muscular attachment of the pterygoid muscles to the plates and the mandible.

Abnormalities of the mandible affect vertical dimension and the envelope of motion. The mandibular skeletal and muscular defects are often unilateral in nature; however, because of the malpositioned mandible, occlusal contact is disrupted in the entire arch.

Maxillofacial patients often do not have a repeatable interocclusal contact, but the clinician can develop a prosthetic occlusion that allows a repeatable interocclusal area of contact dictated by, and in harmony with, the aberrant envelope of mandibular motion.

CHAPTER POINTS

- Skeletal abnormalities of the maxilla affect facial form and vertical dimension, but usually do not disrupt the mandibular envelope of motion.
- Trauma, resections, and reconstructions of the head and neck may disrupt motor innervation, cause muscular fibrosis, and alter the synergy of the muscles of mastication.

- The abnormalities of the muscles of mastication form and function are usually unilateral, and the deviation of the envelope of motion can be predicted by knowing the site and etiology of the congenital or acquired abnormality.
- Disruptions of the muscles of mastication may result in deviation and rotations of the mandible.
- Disruptions of the muscles of mastication may result in the inability to close the mandible into appropriate normal intercuspation; prostheses are required to achieve a stable occlusion.
- The occlusion of the maxillofacial patient may be more of a contact area as compared to a point contact.
- Despite the gross disruptions of occlusion and mandibular position evidenced in the maxillofacial patient, temporomandibular (TM) discomfort is not a common patient complaint.

Maxillofacial prosthetics are defined by the American Academy of Maxillofacial Prosthetics as prosthetic treatments for patients with craniofacial abnormalities as a result of cancer surgery, trauma, or congenital anomalies. The facial skeleton and muscle attachments are often affected, and teeth may be absent, lost, malformed, or malpositioned. Patients often present for dental intervention in various stages of reconstruction of the facial skeleton; ranging from no reconstruction to very complex grafting procedures of the maxilla and mandible. Muscles of mastication and facial expression are usually affected by the etiological factor and the subsequent reconstruction. Likewise, the occlusion and the envelope of motion may be altered.

The movement of the mandible is synergistically choreographed by the many paired muscles of mastication. Excursions, opening, and closing of the mandible involve relaxation of some muscles and contraction of others. The timing, rate, and magnitude are very subtle (Laskin, 2006). In the maxillofacial prosthetic patient, there is often a difference in the structural integrity and innervation of the contralateral and affected ipsilateral muscles. The lack of

balance deviates and rotates the mandible in an altered envelope of motion. The small "hit and slide" that is seen in the normal stomatognathic system between centric relation occlusion and maximum intercuspation pales in comparison to the severe malocclusion or lack of occlusion that occurs in the maxillofacial patient. Knowing the etiology of the patient's diagnosis allows the experienced clinician to predict the resultant malocclusion.

CONGENITAL ANOMALIES

Cleft palate is the most frequent jaw craniofacial anomaly. It may be seen as a definitive diagnosis, but may also be seen in combination with several rare genetic disorders that include multiple organ phenotypic abnormalities.

The anterior aspect of the cleft results in a bony defect in the area of the cuspids. The defect may be bilateral or unilateral, depending on the involvement of the cleft. Surgical treatment during infancy often impairs growth in the maxilla, resulting in reverse articulation or in missing or severely malpositioned anterior dentition. Orthodontic treatment is necessary to achieve maxillary expansion and position teeth. More sophisticated reconstruction may include bone grafting in the alveolar defect to position the cuspid or prepare the site for an implant. Orthodontics and palatal expansion may not be financially feasible or desired by some patients. Even with orthodontic treatment, it is often not possible to counter the scarring that occurred with previous surgical procedures. The patient may still have a hypoplastic anterior maxilla, with anterior open occlusion or complete lack of anterior teeth. The occlusion in the cleft palate patient often results in lack of mutually protected occlusion in the anterior teeth and posterior occlusal wear due to mandibular excursions.

Cleft palate patients may also have complete reverse articulation in anterior and posterior dentition with a closed occlusal vertical dimension (OVD) (Figure 19-1; Box 19.1). Despite these suboptimal occlusal schemes, TM dysfunction is not prevalent in this population.

Partial and total anodontia is a finding in ectodermal dysplasia. When the loss of the OVD is great enough, a removable prosthesis that overlays the entire maxillary dentition will achieve normal OVD and lip support. This prosthesis can offer balanced

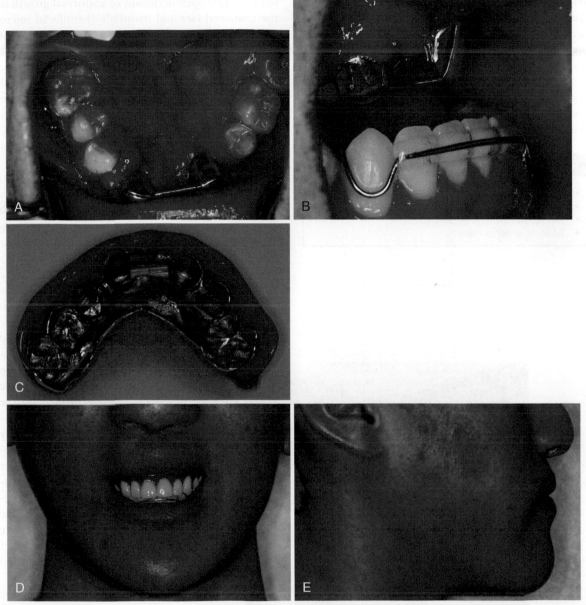

FIG 19-1 A and **B,** This bilateral cleft palate patient has had teeth 7 to 10 and the associated alveolus resected in early childhood. He has a narrowed palate with complete reverse articulation and loss of vertical dimension. **C, D,** and **E,** An acrylic resin prosthesis with a partial prosthesis framework and clasp assemblies incorporated within the acrylic resin supports the lip and restores the occlusal vertical dimension. (Treatment and photographs courtesy of Dr. Jonathan Wiens, Bloomfield, Michigan.)

articulation with the mandible (Figure 19-2). Maintaining these teeth and changing the prosthesis as needed until adulthood will maintain the alveolar processes until a potential implant therapy can be planned.

Other craniofacial anomalies also appear with other organ system malformations (e.g., DiGeorge syndrome). For instance, they can include a long lower third of the face due to excessive mandibular growth with anterior open occlusion or abnormal growth on the ipsilateral face and mandible (hemifacial microsomia). The dentition may achieve strange wear patterns due to the lack of mutually protected occlusion. Orthognathic surgery and orthodontics are often necessary. If the skeletal abnormalities are not surgically corrected, orthodontics alone will rarely achieve normal articulation and facial form. Again, overlay prostheses on the affected dentition may be preferable to fixed restorations that would have unfavorable crown/root ratios.

BOX 19.1 CLEFT PALATE DEFICITS

- Hypoplastic maxilla
- Reverse articulation
- Decreased vertical dimension
- Missing anterior dentition

SURGERY AND TRAUMA TO THE JAWS

A neoplastic diagnosis requiring surgery of the muscles of mastication or the jaws impacts final occlusion.

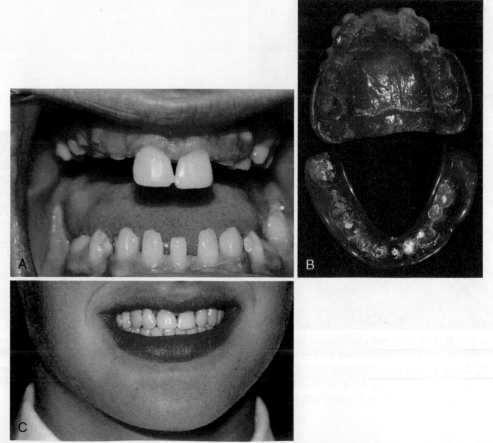

FIG 19-2 The partial anodontia in this adolescent includes missing and malpositioned permanent teeth and worn deciduous dentition. Overdentures can be modified intraorally to continue occlusal contact with the prosthesis and restore occlusal vertical dimension.

Extensive trauma of the jaws will require surgical intervention, and the final reconstructive and occlusal results can be similar to a neoplastic resection.

Alveolar Restorations

Surgery or traumas that involve the alveolus, but leave the form of the mandible and maxilla intact, impact occlusion because of missing teeth, but muscle attachments usually remain intact and therefore the envelope of mandibular motion is within normal limits. Prosthetic replacement of the missing teeth and alveolar bone to achieve facial form is all that is required. These impacts commonly result from avulsion traumas, for instance from motor-vehicle accidents or serious falls avulsing the anterior maxillary teeth and alveolus.

Tumor surgeries that resect teeth and the alveolus are called coronal resections, as they are resections of the alveolar and basal bone in the coronal plane. The usual diagnoses are epithelial tumors of the gingiva and palate. If enough basal bone remains, removable prostheses or implant restorations of fixed or removable prostheses will restore the occlusion in harmony with existing teeth and the normal envelope of motion.

Discontinuity Restorations

Trauma to or resection of the jaws creates a discontinuity defect of bone. Occlusion is not only altered because of missing teeth, but also postoperative function is greatly impacted by the altered envelope of motion due to muscle absence, muscle scarring, loss of muscle attachment, and disruption of synergy of the remaining muscles of mastication (Beumer, 2011).

Maxilla

Resection of the anterior maxilla impacts no muscles of mastication, but resection of the posterior maxilla in the hamular notch area involves the pterygoid plates and attachment of the pterygoid muscles. These neoplasms are usually of salivary gland origin or are epithelial, or bony sarcomas. The pterygoid plates are tenuously attached to the posterior maxilla; even if the plates are not involved in the tumor, the resection of the maxilla detaches or fractures the plates and disrupts some or all of the fibers of the pterygoid muscles. This disruption in turn affects the envelope of motion of the mandible on the ipsilateral (resected) side.

Immediate postoperative findings are an inability to move the mandible to the contralateral (nonresected) side to achieve full intercuspation. Inflammation and surgical disruption of the pterygoid attachments allow the mandible to deviate to the ipsilateral side, due to the action of the contralateral pterygoids. The teeth on the contralateral side contact slightly medial to the intercuspation contact with the cusps, making contacts on the palatal inclines of the maxillary teeth. Because the ipsilateral maxillary teeth are missing, a malocclusion is noted on the contralateral side that is actually a muscle defect at the surgical site. In addition, a decrease in vertical opening of the jaw is common due to pain, the inflammatory process, and surgical damage to the pterygoid muscles.

In the later postoperative course, when swelling and pain subsides, the malocclusion will be less noticeable, and patients usually can approximate the correct mandible closure or guide along the inclined planes and achieve maximum intercuspation. The remaining soft tissues in the infratemporal fossa (including pterygoid muscles) heal in a fibrous attachment to the skin graft and to each other (Figure 19-3). Scarring and shortening of these tissues can lead to limited vertical opening of the mouth. However, if patients perform stretching exercises to increase vertical opening during the formation of this fibrous

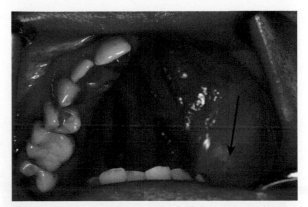

FIG 19-3 The medial pterygoid muscles and remnants of the lateral pterygoid muscles are still attached to the mandible, but have no bony attachments because of loss of the pterygoid plates. The remnants are scarred to each other and to the skin graft within the defect (*arrow*) (Hanasono and Jacob, 2010).

tissue, they can achieve a near-normal envelope of motion.

Patients who have had postoperative radiation therapy after maxillectomy are at high risk for limited vertical opening as the scar tissue forms at the surgical site. The extent of lateral excursions (especially beyond the functional masticatory envelope) is also limited, as the ipsilateral and contralateral pterygoids are not working in harmony (Curtis, 1974).

Mandible

The mandible has many muscle attachments along its course that impact the envelope of motion. These include the muscles attached to the condyle (lateral pterygoid), ramus (temporalis and medial pterygoid), body (masseter and mylohyoid), and anterior mandible (hyoids and digastric). In routine dentistry, the contribution of each muscle group is not as evident and may impact the difference between maximum intercuspation and centric relation occlusion by a few millimeters because of muscle imbalance, but in the maxillofacial patient, loss of muscle attachments can alter tooth contact from the preoperative intercuspation position by centimeters.

Loss of mandibular continuity may be due to avulsion injuries or neoplastic resection. Movement of the mandibular remnants may differ, depending on what portion of the mandible is lost.

Lateral resection of the mandible along the body allows the ipsilateral ramus to be pulled superiorly and medially with the contralateral portion of the mandible deviated and rotated inferiorly to the resected side. The ipsilateral temporalis and pterygoid muscles are responsible for the displacement of the ramus. The smaller the remaining segment of ramus is, the more the condyle can be displaced out of the glenoid fossa. If more of the ramus remains, the coronoid process may be positioned against the maxillary dentition or alveolus, causing pain to the patient and precluding wearing a denture (Figure 19-4). It has long been recognized that this condylar remnant has no value if reconstruction is not immediate, and therefore the ascending ramus is usually resected if the mandibular body is resected.

The deviation toward the defect side will disrupt contact of the contralateral dentition. The deviation is greatest at the anterior mandible and decreases toward the molar area. The only contact may be between the mandibular buccal cusps of the second molar and the maxillary second molar palatal cusps. This contact is unstable and also opens the OVD as evaluated in the anterior region. It may be necessary to recontour/flatten the cusps to allow the correct OVD. Because of the deviation, a maxillary prosthesis will be necessary to give the patient contact palatal to the existing maxillary teeth on the contralateral side.

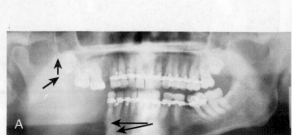

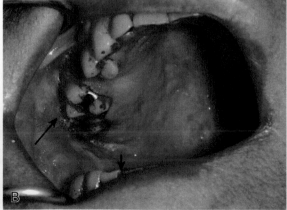

FIG 19-4 A, The arrows point out that the right ramus is displaced medially and superiorly after a right-sided posterior body jaw resection. The anterior mandible is rotated inferiorly and moved to the surgical side. Note the alteration of the mandible midline. **B,** Intraorally there is deviation to the right of the remaining mandible, and the position of the right ramus against the dentition is noted (*arrow*).

In addition to the deviation of the contralateral mandible, there is also rotation of the chin point inferiorly. This is due to hyoid and digastric muscles, gravity, and head position. Some clinicians assume that if the mandibular resection occurs at the mid body that the rotation will be less, but the amount of rotation is not predictable. There may be little facial disfigurement, but an open occlusion on the ipsilateral premolars can be several millimeters (Figure 19-5). When restoring the occlusion in these patients, it may be necessary to overlay the ipsilateral mandibular dentition or increase the height of the teeth with fixed restorations.

When the contralateral posterior dentition makes contact, the contralateral masseter contracts and the mandible can be seen to rotate more inferiorly at the chin point and in the ipsilateral premolar area. This motion will further open the ipsilateral occlusion.

The patient usually gains an increased anterior horizontal overlap due to the deviation of the mandible that moves the chin point posteriorly. The patient will lose anterior tooth contact and become more class II in appearance. Any change in the mandibular occlusion allows the anterior teeth to drift and rotate or hypererupt around the contact points. This is especially objectionable when it occurs in the

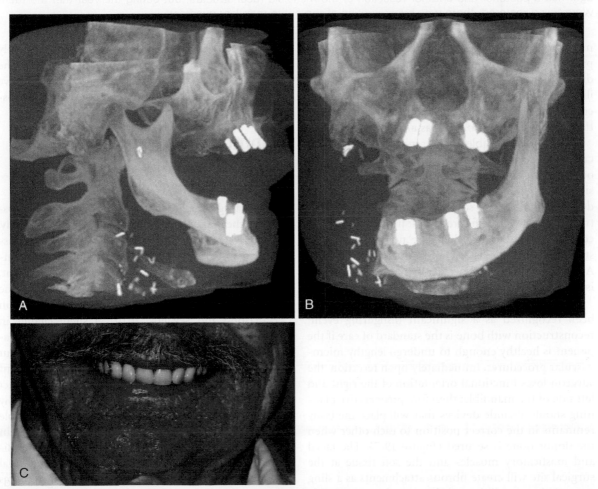

FIG 19-5 A and **B,** The deviation and rotation of the mandible is evident in this posterior lateral resection. **C,** Use of implant-supported dentures allows the decrease of the anterior horizontal overlap and leveling of the occlusal plane, despite the jaw rotation. The chin point is positioned to the right.

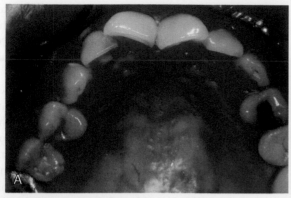
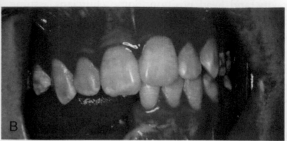

FIG 19-6 A, This patient had a posterior and anterior resection of the mandible that was reconstructed, but dentition was not restored for many months. There was rotation of the incisors during that time. **B,** This teenager had a posterior and anterior resection of the mandible reconstructed, but during the year that the teeth were being restored, there was hypereruption of the entire maxillary quadrant.

maxillary teeth. Patients should be given a lingual or palatal reciprocating retainer immediately after mandibular dentition is disrupted (Figure 19-6). If a maxillary prosthesis is required palatal to the maxillary contralateral teeth to create a functional dentition, this prosthesis will also serve as a retainer.

Loss of the mandible up to or including the midline creates great facial disfigurement because of collapse of the chin, and the width of the face is decreased significantly. The remaining mandible rotates and deviates significantly, so much so that even the contralateral face is disfigured and lip competence is compromised. Because there are no paired muscles still intact, the deviation and rotation is extreme. Achieving a functional occlusion and perioral tissues is almost impossible without bony reconstruction.

The loss of any of the body of the mandible has been recognized as a significant disfiguring event; reconstruction with bone is the standard of care if the patient is healthy enough to undergo lengthy microvascular procedures. Immediately upon resection, the surgeon loses functional orientation of the right and left side of the mandible; therefore preoperative planning should include devices that will place the bony remnants in the correct position to each other when the donor bone is secured (Figure 19-7). The facial and masticatory muscles and the soft tissue at the surgical site will create fibrous attachments as a sling around the mandible and function in a repeatable fashion with the remaining muscles on the contralateral side of the mandible. Failure to maintain this preoperative bony position has been known to severely limit mandibular motion of opening and cause the reconstructed mandible to encroach on restorative space; both of these findings can preclude any prosthetic restoration of these patients.

ADDITIONAL OBSERVATIONS ON MAXILLOFACIAL OCCLUSION

Occlusal Records

An exacting centric relation occlusion is rarely possible in the maxillofacial patient who has any anomaly, trauma, or resection that involves the muscles of mastication and affects the envelope of motion. A repeatable hinge motion of the mandible is not evident; rather a deviated and rotated path of motion is the norm. An articulator cannot mimic this motion (Hanasono and Sevallos, 2010). A slight change in OVD can equate to a much greater change in deviation and rotation. The clinician is less worried about where the mandible is when the mouth is open, but rather has functional concerns upon final contact with the opposing dentition. There is a philosophy that to decrease the deviated position of the mandible at contact and realign the facial form of the chin point, the clinician should guide or push the mandible into the appropriate closing motion and final occlusal contact. Unfortunately, this guidance places the mandible in a position that the patient may not be able to obtain during his or her own closure, because the remaining muscles and tissues have their

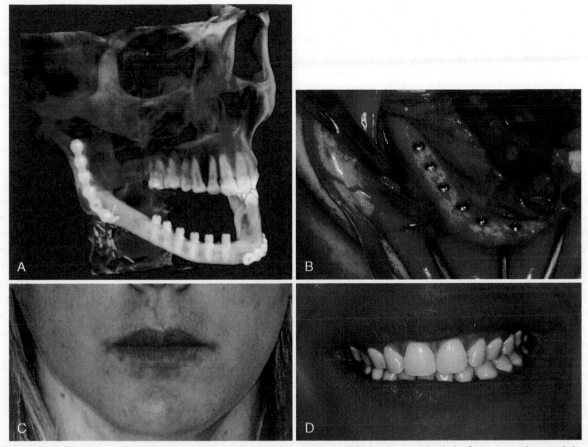

FIG 19-7 A, The bone plates are adapted and secured to the mandible intraoperatively before resection and then repositioned to secure the fibula flap. **B,** Multiple implants are placed in the fibula. **C** and **D,** The patient had normal postoperative occlusion and was restored with a removable implant-retained restoration (Iizuka, 2005).

own envelope of motion and closure. The patient does have proprioception and the envelope of motion, albeit aberrant due to lack of bilateral muscle function, can often be repeatable within an occlusal contact area of a few millimeters. Head position will alter the posture of the mandible and closure of the mandible, again because of lack of bilateral muscle function. Therefore, making a record for occlusal restoration using a head upright position at the OVD which is patient directed rather than clinician forced has the greatest likelihood of ensuring patient comfort. Functionally generated occlusion may be valuable.

Guidance Appliances

A clinician should not underestimate the large forces generated by the muscles of mastication and facial

expression. In the maxillofacial patient, the disrupted envelope of motion and missing teeth before and after the resection (or trauma) create abnormal and unstable contacts on the remaining dentition. There have been published accounts of creating guidance prostheses attached to the teeth that allow the appliance or teeth to interlock during the aberrant closure of the mandible and force the mandible into a more normal path of closure that is counter to the closure path and timing of the remaining muscles. The goal has been to have the patient make full occlusal contact of the remaining dentition and improve the patient's postoperative facial appearance by negating the rotation and deviation of the mandible. These prostheses move the mandible antagonistically to the scarred soft tissues and imbalanced muscle movement. They place very large horizontal forces on the teeth and can orthodontically move the teeth or place the teeth under traumatic forces that can loosen the teeth. To reduce forces on the dentition, it is imperative to restore the dentition in harmony with the new envelope of motion. This would include adjusting the occlusion, creating overlay prostheses to harmonize the tooth contact, and creating a prosthesis to splint or reciprocate the teeth to counter lateral forces.

Closing the Vertical Dimension of Occlusion

Some authors state that the OVD in the mandibular discontinuity patient should be "decreased" to achieve appropriate function. In the routine prosthetic patient, the OVD is determined by speech, lip posture, and overall facial appearance. Similar parameters should be considered in the maxillofacial patient. The discontinuity patient may have an obvious opened OVD due to the mandibular deviation and contacting on the inclined planes of the maxillary posterior dentition. Adjusting these offending contacts will restore the predefect OVD.

Impaired lip competence due to the rotated chin point and deviated mandible tending toward a Class II facial appearance may become apparent in the mandibular discontinuity patient (Table 19.1). Achieving ideal lip competence, speech, and facial appearance are also guiding parameters for establishing the OVD in this patient. The clinician should not consider that there is a prescribed reduction in the OVD from measurement parameters usually used to establish it.

SUMMARY

When restoring occlusion in any dental patient, the clinician is always attempting to establish occlusion in harmony with a repeatable position of the mandible. Restoration of the maxillofacial patient also strives to restore dentition when the mandible is in a repeatable position at a specific OVD.

The right and left condyles may not be seated within the glenoid fossa in similar positions to each other, but the maxillofacial patient usually achieves a near-repeatable position that can be employed for restoration. These positions are often deviated from conventional dental contact, but the primary goal is simultaneous bilateral occlusal contacts. The remaining dentition should be supported with splinting type prostheses or retainers to supplement periodontal support and maintain position.

REFERENCES

Beumer J III, Marunick MT, Esposito SJ, editors: *Maxillofacial Rehabilitation: Prosthodontic and Surgical Management of Cancer-Related, Acquired, and Congenital Defects of the Head and Neck*, ed 3, Chicago, 2011, Quintesssence.

Curtis TA, Cantor R: The forgotten patient in maxillofacial prosthetics, *J Prosthet Dent* 31(6): 662–680, 1974.

Hanasono MM, Jacob RF, Bidaut L, et al: Midfacial reconstruction using virtual planning, rapid prototype modeling, and stereotactic navigation, *Plast Reconstr Surg* 126(6):2002–2006, 2010.

Hanasono MH, Zevallos HP, Skoracki RJ, et al: A prospective analysis of bony versus soft-tissue reconstruction for posterior mandibular defects, *Plast Reconstr Surg* 125(5):1413–1421, 2010.

Hannam AG, Stavness IK, Lloyd JE, et al: A comparison of simulated jaw dynamics in models of segmental mandibular resection versus resection with alloplastic reconstruction, *J Prosthet Dent* 104(3):191–198, 2010.

Iizuka T, Häfliger J, Seto I, et al: Oral rehabilitation after mandibular reconstruction using an osteocutaneous fibula free flap with endosseous implants. Factors affecting the functional outcome in patients with oral cancer, *Clin Oral Implants Res* 16(1):69–79, 2005.

Laskin DM, Greene CS, Hylander WL, editors: *Temporomandibular Disorders: An Evidence-based Approach to Diagnosis and Treatment*, Chicago, 2006, Quintessence.

Table 19.1 Mandibular Discontinuity Deficits	
Rotation of chin point	Ipsilateral
Mandible deviated	Ipsilateral
Open posterior occlusal contact	Ipsilateral
Mandibular contact medial to maxillary dentition	Contralateral
Class II appearance	Anterior
Open occlusion in incisors	Anterior

CHAPTER 20

Occlusal Splints and Management of the Occlusion

Tom Wilkinson

CHAPTER OUTLINE

SYNOPSIS

Occlusal splints have been used for more than a hundred years to manage jaw dysfunction, and they continue to be a common treatment modality. Hypotheses have been suggested to explain their action, but lack scientific validation.

There is general agreement that splints protect against tooth wear and are valuable in preparation for dental treatment, especially with complex restorative procedures including change of occlusal vertical dimension or jaw position. However, it has been difficult to establish the efficacy of splints in the management of temporomandibular disorders (TMDs). Although many studies claim that splints reduce nocturnal bruxism, others have shown that this does not occur, and some patients show increased jaw muscle force while wearing a splint.

The use of better study design in recent years has improved our understanding of splint efficacy. Pain reduction has been shown to occur in treatment and control groups, suggesting a placebo effect as well as the natural regression of symptoms with time. Stabilization (or Michigan) splints and palatal splints (no occlusal coverage, used as a study control) were found to be more effective than using "inactive control" splints (worn only during review visits) or a "no splint" control.

Trials have also shown that there was no apparent difference between a stabilization splint and a nonoccluding palatal appliance, suggesting that pain reduction is not due to a change in mandibular position or sensorimotor feedback, but to a nonspecific behavioral response.

These reviews suggest that there is sufficient evidence to support the use of splints as adjuncts to treatment for localized myalgia or arthralgia. The most common design is the full upper arch, flat plane-stabilization (or Michigan) splint (Figure 20-1).

This chapter details the clinical and laboratory stages of preparing this appliance and procedures for its adjustment and use.

CHAPTER POINTS

- *Impression-taking*: The splint covers all teeth on the upper arch and opposes all lower teeth. Accurate alginate impressions of both arches are required, and these can be taken in stock trays.
- *Transfer records*: A facebow may be used to transfer the relationship of the maxilla to the intercondylar axis and Frankfort horizontal. An interocclusal (or maxillomandibular [MMR]) record documents the relationship of the mandible to the maxilla in centric relation.
- *Mounting casts on the articulator*: A semiadjustable articulator is suitable for splint construction and may be set to average condylar values. The maxillary cast is articulated using the facebow transfer, and the mandibular cast using the occlusal record.
- *Block-out undercuts*: An ideal path of insertion is determined for the splint, and undesirable undercuts are blocked out.
- *Splint fabrication*: Frictional retention is provided by the amount of buccal and labial tooth coverage. The flat occlusal table of the splint provides point contact for the buccal cusps of the lower molars and premolars. The tips of the canines and incisors contact a narrower anterior ledge. An anterior ramp provides guidance for canine or anterior teeth in lateral and protrusive movements.
- *Intraoral adjustment*: Adjustment of the inner surface of the splint after processing may be required to provide a firm and comfortable fit. The occlusal table is adjusted to provide even and simultaneous bilateral contact in retruded contact position (RCP) and then to a "long centric" position. The anterior ramp is then adjusted to provide anterior guidance without molar contacts.
- *Patient instructions*: Patients are instructed to use the splint while sleeping. Good oral hygiene needs to be emphasized, and patients are instructed in the cleaning and storage of their splint.
- *Review of splint*: Reviews are needed as part of a long-term management strategy. The splint may need to be adjusted if dental restorations are placed at a later time.

LITERATURE REVIEW

Early theories of the mode of action of splints were based on the concept that occlusal interferences caused masticatory muscle hyperactivity and parafunction, resulting in muscle pain and, in turn, increased hyperactivity (Travell & Rinzler 1952). This sequence of events was considered to be reduced or eliminated by the splint, as it provided an ideal occlusal scheme (Posselt 1968).

Laskin (1969) suggested that parafunction and the resultant pain and dysfunction were more related to the central effect of stress than to the peripheral role of occlusal irregularities. He described this condition as myofascial pain-dysfunction syndrome (MPD). This theory was reinforced by studies that showed a positive correlation between life events, nocturnal electromyographic (EMG) levels, and masticatory muscle pain (Rugh & Solberg 1979).

Splints have been used to treat the less common muscle conditions described as myositis and myospasm, as well as the more common conditions described as myofascial pain and postexercise muscle soreness associated with bruxism. However, there has been controversy concerning the efficacy of occlusal splints in the treatment of TMDs. A National Institute of Health Conference in 1997 on the management of TMDs reported that "the efficacy of most treatment approaches for TMDs is unknown because most have not been adequately evaluated in long-term studies and virtually none in randomized controlled group trials. Moreover, their superiority to placebo controls or 'no treatment' controls remains undetermined" (Lipton & Dionne 1997).

SPLINTS AND MUSCLE AND JOINT PAIN

Myofascial pain (fulfilling the Research Diagnostic Criteria for Temporomandibular Disorders [RDC/

TMD] criteria of Dworkin & LeResche 1992) has been reported in approximately 50% of patients presenting at a facial pain clinic (Fricton et al. 1985). It is categorized by muscle tenderness, pain that can be made worse by function, and referral of pain to other regions, and it is found in bruxing and non-bruxing patients. There is currently no convincing research-based evidence to explain the etiology of myofascial pain.

Studies have shown the development of jaw muscle myalgia with voluntary clenching (Arima et al. 1999). It has been suggested that subjects demonstrating intermittent bruxing at times of high stress may be exhibiting postexercise muscle soreness, and that this is more likely to occur on waking. However, the majority of bruxers do not exhibit pain, and it has been suggested that their muscles may have adapted with time as a training effect. Studies of resting EMG levels in bruxers with pain were found to not be significantly different from bruxers without pain (Lund 2001). The poor correlation between pain and resting EMG contradicts the earlier "vicious cycle" theory associated with occlusal irregularities.

Self-reports of pain among 19 confirmed nocturnal bruxers in a polysomnographic study were compared with 61 patients in another study with jaw muscle myofascial pain (RDC/TMD criteria) with no evidence of bruxism (Dao et al. 1994a). Only 6 of the 19 bruxers experienced pain, and this typically occurred in the morning, whereas the majority of the myofascial group reported pain in the evening. The authors suggested that bruxism and jaw muscle myofascial pain might be distinct entities with different etiologies.

Patients treated with splints for jaw muscle pain may have myositis or myospasm conditions, myofascial pain, or postexercise muscle soreness. Research evidence is lacking to determine whether these are discrete conditions; their etiology and natural history and the role of bruxism is unclear. There may also be other conditions causing pain that have not yet been identified.

Occlusal splints have been shown to reduce nocturnal EMG levels, but their effect is variable and, in some studies, subjects have shown increases in activity. Clark (1988) reviewed the efficacy of these appliances and concluded that a strong association had been demonstrated between muscle hyperactivity and the symptoms of jaw pain, and that occlusal splints had been used effectively to treat this condition. However, the evidence is weak, and care must be taken in drawing the conclusion that there is a cause-and-effect relationship between bruxism and the different subgroups of TMDs.

Clark also reported on several theories proposed to explain how splints reduce symptoms (Clark 1988), including the provision of an interference-free occlusal scheme, alteration of vertical dimension, correction of the occlusion to centric relation, realignment of the TM joints, and increased cognitive awareness. Dao & Lavigne (1998) reviewed these theories and concluded that the quality of the evidence was questionable and was based on unsubstantiated etiologies.

The best evidence of therapeutic efficacy comes from systematic reviews of well-designed randomized controlled trials (RCTs). The incorporation of a control group is essential, as TMD symptoms fluctuate, there is a high rate of spontaneous remission, and placebo effects may significantly contribute to symptom relief. Random assignment of patients to groups as well as blinded data collection and analysis are essential to limit bias. The majority of past studies do not fulfil these requirements, and hence the true therapeutic value of splint therapy has not been established.

Dao et al. (1994a) completed an RCT with 61 patients with myofascial pain (RDC/TMD criteria), divided into three groups: a treatment group using a stabilization (Michigan) splint 24 hours a day, a passive control group who wore a similar splint but only for 30 minutes at each review appointment, and an active control group who used a nonoccluding palatal splint 24 hours a day. The patients' report of pain using a visual analog scale (VAS) reduced significantly with time for all three groups, and there was no significant difference between groups. They concluded that this study cast doubts on the therapeutic value of occlusal splints, and felt that the reduction in pain may have been due to placebo effects or spontaneous remission. This study caused considerable concern among clinicians, particularly as the results were thought to apply to jaw muscle pain in general.

However, the authors failed to indicate that they excluded patients with a history of bruxism. This only became evident when these same patients were reviewed in a subsequent paper (Dao et al. 1994b). Hence the conclusions of the 1994 study for treatment efficacy are only valid for the TMD subgroup of myofascial pain without bruxism.

The outcome of the 1994 study was further analyzed by the authors, who compared patients' reports at each visit of "pain" (efficacy) with reports of "pain relief" (effectiveness) (Feine et al. 1995). They reported that pain relief scores increased with time for each of the three groups but increased significantly less for the passive control group. They hypothesized that patients in the passive control group may have been increasingly convinced that they had not received "true" treatment, which may have explained why they perceived treatment as being less efficacious. It is interesting to consider that patient satisfaction with treatment depends on factors other than pain relief. It would seem that there may have been differences in the strength of the placebo effect between groups, but this only became obvious when the outcome variable was changed from "pain" to "pain relief." The authors concluded that until the cause of TMDs is known, it was justifiable to provide a treatment that does not necessarily reduce pain but makes the patient feel better.

Ekberg et al. (1998) carried out a similar RCT with a patient group with arthralgia (RDC/TMD criteria) and compared the efficacy of a stabilization (Michigan) splint with a nonoccluding but active palatal splint. Patients were not excluded because of a history of bruxism. VAS scores were used to assess pain intensity, and no statistically significant differences were found between the stabilization and palatal splint. However, when the outcome measure of "perceived relief" was considered, the stabilization splint was statistically superior to the palatal splint. This disagreed with the original study of Dao et al. (1994a), but the authors considered that this was because the study was of patients with arthrogenous pain, whereas Dao's group studied patients with myofascial pain.

Several studies have evaluated (meta-analyses) RCTs of splint therapy. Raphael & Marbach (1997) reviewed the literature on occlusal appliances for TMDs and reported that "most controlled studies conclude that appliances are not effective."

Dao & Lavigne (1998) reviewed similar literature and concluded that the true efficacy of splints is still questionable and that the improvement in pain in most studies may be due to nonspecific effects of treatment such as placebo or regression to the mean. They considered that splints might have a place in changing harmful habits and promoting patients' perception of well-being. They concluded that until the natural history and etiology of the different TMDs are determined and more specific treatment regimens are developed for these conditions, splints should only be used as an adjunct to pain management.

Forssell et al. (1999) carried out a meta-analysis of RCTs of splint therapy and reported that the stabilization splint was found to be superior to 3 and comparable to 12 control treatments and superior or comparable to 4 passive controls, but expressed concern that palatal splints, acupuncture, ultrasound, and transcutaneous electrical nerve stimulation (TENS) had been used as controls when these may have affected muscle function and the subject's cognitive awareness. They concluded that "occlusal splints may be of benefit in the treatment of TMDs."

Kriener et al. (2001) reviewed RCTs of splint therapy. They suggested that differences in the TMD population studied may affect outcomes, with some studies only including myofascial pain patients and others including myogenous and arthrogenous subjects, and that outcomes might vary between bruxer and nonbruxer populations.

They concluded that splints were operating in a similar way to the behavioral interventions of biofeedback and relaxation, not as a medical device that was producing effects through physical changes in the position of the mandible. They felt that there was sufficient evidence to support the use of splints for the management of localized myalgia or arthralgia.

Fricton (2010) conducted a meta-analysis of RCTs of orthopedic appliances for TMDs and reported that hard stabilization appliances have good evidence of modest efficacy in the treatment of TMD pain compared with nonoccluding appliances and no treatment. They were equally effective in reducing pain when compared with physical, behavioral, pharmacological, and acupuncture treatments. They reported that soft appliances, anterior appliances, and repositioning appliances had some RCT evidence of efficacy in reducing pain. However, they reported that the potential for adverse events with these latter appliances was higher and suggested close monitoring with their use.

Anterior bite splits have been promoted to prevent and treat bruxism, TMDs, tension-type headaches, and migraines. A systematic evaluation of RCTs of the efficacy of these appliances (Stapelmann & Turp 2008) reported that for the management of TMDs, these appliances are similarly efficacious when compared to full-arch stabilization splints. They were unable to find support for the statement that the anterior appliance was indicated for the prevention of bruxism, TMDs, tension-type headaches, or migraines. They reported that concern had been expressed by authors that the anterior appliance may lead to unintended occlusal change and that it was crucial that patients were monitored. They concluded that the full-arch stabilization splint remained the "gold standard" for the therapy of patients with TMDs.

SPLINT CONSTRUCTION

Splint Design

Design preferences vary widely between clinicians, who may choose upper or lower appliances, interlocking versus flat plane appliances, appliances with or without anterior guidance, and appliances of various thicknesses, but these preferences are not supported by outcome studies involving RCTs.

There may be differences in the choice of materials between hard and soft appliances. Soft appliances may be preferred by clinicians because of their perceived comfort and for ease of fitting. However, there is evidence to suggest that soft appliances are less effective in reducing bruxism (Kuboki et al. 1997) with a small percentage of patients reporting a "squeezing or trampolining" habit when using these appliances.

The most common appliance used around the world is the stabilization (Michigan) splint. This is a rigid upper appliance with a flat occlusal plane and a ramp providing anterior guidance. It is usually constructed with minimal increase in vertical dimension, consistent with providing strength, and is adjusted to even contact of all lower teeth in retruded contact position (RCP) or centric relation. This is the design that will be described in this text (Figure 20-1).

Preparation of Casts

Upper and lower alginate impressions in stock trays provide suitable casts in dental stone for splint construction.

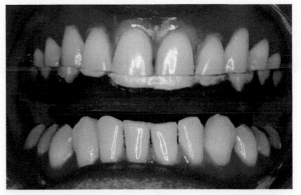

FIG 20-1 Extraoral Photograph of a Stabilizing (Michigan) Splint Seated on the Maxillary Teeth with the Jaw Slightly Opened Frictional retention is provided by 25% coverage of the labial surfaces of the incisors and canines, 33% coverage of the buccal surfaces of premolars, and 50% coverage of the buccal surfaces of molars.

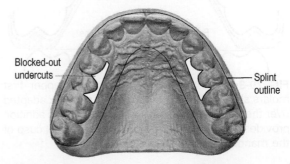

FIG 20-2 The Outline of Splint Extensions and Lingual Undercuts Blocked out with Plaster

A facebow may be used to transfer the relationship of the maxilla to the intercondylar axis and Frankfort horizontal; a maxillomandibular (MMR) record is used to record the relationship of the maxillary and mandibular arches in centric relation to complete the transfer record (see Chapters 1 and 6).

Frictional retention for the splint is provided by 25% coverage of the labial surfaces of the incisors and canines, 33% coverage of the buccal surfaces of premolars, and 50% coverage of the buccal surfaces of molars (Figure 20-1). It is important to block out undercuts on maxillary casts to reduce chairside time when fitting the appliance (Figure 20-2). The appliance extends 5 to 10 mm into the palate beyond the palatal gingival margin.

Splint Fabrication

A 2 mm-thick thermosetting blank may be heated and pressure-molded over the upper cast. Autopolymerizing resin is adapted over the blank, and the articulator is then closed to the determined vertical dimension of the splint. The resin is shaped to provide a flat occlusal plane approximately 5 mm in width to be contacted by the buccal cusps of the lower molar and premolar teeth (Figure 20-3). The canine and incisor teeth contact a narrower 2-mm flat anterior ledge. An anterior ramp with a 45° slope extends from this ledge to provide guidance in lateral and protrusive mandibular movements (Figure 20-4). The

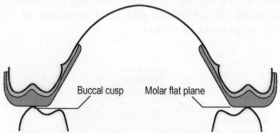

FIG 20-3 A frontal section through the upper first molars showing a 2-mm thermosetting blank adapted over the molar surface and palate. The acrylic addition provides a flat plane against which the buccal cusp of the mandibular molars occludes.

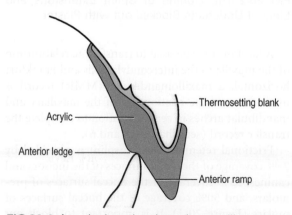

FIG 20-4 A sagittal section through a maxillary central incisor showing a 2-mm thermosetting blank adapted over the maxilary incisor and palate with acrylic resin buildup to provide an anterior ledge and a 45° anterior ramp.

resin is then processed in a pressure flask to reduce porosity.

Laboratory Splint Adjustment

The splint is adjusted on the articulator, with plastic articulating tape, to provide simultaneous RCP contact of incisor and canine tips and premolar and molar buccal cusps in centric relation (Figure 20-5, A). These centric contacts are marked in one color, and the path of the tips of the lower teeth during lateral and protrusive excursions are marked against the anterior ramp in a different color (Figure 20-5, B and C). The splint is adjusted so that the ipsilateral lower canine tip is the only tooth contacting during lateral excursion and the incisor and canine tips are the only teeth contacting the splint in protrusion, eliminating any contralateral or protrusive contacts on molars or premolars.

The splint is then removed from the cast and the palate removed. The labial, buccal, and palatal extensions are polished (Figure 20-6). The occlusal surface is left unpolished so that articulating tape leaves clear marks during splint adjustment in the mouth.

Intraoral Adjustment

Judicious blocking out of undercuts during construction reduces chairside time in fitting the splint. Pressure indicator paste may be used to disclose any points on the fitting surface that are preventing the splint from fully seating or causing rocking.

The occlusal surface of the splint is then adjusted to even and simultaneous contact of the tips of all lower anterior teeth and all buccal cusps of molar and premolar teeth in centric relation. Miller holders that support articulating paper assist these adjustments. Some clinicians may allow the patient "freedom in centric" by adjusting the occlusal surface to even contact of lower teeth at median occlusal position (MOP)—a "snap jaw closure" that brings the mandible slightly forward from RCP.

The anterior ramp is then adjusted to provide smooth incisal and canine guidance in lateral movement and incisal guidance during protrusion.

Patient Instructions

Patients are instructed to use the appliance only during sleep. They are advised that some patients occasionally take splints out during sleep without

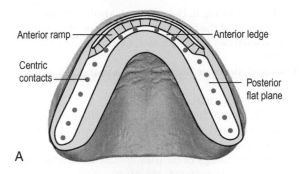

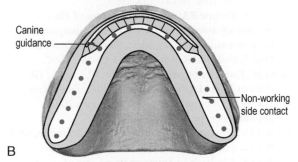

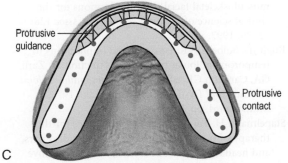

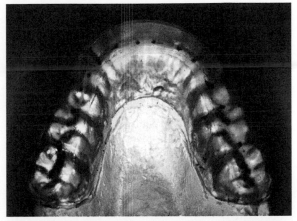

FIG 20-6 An Intraoral Occlusal View of a Stabilizing (Michigan) Splint Showing a Flat Plane Occlusal Surface with an Anterior Ramp Articulator tape markings show right and left canine guidance on the anterior ramp and the centric contacts of the lower teeth.

FIG 20-5 An Occlusal Splint A, A horizontal flat plane contacted by the buccal cusps of the lower molar and premolars and the narrower horizontal anterior ledge contacted by the mandibular canines and incisors. The 45° anterior ramp arises immediately from the point of contact of the mandibular anterior teeth. **B,** The laterotrusive path of the mandibular right canine tooth against the anterior ramp during a right-sided lateral excursion. The mediotrusive path of the mandibular left first molar is shown as a mediotrusive or nonworking side contact. **C,** The path of the mandibular incisor and canine teeth against the anterior ramp during a protrusive movement. The path of the mandibular left first molar is shown as a protrusive contact.

waking, and that splints may increase or decrease salivation during sleep. They may find that the splint may be tight on different teeth from time to time, but this discomfort will decrease with continued use. Patients are instructed to monitor their oral hygiene because of the risk of increased plaque accumulation around their teeth and inside the splint.

Review of Splint

Review appointments check that occlusal contacts on the splint are stable and are used to reinforce avoidance of daytime parafunction habits. Reviews every 2 months over the first 6 months are desirable to determine when symptoms improve, indicating that patients may start to reduce the frequency of splint wear. There may be a need to return to using the splint if symptoms worsen or if they realize from their self-monitoring that there has been an increase in clenching, particularly at times of stress.

Patients should be informed that teeth might move slightly if they cease using the splint for a period and that any initial discomfort or tightness will settle on resuming splint use. Patients using splints on a long-term basis should be reviewed every 12 months to ensure there is no occlusal or periodontal change. Splints may need to be adjusted after new restorations.

251

REFERENCES

Arima T, Svensson P, Arendt-Nielsen L: Experimental grinding in healthy subjects: a case for postexercise jaw muscle soreness, *J Orofac Pain* 13:104–114, 1999.

Clark GT: Interocclusal appliance therapy. In Mohl ND, Zarb GA, Carlsson GE, et al, editors: *A Textbook of Occlusion*, Chicago, 1988, Quintessence, pp 271–284.

Dao TT, Lavigne GJ: Oral splints: the crutches for temporomandibular disorders and bruxism? *Crit Rev Oral Biol Med* 9:345–361, 1998.

Dao TT, Lavigne GJ, Charonneau A, et al: The efficacy of oral splints in the treatment of myofascial pain of the jaw muscles; a controlled clinical trial, *Pain* 56:85–94, 1994a.

Dao TT, Lund JP, Lavigne GJ: Comparison of pain and quality of life in bruxers and patients with myofascial pain of the masticatory muscles, *J Orofac Pain* 8:350–355, 1994b.

Dworkin SF, LeResche L: Research diagnostic criteria for temporomandibular disorders: review, criteria, examinations and critique, *J Craniomandib Disord* 6:301–355, 1992.

Ekberg EC, Vallon D, Nilner M: Occlusal appliance therapy in patients with temporomandibular disorders: a double-blind controlled study in a short-term perspective, *Acta Odontol Scand* 56:122–128, 1998.

Feine JS, Lavigne GJ, Lund JP: Assessment of treatment efficacy for chronic orofacial pain. In Morimoto T, Matsuya T, Takada K, editors: *Brain and Oral Functions*, Amsterdam, 1995, Elsevier, pp 257–264.

Forssell H, Kalso E, Koskela P, et al: Occlusal treatments in temporomandibular disorders: a qualitative systematic review of randomised controlled trials, *Pain* 83:549–560, 1999.

Fricton J: Systematic review and meta-analysis of randomized controlled trials evaluating intraoral orthopedic appliances for temporomandibular appliances, *J Orofac Pain* 24:237–254, 2010.

Fricton JR, Kroenig R, Haley D, et al: Myofascial pain syndrome of the head and neck: a review of clinical characteristics of 164 patients, *Oral Surg* 60:615–623, 1985.

Kriener M, Betancor E, Clark GT: Occlusal stabilisation appliances: evidence of their efficacy, *J Am Dent Assoc* 132:770–777, 2001.

Kuboki T, Azuma Y, Orsini M, et al: The effect of occlusal appliances and clenching on the temporomandibular joint space, *J Orofac Pain* 11:67–77, 1997.

Laskin DM: Etiology of the pain-dysfunction syndrome, *J Am Dent Assoc* 79:147–153, 1969.

Lipton JA, Dionne RA: National Institutes of Health technology assessment conference on management of temporomandibular disorders, *Oral Surg Oral Med Oral Pathol Oral Radiol Endod* 83:49–183, 1997.

Lund JP: Pain and movement. In Lund JP, Lavigne GJ, Dubner R, et al, editors: *Orofacial Pain: From Basic Science to Clinical Management*, Chicago, 2001, Quintessence, pp 151–163.

Posselt U: *Physiology of Occlusion and Rehabilitation*, ed 2, Philadelphia, 1968, FA Davis.

Raphael K, Marbach JJ: Evidence-based care of musculoskeletal facial pain. Implications for the clinical science of dentistry, *J Am Dent Assoc* 128: 73–79, 1997.

Rugh JD, Solberg WK: Psychological implications in temporomandibular pain and dysfunction. In Zarb GA, Carlsson GE, editors: *Temporomandibular Joint Function and Dysfunction*, Copenhagen, 1979, Munksgaard, pp 239–258.

Stapelmann H, Turp JC: The NTI-tss device for the therapy of bruxism, temporomandibular disorders, and headaches—where do we stand? A qualitative systematic review of the literature, *BMC Oral Health* 8:22, 2008.

Travell JG, Rinzler SH: The myofascial genesis of pain, *Postgrad Med* 11:425–434, 1952.

CHAPTER 21

Occlusal Adjustment in Occlusion Management

Anthony Au and Iven Klineberg

SYNOPSIS

Occlusal adjustment is important in prosthodontic pretreatment and has been used for selected cases of temporomandibular disorders (TMDs). The clinical procedure involves tooth surface reduction and tooth surface addition with an appropriate restorative material. Occlusal adjustment is distinguished from occlusal equilibration and selective grinding by distinct indications and aims. A systematic preclinical and clinical approach has clear advantages for long-term stability of treatment. There is, however, disagreement regarding terminology and the scientific justification of this procedure in the management of TMDs and, in particular, chronic orofacial pain. This chapter aims to clarify definitions and examines research evidence available for the application of occlusal adjustment.

CHAPTER POINTS

- Occlusal adjustment may involve tooth surface reduction and/or tooth surface addition.
- Occlusal adjustment is different from occlusal equilibration and selective grinding.
- Specific aims and indications are described for occlusal adjustment.
- Occlusal adjustment should only be used where there is a justifiable indication.
- There is no strong evidence to indicate that it is more effective than conservative reversible procedures in treatment of TMDs. Nor is there evidence for its use in the management of chronic orofacial pain
- It is recommended that occlusal adjustment be planned on articulated study casts before being attempted clinically.
- The use of a vacuum-formed template allows accurate implementation of preplanned occlusal adjustment.

INTRODUCTION

Occlusal adjustment is a procedure whereby selected areas of tooth surface, in either dentate or partially dentate patients, are modified to provide improved tooth and jaw stability and to direct loading to appropriate teeth during lateral excursions. This may involve tooth surface reduction and tooth surface addition with a restorative material. Where tooth surface reduction is required, this is completed with minimal adjustment. There is evidence from case-controlled studies that reduction of tooth contact interferences may reduce specific signs and symptoms of TMDs, such as temporomandibular (TM) joint clicking (Pullinger et al. 1993, Au et al. 1994). However, these are not prospective controlled studies. Where tooth surface addition is required, a restorative material may be added to enhance buccolingual and mesiodistal stability of strategic teeth or to provide more definite guiding inclines for lateral guidance.

Occlusal adjustment is distinguished from occlusal equilibration and selective grinding.

Occlusal equilibration: This is carried out to produce a specific occlusal scheme, generally in severely debilitated dentitions, requiring extensive restorative treatment. It is usually designed to achieve:

- Coincidence between retruded contact position (RCP) and intercuspal contact position (ICP)
- Precise cusp-to-fossa or cusp-to-marginal ridge contacts
- Anterior guidance resulting in disclusion of posterior teeth with lateral jaw movement

Occlusal equilibration may require extensive tooth modification to develop the prescribed occlusal scheme. Those features may be achieved with fixed restorative procedures.

Selective grinding: This is the reshaping of one or more teeth to reduce or alter specific undesirable occlusal contacts or tooth inclinations. It may be carried out to reduce plunger cusps, over-erupted posterior teeth with unopposed contacts, wedging or locking effects of restorations, or extruded teeth, each of which may prevent freedom of the jaw to move anteriorly and laterally without tooth contact interferences. Selective grinding has also been used as an adjunct treatment in different disciplines, including periodontics, orthodontics, general restorative dentistry, and endodontics, but is often incorrectly termed *occlusal adjustment* in the literature. The references listed under "Further Reading" provide examples of its use in different dental disciplines.

Aims of Occlusal Adjustment

- To maintain intraarch stability by providing an occlusal plane with minimal curvature anteroposteriorly and minimal lateral curve. This minimizes the effect of tooth contact interferences.

- To maintain interarch stability by providing bilateral synchronous contacts on posterior teeth in RCP and ICP at the correct occlusal vertical dimension (OVD). Supporting cusps of posterior teeth are in a stable contact relationship with opposing fossae or marginal ridges.
- To provide guidance for lateral and protrusive jaw movements on mesially directed inclines of anterior teeth, or as far anteriorly as possible. Posterior guiding contacts are modified so as not to be a dominant influence in lateral jaw movements. This is a commonly accepted practice in developing a therapeutic occlusion as it is clinically convenient. However, there is inadequate evidence from controlled studies to justify its routine use in the natural dentition.
- To allow optimum disk-condyle function along the posterior slope of the eminence, by encouraging smooth translation and rotation of the condyle.
- To provide freedom of jaw movement anteriorly and laterally. This overcomes a restricted functional angle of occlusion (FAO) caused by inlocked tooth relationships. A restricted FAO arises in the following types of tooth arrangements: deep anterior overbite that is not in harmony with the condylar pathway, undercontoured restorations with loss of OVD, extruded teeth, and plunger cusps. This has been a traditionally accepted practice in restorative dentistry. Although there appear to be subjective benefits for the patient, these are not verified by controlled clinical trials.

Indications for Occlusal Adjustment

- As a pretreatment in prosthodontics and general restorative care:
  - to improve jaw relationships and provide stable tooth contacts for jaw support in ICP
  - to improve the stability of individual teeth
- To enhance function by providing smooth guidance for lateral and protrusive jaw movements. This may involve modification of plunger cusps, inlocked cuspal inclines, and mediotrusive, laterotrusive, and protrusive tooth contact interferences.
- To modify a traumatic occlusion where tooth contact interferences are associated with excessive tooth loading, such as may occur in parafunctional clenching, resulting in tooth sensitivity, abfractions or fractures, and/or increased tooth mobility.

Occlusal adjustment will direct loading to appropriate teeth in an optimal direction and, where possible, along their long axes.

- To stabilize orthodontic, restorative, or prosthodontic treatment. In such cases where it is decided that existing restorations are to be retained, an occlusal adjustment may be indicated. Alternatively, adjustment in conjunction with occlusal build-up on selected teeth may be required.

Occlusal adjustment has been used both as a pretreatment restorative procedure involving fixed and removable prosthodontics and as adjunctive therapy in the treatment of TMDs. Improved neuromuscular harmony as well as signs and symptoms of TMDs following occlusal adjustment procedures have been described in a randomized controlled study by Forssell et al. (1987), but the evidence is weakened by the presence of non-homogenous study groups and mixed therapies. It should be emphasized that the same group of researchers concluded in subsequent systematic reviews of the literature that the evidence to support occlusal adjustment as a reasonable treatment modality for TMD is lacking (Forssell et al. 1999, Forssell & Kalso 2004). The effect of occlusal adjustment on sleep bruxism has also been investigated in uncontrolled studies (Bailey & Rugh 1980). Clark et al. (1999) reviewed articles that described the effect of experimentally induced occlusal interferences on healthy, non-TMD subjects. Symptoms including transient tooth pain and mobility were reported, and changes in postural muscle tension levels and disruption of smooth jaw movements were noted. Occasional jaw muscle pain and TM joint clicking were also observed. However, the data do not strongly support a link between experimentally induced occlusal interferences and TMDs. Tsukiyama et al. (2001) provided a critical review of published data on occlusal adjustment as a treatment for TMDs and concluded that current evidence does not support the use of occlusal adjustment in preference to other conservative therapies in the treatment of bruxism and nontooth-related TMDs. Several systematic reviews of the literature (Forssell et al. 1999, Koh & Robinson 2003, Forssell & Kalso 2004, List & Axelsson 2010), collectively covering the years 1966 to 2009, concluded that the available randomized controlled trials showed no evidence that occlusal adjustment relieved the symptoms of or prevented TMD.

This is not surprising as there are no randomized controlled trials demonstrating a link between tooth contact interferences and bruxism or chronic orofacial pain. There is some evidence that tooth contact interferences may be related to jaw muscle pain and TMDs through their effects on directional guidance of teeth in function. However, evidence from current studies is weak, as direct comparison between the studies is not possible because of:

- Difference in philosophy between various researchers regarding mandibular and condylar position and the method of achieving RCP during occlusal adjustment
- Difference in philosophy of the occlusal contact scheme
- Lack of a standardized approach to the measurement of the study and outcome factors
- Lack of clearly defined TMD diagnostic subgroups in treatment subjects
- Lack of adequate blinding during the experiments
- Small sample size with sometimes high subject loss to followup
- Short follow-up periods
- Non-standardized control treatments
- Poorly defined study bases (hospital or pain clinic populations)
- No adjusting for potential confounders or effect modifiers

If the efficacy of occlusal adjustment is to be demonstrated, well-designed multicenter studies using clearly defined diagnostic subgroups, with large sample sizes and long follow-up periods, are necessary. Until then, the recommendations of the Neuroscience Group of the International Association for Dental Research, through its consensus statement on TMDs (2002), should be heeded: "it is strongly recommended that, unless there are specific and justifiable indications to the contrary, treatment should be based on the use of conservative, reversible and preferably evidence-based therapeutic modalities. While no specific therapies have been proven to be uniformly effective, many of the conservative modalities have proven to be at least as effective in providing palliative relief as various forms of invasive treatment, and they present much less risk of producing harm." Ten years on, there has been no further scientific evidence to suggest otherwise, and Turp & Schindler

(2012) recommended that treatment should focus on nonocclusal factors. In addition, it needs to be acknowledged that the American Association of Dental Research confirmed its support for this clinical approach.

CLINICAL PRACTICE

Clinical occlusal adjustment is facilitated by carrying out the procedure initially on study casts, articulated on an adjustable articulator by accurate transfer records (Figure 21-1). There are advantages in treatment planning in this way:

- Clinical time is reduced, as treatment planning decisions have been made concerning the optimum areas of tooth structure to be adjusted, following analysis and adjustment of study casts. It is then relatively easy to follow the pattern of adjustment determined on casts when completing an adjustment clinically.
- Diagnostic occlusal adjustment on articulated study casts also allows assessment of the amount of tooth surface reduction required. If the diagnostic adjustment indicates that removal of tooth structure is excessive, other forms of management such as tooth surface addition, orthodontic treatment, or onlay prostheses may be indicated.
- Areas of tooth adjustment are carefully selected, as failure to do so may undermine occlusal stability, leading to further deterioration of the existing clinical situation.

Equally important is the presentation of the proposed diagnostic adjustment to the patient, illustrating the reason for the procedure and the teeth to be modified, to ensure that informed consent is obtained. This may be of importance in one's defence should a dentolegal problem arise. The following text describes an accurate method for transposing the preplanned occlusal adjustment, as already performed on articulated casts, to the correct areas of tooth structure in the mouth.

Preclinical Preparation

The preclinical sequence to be followed includes verification of the articulation of casts when transfer records are taken. Kerr occlusal indicator wax (Kerr, Emeryville, California) is used to record RCP contacts. This record is chilled, removed from the mouth, and taken to the laboratory, where the perforation points are checked against the initial contact points of the articulated casts. Coincidence of these indicates an accurate articulation of casts. Tru-fit dye spacer (George Taub Products and Fusion Co. Inc., Jersey City, New Jersey) or a text highlighting pen in a different color from the stone cast may be used to cover contacting surfaces of all upper and lower teeth (Figure 21-2). The occlusal adjustment sequence is carried out on the articulated casts as follows:

- RCP contacts are adjusted to provide well-distributed bilateral synchronous contacts, providing optimum jaw support.

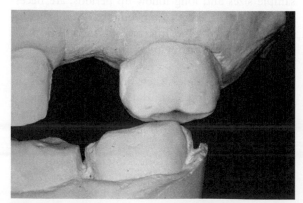

FIG 21-1 Mediotrusive interference on the palatal cusp of the upper second molar demonstrated on articulated casts.

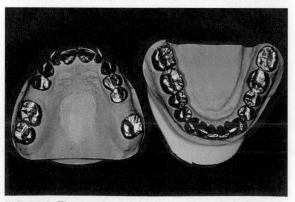

FIG 21-2 The teeth of the upper and lower duplicate casts painted with die spacer in preparation for preclinical laboratory occlusal adjustment.

- ICP contacts are adjusted to provide well-distributed bilateral synchronous points of tooth contact.
- The slide between RCP and ICP will be reduced or eliminated; however, routine elimination of this slide is not an essential requirement.
- Mediotrusive interferences are eliminated to allow laterotrusive guidance on canines (canine guidance); canines and bicuspids; or canines, bicuspids, and molar teeth (group function).
- Laterotrusive adjustment is completed when it is possible to move the maxillary cast in a lateral and lateroprotrusive direction without interference, with the canines or the canines in conjunction with posterior teeth providing guidance.
- Protrusive contacts are adjusted to allow canines and incisors to provide protrusive guidance. The adjustment is restricted to regions between cusps where possible. Care is taken to preserve supporting cusp tips and to recontour cuspal inclines, opposing fossae, or marginal ridges, thus providing cusp tip to fossa or marginal ridge contacts.

Minimal tooth adjustment is emphasized, and to simplify the procedure, adjustments are confined where possible to the maxillary arch. The adjusted areas of the casts are then marked with ink to allow clear identification. A clear thermoplastic vacuum-formed template (Bego adaptor foils, 0.6 mm thickness) is drawn down over the original cast (Figure 21-3) and then placed over the adjusted cast (Figure

21-4). With the use of a sharp scalpel or a flat fissure bur, areas on the template corresponding to the adjusted areas on the cast are carefully removed. The template is trimmed (Figure 21-5) around its entire periphery to restrict its extensions to only 2 mm beyond the gingival margins. The peripheries are smoothed to remove sharp edges that may traumatize intraoral soft tissues.

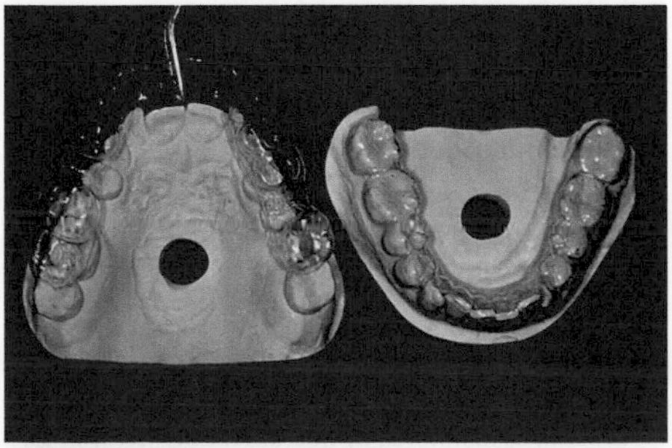

Clinical Procedures

The template is seated over the teeth and examined for accuracy of fit around the teeth. It should not

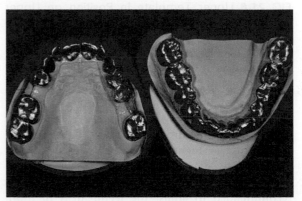

FIG 21-4 Templates Placed Over Adjusted Duplicate Casts Adjusted areas are highlighted with ink to allow clear identification. Wax has been added to the palatal surface of tooth 13 to represent the area where composite resin will be placed to provide an occlusal contact.

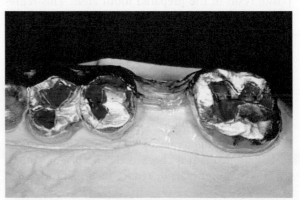

FIG 21-3 Clear Thermoplastic Templates Made Over Unadjusted Casts The center vent hole in the casts allows improved adaptation of the thermoplastic material to the casts.

FIG 21-5 Trimmed Templates Over Adjusted Casts (Palatal view) Perforations in the template correspond to adjusted areas of tooth cusps on the cast.

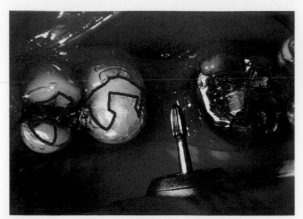

FIG 21-6 Upper Template in Position on Upper Teeth Areas of tooth to be adjusted protrude through the prepared template perforations and are indicated by the highlighted outlines.

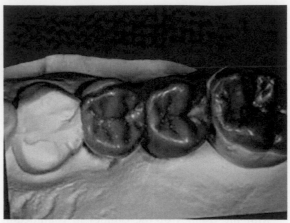

FIG 21-7 Diagnostic wax-up of a planned three-unit bridge in quadrant one is shown. The completed occlusal adjustment is a preparatory step for three-unit bridgework in the upper posterior quadrants. If no further treatment was required, adjusted tooth areas would be polished and fluoride applied to complete treatment.

cause discomfort to soft tissues. The areas of tooth cusp or marginal ridge to be adjusted are clearly visible protruding through the prepared perforations of the template (Figure 21-6). A pear-shaped composite finishing diamond (Komet 8368.204.016) or 12-fluted tungsten carbide burr (Komet H46.014) is recommended to adjust the teeth. Areas of tooth structure protruding beyond the perforations in the template are removed (Figure 21-6). Where addition of a restorative material is required, a thermoplastic vacuum-formed template can be made over a duplicate of the diagnostic wax-up. The template can be used clinically to assist the precise placement of composite resin in the prepared tooth areas. This represents the initial adjustment stage.

The occlusal adjustment may then be refined and completed. The adjustments are checked repeatedly using plastic articulating tape (GHM foil—Gebr. Hansel-Medizinal, Nurtingen, Germany; Ivoclar/Vivadent, Schaan, Liechtenstein) as well as the clinician's tactile sense:

- RCP adjustment is checked to ensure well-distributed bilateral stops on supporting cusps.
- ICP adjustment is checked also for bilateral stops. This may eliminate or reduce the magnitude of an RCP/ICP slide.
- Mediotrusive interferences are refined to ensure canine or anterior guidance or group function in laterotrusion.

- Protrusive interferences are refined to allow guidance on canines or canine and incisor teeth.
- All adjusted tooth surfaces are polished and topical fluoride applied.
- If required as part of further treatment, impressions of the adjusted dental arches are taken and casts prepared for a diagnostic wax-up of planned restorations are made on articulated study casts of the adjusted occlusion (Figure 21-7).

ACKNOWLEDGMENTS

We would like to express our thanks to Mr. Charles Kim for his preparation of the laboratory technical work.

REFERENCES

Au A, Ho C, McNeil DW, et al: Clinical occlusal evaluation of patients with craniomandibular disorders, *J Dent Res* 73:739, 1994. (abstract).

Bailey JO, Rugh ID: Effect of occlusal adjustment on bruxism as monitored by nocturnal EMG recordings, *J Dent Res* 59:317, 1980. (abstract).

Clark GT, Tsukiyama Y, Baba K, et al: Sixty-eight years of experimental occlusal interference studies: what have we learned?, *J Prosth Dent* 82:704–713, 1999.

Forssell H, Kalso E: Application of principles of evidence-based medicine to occlusal treatment for temporomandibular disorders: are there lessons to be learned?, *J Orofac Pain* 18:9–22, 2004.

Forssell H, Kalso E, Koskela P, et al: Occlusal treatments in temporomandibular disorders: a qualitative systematic review of randomized controlled trials, *Pain* 83:549–560, 1999.

Forssell H, Kirveskari P, Kangasdniemi P: Response to occlusal treatment in headache patients previously treated by mock occlusal adjustment, *Acta Odont Scand* 45:77–80, 1987.

Koh H, Robinson P: Occlusal adjustment for treating and preventing temporomandibular joint disorders, *Cochrane Syst Rev* CD003812, 2003.

List T, Axelsson S: Management of TMD: evidence from systematic reviews and meta-analyses, *J Oral Rehabil* 37:430–451, 2010.

Pullinger AG, Seligman DA, Gornbein JA: A multiple logistic regression analysis of the risk and relative odds of temporomandibular disorders as a function of common occlusal features, *J Dent Res* 72:968–979, 1993.

Tsukiyama Y, Baba K, Clark GT: An evidence-based assessment of occlusal adjustment as a treatment for temporomandibular disorder, *J Prosth Dent* 86:57–66, 2001.

Turp JC, Schindler H: The dental occlusion as a suspected cause for TMDs: epidemiological and etiological considerations, *J Oral Rehabil* 39:502–512, 2012.

Further Reading

Branam SR, Mourino AP: Minimizing otitis media by manipulating the primary dental occlusion: case report, *J Clin Pediatr Dent* 22:203–206, 1998.

Davies SJ, Gray RMJ, Smith PW: Good occlusal practice in simple restorative dentistry, *Brit Dent J* 191:365–381, 2001.

Foz AM, Artese HPC, Horliana CRT, et al: Occlusal adjustment associated with periodontal therapy—a systematic review, *J Dent* 40:1025–1035, 2012.

Gher ME: Changing concepts. The effects of occlusion on periodontitis, *Dent Clin North Am* 42:285–297, 1998.

Greene CS, Laskin DM: Temporomandibular disorders: moving from a dentally based to a medically based model, *J Dent Res* 79:1736–1739, 2000.

Hellsing G: Occlusal adjustment and occlusal stability, *J Prosth Dent* 59:696–702, 1988.

Karjalainen M, Le Bell Y, Jamsa T, et al: Prevention of temporomandibular disorder-related signs and symptoms in orthodontically treated adolescents. A 3-year follow-up of a prospective randomized trial, *Acta Odont Scand* 55:319–324, 1997.

Kopp S, Wenneberg B: Effects of occlusal treatment and intra-articular injections on temporomandibular joint pain and dysfunction, *Acta Odont Scand* 39:87–96, 1981.

Luther F: Orthodontics and the temporomandibular joint: where are we now? Part 2. Functional occlusion, malocclusion, and TMD, *Angle Orthod* 68:305–316, 1998.

Marklund S, Wänman A: A century of controversy regarding the benefit or detriment of occlusal contacts on the mediotrusive side, *J Oral Rehabil* 27:553–562, 2000.

Minagi S, Ohtsuki H, Sato T, et al: Effect of balancing-side occlusion on the ipsilateral TMJ dynamics under clenching, *J Oral Rehabil* 24:57 62, 1997.

Rosenberg PA, Babick PJ, Schertzer L, et al: The effect of occlusal reduction on pain after endodontic instrumentation, *J Endod* 24:492–496, 1998.

Tsolka P, Morris RW, Preiskel HW: Occlusal adjustment therapy for craniomandibular disorders: a clinical assessment by a double-blind method, *J Prosthet Dent* 68:957–964, 1992.

Vallon D, Ekberg EC, Nilner M, et al: Short-term effect of occlusal adjustment on craniomandibular disorders including headaches, *Acta Odont Scand* 53:55–59, 1995.

Specialty programs must undergo a demanding process of accreditation to ensure that the educational standards to which all programs are held accountable are appropriately representative of the specialty. The most rigorous didactic standards in the specialty of prosthodontics are found in the areas of fixed, removable, and implant prosthodontics and in the area of occlusion.

Although different countries address education differently, it is recognized that occlusion remains one of the most important topics in dental education. It is unlikely that dentistry case management could be discussed appropriately without an understanding of occlusion. Moreover, it is impossible to consider clinical research without defining the management of the occlusion for those participating in the research programs. Failure to do so would create variables that would undermine the relevance of such investigation.

Clinicians have pondered why occlusion was separated from the other aspects of prosthodontic treatment. Because occlusion is considered integral to all disciplines in prosthodontics, if occlusion is separated from fixed, removable, and implant prosthodontics, how would prosthodontic care be provided?

This has been a perplexing interpretation on the part of our colleagues. It seems that the knowledge base about occlusion is perceived to be stronger if occlusion stands on its own as a foundation of prosthetic care. Our perception differs on this point. The importance of occlusion is that it is irreversibly linked to all aspects of prosthodontic care. The understanding that occlusion changes as patients age, as specific therapeutic intervention is provided, as prostheses change, and as muscles and bones respond to the demands placed upon them leads the clinician, the educator, and the investigator to a deeper respect for this complex interpretation of occlusion.

This book has provided a breadth of information and contemporary knowledge about occlusion, disease, and therapy in dentistry. The editors hope that the information provided has opened new insights into a deeper understanding of the interconnections of occlusion and dental care.

Steven E. Eckert and Iven Klineberg

Note: Page numbers followed by "*f*" refer to illustrations; page numbers followed by "*t*" refer to tables; page numbers followed by "*b*" refer to boxes.

Printed and bound by CPI Group (UK) Ltd, Croydon, CR0 4YY

03/10/2024

01040365-0001